$4.00

THE STRESS OF LIFE

revised edition

OTHER BOOKS BY HANS SELYE

THE STEROIDS. 4 vols., in *Encyclopedia of Endocrinology*. Montreal: A. W. T. Franks Publ. Co., 1943.

OVARIAN TUMORS. 2 vols., in *Encyclopedia of Endocrinology*. Montreal: Richardson, Bond & Wright, 1946.

TEXTBOOK OF ENDOCRINOLOGY. First ed., 1947; Second ed., Montreal: Acta Endocrinologica, Université de Montréal, 1949.

ON THE EXPERIMENTAL MORPHOLOGY OF THE ADRENAL CORTEX (in collaboration with H. Stone). Springfield, Ill.: Charles C. Thomas Publ., 1950.

STRESS. Montreal: Acta Inc., Med. Publ., 1950.

FIRST ANNUAL REPORT ON STRESS, 1951. Montreal: Acta Inc., Med. Publ., 1951.

SECOND ANNUAL REPORT ON STRESS, 1952. Montreal: Acta Inc., Med. Publ., 1952.

*THE STORY OF THE ADAPTATION SYNDROME (told in the form of informal illustrated lectures). Montreal: Acta Inc., Med. Publ., 1952.

THIRD ANNUAL REPORT ON STRESS, 1953. Montreal: Acta Inc., Med. Publ., 1953.

FOURTH ANNUAL REPORT ON STRESS, 1954. Montreal: Acta Inc., Med. Publ., 1954.

FIFTH ANNUAL REPORT ON STRESS, 1955−56. Montreal: Acta Inc., Med. Publ., 1956.

THE CHEMICAL PREVENTION OF CARDIAC NECROSES. New York: The Ronald Press Co., 1958.

THE PLURICAUSAL CARDIOPATHIES. Springfield: Charles C. Thomas Publ., 1961.

CALCIPHYLAXIS. Chicago: The University of Chicago Press, 1962.

SYMBOLIC SHORTHAND SYSTEM (SSS) FOR PHYSIOLOGY AND MEDICINE. Montreal: Acta Inc., Med. Publ., First ed., 1956; Second ed., 1958 (in collaboration with M. Nadasdi); Third ed., 1960 (in collaboration with P. Prioreschi). Montréal:

IMCE, Université de Montréal, 1964, Fourth ed. (in collaboration with G. Ember).

THE MAST CELLS. London: Butterworths Inc., 1965.

THROMBOHEMORRHAGIC PHENOMENA. Springfield: Charles C. Thomas Publ., 1966.

*IN VIVO. THE CASE FOR SUPRAMOLECULAR BIOLOGY. New York: Liveright, 1967.

ANAPHYLACTOID EDEMA. St. Louis: Warren H. Green, 1968.

EXPERIMENTAL CARDIOVASCULAR DISEASES. Berlin/ Heidelberg/ New York: Springer-Verlag, 1970.

HORMONES AND RESISTANCE. Berlin/Heidelberg/ New York: Springer-Verlag, 1971.

*STRESS WITHOUT DISTRESS. New York: J. B. Lippincott Co., 1974.

*FROM DREAM TO DISCOVERY. New York: McGraw-Hill, 1964; Second printing, New York: Arno Press, 1975.

*THE STRESS OF LIFE. New York: McGraw-Hill, 1956; revised ed., 1975.

STRESS IN HEALTH AND DISEASE. Reading, Mass.: Butterworths Inc., 1976.

*Written in nontechnical language for the general reader.

THE
STRESS OF
LIFE

by
Hans Selye, M.D.

revised edition

McGRAW-HILL BOOK CO.

New York   St. Louis   San Francisco   Bogotá   Düsseldorf
Madrid   Mexico   Montreal   Panama   Paris   São Paulo
Tokyo   Toronto

Book design by Elaine Gongora

THE STRESS OF LIFE, revised edition

Paperback Edition, 1978

Library of Congress Cataloging in Publication Data

Selye, Hans, date
   The stress of life.

   Bibliography: p.
   Includes index.
   1. Stress (Physiology)   2. Adaptation
(Physiology)   I. Title.
QP82.2.S8S44   1978   616.07   77–14023
ISBN 0–07–056212–1
   678910   MUMU   8987654321

"This book is dedicated to those who are not afraid to enjoy the stress of a full life, nor so naïve as to think that they can do so without intellectual effort." H.S.

*It is highly dishonorable for
a Reasonable Soul to live in so
Divinely built a Mansion as the
Body she resides in, altogether
unacquainted with the exquisite
structure of it.*
—Robert Boyle, 1627–1691

*Not only will men of science have to grapple with
the sciences that deal with man, but—and this is
a far more difficult matter—they will have to
persuade the world to listen to what they have
discovered. If they cannot succeed in this difficult
enterprise, man will destroy himself by his
halfway cleverness.*
—Bertrand Russell, 1872–1970

Preface to the
Revised Edition

Since the publication of "A Syndrome Produced by Diverse Nocuous Agents" in 1936, approximately 110,000 articles and books have been written on what is now known as the "general adaptation syndrome" (G.A.S.) or "Stress Syndrome," and on the "Diseases of Adaptation," in which nonspecific bodily or mental stress plays a decisive role. I myself have written thirty books and about 1,500 technical articles in scientific journals on various special aspects of this subject. Though untrained in philosophy, psychology and sociology, I have even had the temerity recently of compiling a brief résumé under the title *Stress without Distress*. This semipopular book outlines the behavioral implications of what the laboratory has taught us about stress in relation to the creation of a code of conduct based not upon purely philosophic considerations or traditions but upon demonstrable biologic laws.

Despite the many recent developments in the field I should like *The Stress of Life*, first published in 1956, to continue its role as a simplified summary of contemporary views on the scientific basis of the entire stress concept as it applies to any field. Judged by the number of references to it, both in scientific and lay literature, the original edition appears to have satisfied this need fairly well in the past. However, until now, it has always been reprinted in English and in all its translations without ever having been revised and brought up to date.

The purpose of the present volume is to remedy this situation. The fundamental principle of a stereotyped nonspecific reaction of the body to any kind of demand made upon it, the important roles of nervous and endocrine factors, particularly of the "hypothalamus-pituitary-adrenocortical axis," as well as the participation of stress, either as a cause or a result of disease, will merely require restating. These concepts have undergone no major modifications in the course of time, and the best we can hope to do is to polish their presentation in the light of the responses to many lectures, publications and round-table discussions, which have shown me where greater clarity and precision would help to avoid misunderstandings. In Books I and II of the revised volume, I have clarified the organization of the text by combining and condensing some chapters.

I have tried to retain the most amusing and instructive anecdotal material concerning the history of the stress concept. However, for the sake of conciseness, I omitted many of the lengthy discussions of subjects which caused animated polemics at the time of the first edition but which are now undisputed textbook material. Among these are such problems as the definition of stress, the justification of distinguishing between stress and stressors or between essentially distinct types of adrenocortical hormones (mineralocorticoids and glucocorticoids); thus, we have gained space for some currently much-discussed concepts, such as the role of stress in the so-called "pluricausal diseases" (maladies elicited by a constellation of potentially pathogenic agents), psychosomatic medicine, life under today's abnormal conditions (pollution of the environment by chemicals, noise, crowding), etc. Finally, I have tried to develop my views on stress in interpersonal relations, which is probably the most common problem we meet nowadays.

As in the first edition, I have attempted to limit the purely technical aspects (especially those concerning biochemistry, biophysics, histology)— important though they all are—because a meaningful discussion of them would require the presentation and explanation of too many complex scientific terms, most of which are of no practical interest to the average reader. Yet, I have at least mentioned a few important and essentially new biochemical facets of stress (e.g., the actions of syntoxic and catatoxic steroids, glucagon, and somatotrophic hormones), because this should never become a merely "inspirational book," based on blind belief in the author's competence to make recommendations for daily life. It has to enable the educated nonmedical reader and the practicing physician not specially trained in research, to make up his own mind about the validity of our applications of laboratory experience to everyday problems.

Hans Selye

Université de Montréal
Montreal, 1975

Preface

The main purpose of this book is to tell, in a generally understandable language, what medicine has learned about stress.

No one can live without experiencing some degree of stress all the time. You may think that only serious disease or intensive physical or mental injury can cause stress. This is false. Crossing a busy intersection, exposure to a draft, or even sheer joy are enough to activate the body's stress mechanism to some extent. Stress is not even necessarily bad for you; it is also the spice of life, for any emotion, any activity causes stress. But, of course, your system must be prepared to take it. The same stress which makes one person sick can be an invigorating experience for another.

It is through the *general adaptation syndrome*, or G.A.S. (the main subject of this book), that our various internal organs—especially the endocrine glands and the nervous system—help us both to adjust to the constant changes which occur in and around us and to navigate a steady course toward whatever we consider a worthwhile goal.

Life is largely a process of adaptation to the circumstances in which we exist. A perennial give-and-take has been going on between living matter and its inanimate surroundings, between one living being and another, ever since the dawn of life in the prehistoric oceans. The secret of health and happiness lies in successful adjustment to the ever-changing conditions on this globe; the penalties for failure in this great process of adaptation are disease and unhappiness. The genetic evolution through endless centuries from the simplest forms of life to complex human beings was the greatest adaptive adventure on earth. The realization of this has fundamentally influenced our thinking, but there is not much we can do about it. Here we are, such as we are; and whether or not man is pleased with the result, he has not—at least up to now—learned to change his own inherited structure.

But there is another type of evolution which takes place in every person during his own lifetime from birth to death: this is adaptation to the stresses and strains of everyday existence. Through the constant interplay between his mental and bodily reactions, man has it in his power to influence this second type of evolution to a considerable extent, especially if he understands its mechanism and has enough will power to act according to the dictates of human intellect.

Stress is essentially reflected by the rate of all the wear and tear caused by life. It will take a whole book to explain the complex mechanisms through which the body can reduce this type of wear and tear and to define the concept more precisely. But let me say here, by way of an introduction, that although we cannot avoid stress as long as we live, we can learn a great deal about how to keep its damaging side-effects, "distress," to a minimum. For instance, we are just beginning to see that many common diseases are largely due to errors in our adaptive response to stress, rather than to direct damage by germs, poisons, or life experience. In this sense many nervous and emotional disturbances, high blood pressure, gastric and duodenal ulcers, and certain types of sexual, allergic, cardiovascular, and renal derangements appear to be essentially *diseases of adaptation*.

In view of all this, stress is undoubtedly an important personal problem for everybody. So much has been written for the general public by others about my work on stress that I gradually came to feel the need of telling the story in my own words. Writing this book certainly helped me. I hope it will also help you. It helped me because it was the first chance I had to put the really salient points together and get a bird's-eye view, not only of the facts discovered in the laboratory, but also of the thoughts and emotions inspired by constant preoccupation with the nature of stress in health and disease.

The urge to share with others the thrill of adventure which comes from penetrating, even if ever so slightly, into hitherto unknown depths of life can become a major source of stress in itself.

In a similar sense, I hope this account will help my readers—physicians and laymen alike—who do not have an opportunity of experiencing at first hand all those manifold satisfactions which come from designing experimental plans and acquiring the techniques necessary to solve some of those problems of life which concern us all.

But I should like to think that this book may offer an even more practical kind of help. Psychoanalysis has shown that knowledge about oneself has a curative value. I think this is also true of psychosomatic, and perhaps even of what we call purely somatic, or bodily, derangements. The struggle for understanding is one of the most characteristic features of our species; that is why man is called *Homo sapiens.* The satisfaction of this urge is our destiny.

It may help you to enter into the spirit of this volume if you keep in mind that I wanted to tell not only what we know about stress but also how we found out about it. This dual task determined the structure of my account and particularly its presentation in the form of five Books.

Book I: The discovery of stress describes the evolution of the stress concept from the earliest records of medical thought on the subject up to the present time.

Book II: The dissection of stress attempts to analyze the mechanism through which our body is attacked by, and can defend itself against, stress-producing situations.

Book III: The diseases of adaptation deals with maladies (cardiovascular diseases, digestive disorders, mental derangements) which we consider to result largely from failures in the stress-fighting mechanism.

Book IV: Sketch for a unified theory explores how our knowledge of stress might help us to appraise those elementary forms of reaction which constitute the mosaic of life in health and disease.

Book V: Implications and applications presents the principal lessons to be learned from the study of the stress of life, and discusses the prevention and cure of disease, not only by medical means, but also through man's ability to devise a natural and healthy philosophy of life. Such a philosophy, it is concluded, must be based primarily on what we have called "altruistic egoism," which maximizes eustress and minimizes distress in our lives.

Readability

In writing this account it seemed logical to proceed from the discovery of stress (Book I) to the analysis of its mechanism in health (Book II) and disease, emphasizing the signs by which you can recognize its threats (Book III); then to explore how this knowledge could further our understanding of life in theory (Book IV) and in practice when faced with the agents that cause the stress of life (Book V). But the most logical structure is not necessarily the most readable sequence for a general reader.

By dealing with my topics in this sequence, I had to intersperse highly technical data between the more easily readable, and perhaps more entertaining, parts of the narrative. If you are totally unacquainted with this field, you may wish to start with Book V (the practical implications and applications of the stress concept in everyday life), using the Glossary as a guide to technical terms, and perhaps looking up occasional earlier passages to which reference is made. If you turn to Book I after this, you will be able to read about the discovery of stress with more understanding. I would recommend that you then peruse at least the Summary of Book II, all of Book III, and the Summary of Book IV. Books II and IV are particularly technical, and even with-

out them, the essence of the volume is quite understandable, although they had to be included to complete the picture for the scientifically and medically
minded reader.

But before I discourage you with too many admo-
nitions, let us now start with the story.

Hans Selye

Université de Montréal
  Montreal, 1956

Acknowledgments

My work on stress is but one small step toward a better comprehension of man's nature, and my desire to share this experience with others was largely prompted by the pleasure and inspiration I personally derived from such remarkable works as:

Bernard, Claude: *Introduction to the Study of Experimental Medicine*, Flammarion, Paris, 1945.

Cannon, W. B.: *The Wisdom of the Body*, W. W. Norton & Company, Inc., New York, 1939.

———: *The Way of an Investigator*, W. W. Norton & Company, Inc., New York, 1945.

Carrel, Alexis: *Man the Unknown*, Harper & Brothers, New York, 1935.

Conant, James B.: *On Understanding Science*, New American Library, New York, 1951.

Darwin, Charles: *The Origin of the Species and the Descent of Man*, Modern Library ed., Random House, Inc., New York, 1955.

Dubos, René: *Man Adapting*, Yale University Press, New Haven, London, 1965.

Einstein, Albert: *Ideas and Opinions*, Crown Publishers, Inc., New York, 1953.

Freud, Sigmund: *Psychopathology of Everyday Life*, New American Library, New York, 1951.

Gamow, George: *The Birth and Death of the Sun*, New American Library, New York, 1953.

Jeans, Sir James: *Stars in Their Courses*, Cambridge University Press, New York, 1931.

Levi, Lennart, ed.: *Society, Stress and Disease. Vol. I. The Psychosocial Environment and Psychosomatic Diseases (Proc. Int. Interdisciplinary Symp., Stock-*

holm, 1970, Oxford University Press, London, New York, Toronto, 1971.

Monod, Jacques: *Chance and Necessity: An Essay on the Natural Philosophy of Modern Biology,* Alfred A. Knopf Inc., New York, 1971.

Sherrington, Sir Charles: *Man on His Nature,* Anchor Book ed., Doubleday & Company, Inc., New York, 1953.

Vallery-Radot, Pasteur: *The Most Beautiful Pages of Pasteur,* Flammarion, Paris, 1943.

Zinsser, Hans: *As I Remember Him,* Little, Brown & Company, Boston, 1940.

May I recommend, therefore, that those who are interested not only in stress but also in understanding the different aspects of Nature consult some of these great examples of writing about science by those who made it. None of them can be read easily in bed after a busy day, but their message is accessible to any educated person, whatever his background, and they can give us an understanding of the highest aspirations of man: to know himself and to devise a purposeful way of life.

I wish to express my particular gratitude to Mr. Daniel Saykaly for his valuable aid and advice concerning the organization of this new edition, and for his editorial work in the preparation and polishing of the text. The assistance of Mr. Ovid Da Silva, Chief of the Editorial Department, and his colleagues, Mr. Geoff Languedoc, Mrs. Cynthia Alperowicz and Ms. Linda Vance is also gratefully acknowledged.

Equal gratitude is due to Mr. Frederic Hills, whose creative editorial work played an essential role in putting the manuscript into a publishable form, and whose supervision guided it safely through the innumerable perils of production and into print. Thanks, too, go to Ms. Peggy Tsukahira, whose contributions as copy editor enhanced the manuscript in countless ways.

My sincere thanks are also due to Acta, Inc., Med. Publ. (Montreal) and Butterworths (London, Reading, Mass.) who permitted me to use a number of passages, as well as illustrations, which first appeared in my more technical books on stress. Other illustrations are reproduced by courtesy of the *Journal of the American Medical Association*, the *British Medical Journal*, the *Canadian Medical Association Journal*, and the *Journal of Clinical Endocrinology and Metabolism*.

All the professional-looking drawings in this volume were prepared by Miss Samia Iskander; the amateurish ones were committed by myself. Mr. Kai Nielsen took the photographs.

Contents

Stress and adaptation. Stress and growth. Stress and speci-
ficity. The structural unit of life: the cell. The functional unit
of life: the reacton. Analysis and synthesis of cellular disease.
Possibilities and limitations of the reacton hypothesis. The
continued importance of in vivo research.

BOOK I

The Discovery of Stress

Summary

In its medical sense, *stress is essentially the rate of wear and tear in the body.* Anyone who feels that whatever he is doing—or whatever is being done to him—is strenuous and wearing, knows vaguely what we mean by *stress.* The feelings of just being tired, jittery, or ill are subjective sensations of stress. But stress does not necessarily imply a morbid change: normal life, especially intense pleasure and the ecstasy of fulfillment, also cause some wear and tear in the machinery of the body. Indeed, stress can even have curative value, as in shock therapy, bloodletting, and sports. In any event, wear and tear is only the result of all this; hence now we define stress as *the nonspecific response of the body to any demand.*

Research on stress was greatly handicapped because we had no objective, measurable indices to assess it, until it was found, some forty years ago, that stress causes certain changes in the structure and chemical composition of the body which can be accurately appraised. Some of these changes are merely signs of *damage;* others are manifestations of the body's *adaptive reactions,* its mechanism of defense against stress. The totality of these changes—the *stress syndrome*—is called the *general adaptation syndrome* (G.A.S.). It develops in three stages: (1) the alarm reaction; (2) the stage of resistance; (3) the stage of exhaustion.

The *nervous system* and the *endocrine* (or *hormonal*) *system* play particularly important parts in maintaining resistance during stress. They help to keep the structure and function of the body steady, despite exposure to stress-producing or *stressor* agents, such as nervous tension, wounds, infections, poisons. This steady state is known as *homeostasis*.

In this section we shall discuss the *evolution of the stress concept*, from antiquity to the present time, and the *psychologic* and *linguistic problems* met when chance observations, made at the bedside of patients or in the research laboratory, are to be translated into a precise science.

chapter 1

Precursors of the Stress Concept

What is stress?   Pónos—the toil of disease.
"Homeostasis"—the staying power of
the body.

What Is Stress?

The soldier who sustains wounds in battle, the mother who worries about her soldier son, the gambler who watches the races—whether he wins or loses—the horse and the jockey he bet on: they are all under stress.

The beggar who suffers from hunger and the glutton who overeats, the little shopkeeper with his constant fears of bankruptcy and the rich merchant struggling for yet another million: they are also all under stress.

The mother who tries to keep her children out of trouble, the child who scalds himself—and especially the particular cells of the skin over which he spilled the boiling coffee—they, too, are under stress. What is this one mysterious condition that the most different kinds of people have in common with animals and even with individual cells, at times when much—much of anything—happens to them? What is the nature of stress?

This is a fundamental question in the life of everyone; it touches closely upon the essence of life and disease. Understanding the mechanism of stress gave physicians a new approach to the treatment of illness, but it can also give us all a new way of life, a new philosophy to guide our actions in conformity with natural laws.

Perhaps the simplest way to enter into the spirit of this concept will be to follow it through its historical evolution. But I wonder where to begin. It would be natural to start with the discovery of stress, yet it seems as though, in a sense, man always knew about this condition and even now still fails to grasp its essence completely.

Perhaps this is true of every fundamental concept; it is not easy to recognize discovery.

It seems to me that most people do not fully realize to what extent the spirit of scientific research and the lessons learned from it depend upon the personal viewpoints of the discoverers at the time basic observations are made. The painter and the message on his canvas, the musician or poet and the emotional impact of their creations are but different aspects of single natural phenomena. It is surprising to what extent the inseparability of this relationship between work and worker has been overlooked as regards the seemingly more impersonal results of scientific investigation. In an age so largely dependent upon science and scientists, this fundamental point deserves special attention.

My book must, therefore, serve the dual purpose of describing not only what has been learned about stress, but also the psychologic processes which led to its discovery. This twin objective is my apology for the many seemingly irrelevant digressions in which I have tried to analyze my own mental reactions to personal laboratory observations.

Was America discovered by the Indians, who were here from time immemorial, by the Norsemen who came in the tenth century, or by Christopher Columbus who arrived in 1492? Is it still being discovered, now every day, by anyone who drills a new oil well or finds another deposit of uranium on this continent? It depends upon the particular aspect of America and upon the extent of exploration to which you attach the greatest importance. Discovery is always a matter of viewpoint and degree. Whenever we single out an individual as *the* discoverer of anything, we merely mean that for us he discovered it more than anybody else.

The historian of any exploration is faced with these confusing facts. Usually, the subject of the discovery has been suspected and even more or less fleetingly seen from many angles by many people long before it was "actually discovered." For practical purposes, it is unimportant who made a scientific discovery, as long as we can enjoy its fruits. But it does matter, if we want to share the thrill of a true adventure story or profit by the practical lessons that can be learned from it. The relativity of discovery has impressed many a scientist. For instance, the great American bacteriologist, Hans Zinsser, said: "So often, in the history of medicine, scientific discovery has merely served to clarify and subject to purposeful control facts that had long been empirically observed and practically utilized. The principles of contagion were clearly outlined and invisible microorganisms postulated by

Fracastorius over a hundred years before the most primitive microscopes were invented; and the pre-Pasteurian century is rich with clinical observations that now seem a sort of gestation period leading to the birth of a new science." (*As I Remember Him*, p. 139.)

We can learn many things by analyzing discoveries, quite apart from the fact that we find out much about the discovered object itself. It is of definite practical value to learn, by studies in retrospect, what makes a discovery little or great, for this will help to guide our efforts in our own fields; and there is room for discovery in any field of human endeavor. For man it is doubly instructive to analyze explorations into the depths of man's nature, for here he is both the explorer and the explored.

It is not to see something first, but to establish solid connections between the previously known and the hitherto unknown that constitutes the essence of scientific discovery. It is this process of tying together which can best promote true understanding and real progress.

With this in mind, let us now take a look at certain early medical concepts about *stress* as a factor in the production of disease. For many centuries, disease was considered to be something caused by evil spirits or demons. Consequently— for instance in primitive Aztec medicine, and in Babylonian medicine thousands of years B.C.—disease was treated by *incantations*, and *dances*, or by *strong drugs*, *poultices*, and *painful bandages*, which were applied by awe-inspiring witch doctors or priest-physicians to frighten and expel the responsible vicious demons.

Bloodletting was another time-honored remedy for a number of diseases. It is difficult to establish precisely when it was used first. In any event, the process of *venesection* (cutting into a vein to draw blood) is clearly depicted on some Greek vases made around 150 B.C.; and it remained an undoubtedly useful standard procedure in medicine until quite recently. In fact, I remember that when I was a boy, my grandfather and even my father, both of whom were physicians, still punctured veins and applied leeches to treat the most diverse diseases by loss of blood.

Flogging of the insane was a common procedure during antiquity and the Middle Ages to drive the demon or devil out of people who suffered from various mental aberrations.

Paracelsus (whose true, but somewhat bombastic, name was Theophrastus Bombastus von Hohenheim) was a famous Swiss physician who lived during the sixteenth century. In his treatise on "Diseases Which Deprive Man of His Reason," he stated that "the best cure and one which rarely fails is to throw such persons into *cold water*."

About 100 A.D. the eminent Greek physician, Rufus of Ephesus, made the important discovery that strong *fever* can cure many diseases. From his descriptions, it is obvious that he dealt mainly with malarial fevers; these he found to be beneficial in melancholia and other mental disorders, as well as in certain diseases of the skin, and also in asthma, convulsions, and epilepsy. Fever treatment was not altogether original with him; certain peoples of Africa, he said, drank the urine of a goat to produce fever, and, "I know also that a Greek physician,

Euenor, employed this remedy." (Ralph H. Major: *A History of Medicine*, p. 184.)

These observations were soon forgotten and it was not until about seventeen centuries later that the great value of treatment with fever was redis-covered and applied to modern medicine. In 1883 Julius Wagner von Jauregg, a Viennese psychia-trist, had noted the disappearance of mental symp-toms in certain patients who accidentally con-tracted typhoid fever. This made such a great impression upon the young doctor that he contin-ued to think and write about the possibilities of fever-cures for insanity until, ten years later, he decided to infect insane persons with various germs, on purpose. He obtained the most spectacu-lar results in patients suffering from a syphilitic mental derangement, general paresis, when he inoculated them with malaria germs. The method was then successfully applied by various other phy-sicians throughout the world.

This was soon followed by the development of various types of *shock therapy* for mental patients. Treatments of this kind depend upon the produc-tion of a shock by electric current or by certain drugs, such as Metrazol or insulin. These proce-dures are still in wide use today.

Nobody really knew how these shock therapies worked. They grew out of chance observations on people in whom diseases were cured after acciden-tal exposure to some kind of shock. It seemed as though the patient was somehow "shaken out of his disease," very much as a child can be made to snap out of a temper tantrum if you suddenly splash a glass of cold water into its face.

The most peculiar thing about all these treatments was a lack of any detectable relationship between the cause of the disease and the way it was treated. It stands to reason that an infection can be cured by a remedy that kills the causative germs; but why should an infection with malaria or treatment with electric shocks cure a mental derangement that was caused, say, by syphilis? This uncertainty about the way these treatments worked created much uneasiness; but they did work—and often in conditions which could not otherwise be treated—and so they enjoyed considerable popularity.

Then, during the first half of this century, a variety of so-called *nonspecific therapies* had a great vogue. These were not so far removed from fever therapy and shock therapy as one might think. They were based upon the observation that the condition of patients suffering from various kinds of chronic diseases—say, rheumatism—is often improved by injections with various foreign materials (for instance, milk, foreign blood, or certain heavy-metal preparations) which stimulate a strong reaction on the part of the body.

The mystic exorcisms of a fear-inspiring priest-physician, the loss of blood, the painful whip, the exhausting fever, the shock of an electric current, and the strong bodily reaction against injections with foreign substances have one thing in common: they all cause wear and tear, making demands for adaptation; they all cause stress.

Could a sudden stress, or push, force the body to "snap out of disease"? One wonders: perhaps it could. If, for instance, the compulsory repetition of

certain defensive bodily actions could force some of
our vital mechanisms "into a groove," so to speak,
an often inappropriate habitual reaction form, a
good push might get us out of it. Everyone has had
experience with a watch, a radio set, or some other
machine: when it suddenly stops, you can often get
it to work again by simply shaking it a bit. The
same is true of a gramophone that suffers from
"compulsory repetition" because the needle has
made itself a wrong groove. If this can happen in a
machine, why not in a living body?

Quite apart from this passive being-pushed-into-
place, in man an extremely threatening treatment
might even stimulate active mechanisms of
defense. These could be intensified to such an
extent that they would overcome not only the damage of the treatment which mobilized them, but,
incidentally, also a disease.

Either of these two possible mechanisms could
explain the nonspecific nature of all these treatments. By *nonspecific treatment* we mean one
whose benefits are not limited to a single disease.
Significantly, none of the treatments so far mentioned are specific for any one malady. They may
not be particularly effective, but they can do some
good in various apparently unrelated diseases. For
instance, an artificially produced fever can
improve a mental disease as well as an inflammation of the eyes or a rheumatoid arthritis.

However, we must admit that these are only
illustrations, not explanations. The fact that a sudden push could set some derailment right in a
machine just helps one to imagine, not to understand, how nonspecific shock treatments and the
like might work.

We shall come back to this later, after having studied the actual mechanism of stress in man, as revealed by scientific inquiry. But, until recently, this much was all we knew—or, perhaps I should say, felt—about the way nonspecific cures might act. This is why all these types of treatment have gone in and out of fashion throughout history, without ever being able to establish themselves as recognized procedures. Scientifically-minded physicians do not like to employ methods which they cannot understand, because such procedures are usually unreliable and sometimes even dangerous. If we do not know through what pathways (nervous, hormonal, or other) a treatment works in the body, we may unwittingly overstrain some weak spot in the patient's system. If we know the mechanism of a treatment, at least we can withhold it from persons who probably could not take it.

I think this gives us a fair picture of what was known about the nonspecific element—or, as we now call it, *stress*—in medical treatment. Let us now have a look at what was known about nonspecific factors in the production of disease.

Pónos—the Toil of Disease

Twenty-four centuries ago, Hippocrates, the Father of Medicine, told his disciples in Greece that disease is not only suffering *(pathos)*, but also toil *(pónos)*, that is, the fight of the body to restore itself toward normal. There is a *vis medicatrix naturae*, a healing force of Nature, which cures from within.

Some 180 years ago, John Hunter pointed out that "There is a circumstance attending accidental injury which does not belong to disease—namely, that the injury done has in all cases a tendency to produce the disposition and the means of cure."

This is an important point and one which, despite being constantly rediscovered during the intervening centuries, is not yet generally understood even today. Disease is not mere surrender to attack but also fight for health; unless there is fight there is no disease.

Not every deviation from the normal condition of the body is disease. Just because a man has lost a leg as a child, he is not ill for the rest of his life. A cripple may be in perfect health despite his physical handicap. A woman born with a malformation, such as a harelip, may be disfigured, but she is not sick. Why? Because there is no *pónos*, no toil; the fight was lost long ago and now there is peace in the body, although it is a scarred body. The very concept of illness presupposes a clash between forces of aggression and our defenses.

"Homeostasis"—the Staying Power of the Body

During the second half of the nineteenth century, the great French physiologist, Claude Bernard, at the Collège de France in Paris, taught that one of the most characteristic features of all living beings is their ability to *maintain the constancy of their internal milieu*, despite changes in the surroundings. The physical properties and the chemical composition of our body fluids and tissues tend to remain remarkably constant despite all the changes around us. For instance, a man can be exposed to great cold or heat without varying his own temperature. He can eat large amounts of one substance or another without greatly influencing the composition of his blood. Whenever this self-regulating power fails, there is disease or even death.

Walter B. Cannon, the famous Harvard physiologist, subsequently called this power to maintain constancy in living beings *homeostasis* (from the Greek *homoios*, like, similar, and *stasis*, position, standing), the ability to remain the same, or static. You might roughly translate it as "staying power." The word *thermostat* (from Greek *thermē*, heat, and *stasis*), which is in common use, refers to a gadget that maintains the temperature static—for instance, in a room or oven—by automatically cutting down heat production when it threatens to become excessive, and vice versa. *Thermostasis* is then the maintenance of a steady temperature; and *homeostasis* is organic stability, or the maintenance of steadiness in every respect.

Apparently, disease is not just suffering, but a fight to maintain the homeostatic balance of our tissues, despite damage. There must be some element of stress here, at least in the sense in which the engineer speaks of stress and strain in connection with the interaction of force and resistance. What we have seen up to now, however, gives us no reason to believe that *nonspecific* stress plays any role in this. As far as we can see at this point, each damaging agent—every germ or poison—may be opposed by a special, highly specific defense mechanism. Examples would be the production of antisera which are good only against certain germs, or the manufacture by the body of some antidotes specifically inactivating certain poisons but not others.

All this does not help us as yet to define biologic stress or disease in precise terms; still, it does leave us with a vague feeling that various types of treatment and many, if not all, diseases have certain things in common, have certain nonspecific, stereotyped features.

Could all this vagueness be translated somehow into measurable terms? Could it point a way to explore whether or not there is some nonspecific defense system built into our body, a mechanism to fight any kind of disease? Could it lead us to a *unified theory of disease?*

Throughout the world and throughout the ages, many physicians must have wondered about this. I am just one of them.

chapter 2

My First Glimpse
of Stress

*How to question Nature.   Great hopes.   Great
disappointment.*

In 1925 I was a student at the Medical School of the
ancient University of Prague. I had just completed
my courses in anatomy, physiology, biochemistry,
and the other preclinical subjects which were
required as a preparation before we saw a patient.
I had stuffed myself full of theoretical knowledge
to the limit of my abilities and was burning with
enthusiasm for the art of healing, but I had only
vague ideas about how clinical medicine worked in
practice. Then came the great day, which I shall
never forget, when we were to hear our first lecture
in internal medicine and see how one examines a
patient.

It so happened that, on that day, by way of an
introduction, we were shown several cases in the
earliest stages of various infectious diseases. As
each patient was brought into the lecture room, the
professor carefully questioned and examined him.
It turned out that each of these patients felt and
looked ill, had a coated tongue, complained of more
or less diffuse aches and pains in the joints, and of
intestinal disturbances with loss of appetite. Most
of them also had fever (sometimes with mental
confusion), an enlarged spleen or liver, inflamed

tonsils, a skin rash, and so forth. All this was quite evident and the professor seemed to attach very little significance to any of it.

Then, he enumerated a few "characteristic" signs which might help in the diagnosis of the disease. These I could not see. They were absent or, at least, so inconspicuous that I could not distinguish them; yet these, we were told, were the important changes to which we would have to give all our attention. At present, our teacher said, most of the characteristic signs happened to be absent, but until they appeared, not much could be done. Without them it was impossible to know precisely what the patient suffered from, and hence it was obviously impossible to recommend any efficient treatment against the disease. It was clear that the many features of disease which were already manifest did not interest our teacher very much because they were "nonspecific," and hence "of no use," diagnostically, to the physician.

Since these were my first patients, I was still capable of looking at them without being biased by current medical thought. Had I known more I would never have asked myself questions, because everything was handled "just the way it should be," that is, "just the way every good physician does it." Had I known more, I would certainly have been stopped by the biggest of all blocks to improvement: the certainty of being right. But I did not know what was right.

I could understand that our professor had to find specific disease manifestations in order to identify the particular cause of disease in each of these patients. This, I clearly realized, was necessary so that suitable drugs might be prescribed, medicines having the specific effect of killing the germs or neutralizing the poisons that made these people sick.

I could see this all right, but what impressed me, the novice, much more was that so few signs and symptoms were actually characteristic of any one disease; most of the disturbances were apparently common to many, or perhaps even to all, diseases.

Why is it, I asked myself, that such widely different disease-producing agents as those which cause measles, scarlet fever, or the flu, share with a number of drugs, allergens, etc., the property of evoking the nonspecific manifestations which have just been mentioned? Yet evidently they do share them; indeed, they share them to such an extent that, at an early stage, it might be quite impossible, even for our eminent professor, to distinguish between various diseases.

Even now—after half a century—I still remember vividly the profound impression these considerations made upon me at the time. I could not understand why, ever since the dawn of medical history, physicians should have attempted to concentrate all their efforts upon the recognition of *individual* diseases and the discovery of *specific* remedies for them, without giving any attention to the much more obvious "syndrome of just being sick." I knew that a syndrome is usually defined as "a group of signs and symptoms that occur together and characterize a disease." Well, the patients we had just seen had a syndrome, but this seemed to be the syndrome that characterized disease as such, not any one disease.

Surely, if it is important to find remedies which help against one disease or another, it would be even more important to learn something about the mechanism of being sick and the means of treating this "general syndrome of sickness," which is apparently superimposed upon all individual diseases!!

As an apology for the two exclamation marks, let me point out that I was only nineteen years old at that time. Because of the confusion created in central Europe by the aftermath of World War I, I was allowed to complete my premedical studies as fast as I could pass the exams, and, with the help of an excellent private tutor, I got to Medical School at an unusually impressionable age.

In view of this I might perhaps also be forgiven for having thought that I could solve all these problems in a jiffy by applying classical research techniques to my problem. For several days, I intended to ask our professor of physiology for some lab space, so that I might analyze the "general syndrome of being sick" with the techniques of physiology, biochemistry, and histology which we had learned in our courses. If these methods could be used to clarify such specific things as the normal mechanisms of blood circulation or nervous conduction, I saw no reason why they could not be used with equal success to analyze the "general syndrome of disease" which interested me so much.

My immediate plans to dissect the general from the specific did not materialize, however. I was soon confronted with a problem which did not have the same general importance, but was more urgent specifically for me—the necessity of passing exams. Moreover, when I presented my idea to the professor of physiology, he merely laughed about it. After all, I really had no precise plan; I had no blueprint to guide the work I wanted to do. Besides, it seemed trivial and obvious to him that if someone was sick he would look sick.

Then, as time went by, this whole problem lost its meaning for me. As I learned more and more about medicine, the many classic textbook subjects of specific diagnosis and treatment began to blur my vision for the nonspecific. The former gradually assumed an ever-increasing importance and pushed the "syndrome of just being sick," the problem of "what is disease in general?" out of my consciousness into that hazy category of all those purely abstract arguments which are blind alleys not worth bothering about.

How to Question Nature

What is disease—not any one disease, just disease in general? This question lingered on in my mind, as it undoubtedly has in the minds of most physicians of all nations throughout history. But there was no hope of an early answer, for Nature—the source of all knowledge—rarely replies to questions unless they are put to her in the form of experiments to which she can say "yes" or "no." She is not loquacious; she merely nods in the affirmative or in the negative. "What is disease?" is not a question to which one can reply in this way.

Occasionally, if we ask, "What would you do in these circumstances?" or, "What is in such and such a place?" she will silently show us a picture. But

she never explains. You have to work things out
yourself first, aided only by instinct and the feeble
powers of the human brain, until you can ask precise questions, to which Nature can answer in her
precise but silent sign language of nods and pictures. Understanding grows out of a mosaic of such
answers. It is up to the scientist to draw a blueprint of the questions he has to ask before the
mosaic makes sense.

It is curious how few laymen, or even physicians,
understand this.

If you want to know whether a certain endocrine
(that is, hormone-producing) gland is necessary for
growth, you remove it surgically from the body of a
growing young experimental animal. If growth
stops, the answer is "yes." If you want to know
whether a certain substance extracted from this
gland is a growth-promoting hormone, you inject it
into the same animal, and, if now the latter begins
to grow again, the answer is "yes."

These are the nods of Nature.

If you want to know what is in the fat tissue
around the kidney, you dissect it and find the adrenal. If your question concerns the shape, size, or
structure of this gland, just look at it; you can even
examine the finest details of its appearance under
a powerful electron microscope.

Such are the pictures of Nature.

But if now you ask, "What is an adrenal?" you
will get no reply. This is the wrong question; it
cannot be answered by nods or pictures.

Only those blessed with the understanding that
comes from a sincere and profound love of Nature
will, by an intuitive feeling for her ways, succeed in

constructing a blueprint of the many questions that need to be asked to get even an approximate answer to such a question.

Only those cursed with a consuming, uncontrollable curiosity for Nature's secrets will be able to—because they will have to—spend their lives working out patiently, one by one, the innumerable technical problems involved in performing each of the countless experiments required.

What is disease?—What is stress?

I did not know how to ask the first of these questions; I did not even think of asking the second.

Great Hopes

Not until about ten years after hearing my first lecture on internal medicine did these same problems confront me again, although now under entirely different circumstances. At the time, I was working as a young assistant in the Biochemistry Department of McGill University in Montreal, engaged in research on sex hormones. I injected rats with various ovarian and placental extracts to see whether the organs of these animals would show such changes as could *not* be due to any *known* sex hormone.

> A *hormone* is a specific chemical messenger-substance, made by an endocrine gland and secreted into the blood, to regulate and coordinate the functions of distant organs. Sex hormones are coordinators of sexual activities, including reproduction.
>
> An *extract* is made by mixing tissue (say, the ovaries of cows) with solvents (water, alcohol, etc.)

and taking what goes into solution. The extract is pure when it contains only the desired substance (for instance, a hormone) and impure when it also contains contaminants (for instance, unwanted and perhaps damaging ovarian substances).

Much to my satisfaction, such changes were produced in my rats even by my first and most impure extracts:

1. There was a considerable enlargement of the *adrenal cortex*.

The *adrenals* are two little endocrine glands which lie just above the kidneys, on both sides. Each of them consists of two portions, a central part, the medulla, and an outer rind, the cortex. Both of these parts produce hormones, but not the same kind. My extracts seemed to stimulate the cortex, without causing much of a change in the medulla. The cortical portion of the adrenals was not only enlarged, but it also showed the microscopic features of increased activity (such as cell-multiplication and discharge of stored fatty secretion-droplets into the blood).

2. There was an intense shrinking (or atrophy) of the *thymus*, the *spleen*, the *lymph nodes*, and of all other *lymphatic structures* in the body.

The *lymphatic structures* are made up of innumerable, small white blood cells, similar to the *lymphocytes*, which circulate in the blood. What a lymphocyte does in solid lymphatic tissue or in the blood is not yet very well known, but it certainly plays an important role in immunologic defense.

For instance, in people exposed to x-rays, the lymphocytes tend to disappear, and then resistance against all kinds of germs and poisons is much impaired.

The *lymphocytes* are made in the lymph nodes, little nodules in the groins, under the armpits, along the neck, and in various other parts of the body. Lymphocytes also make up most of the tissue in the *thymus* and *spleen:* that is why these organs are called *lymphatic tissues* or the *thymicolymphatic system.* The thymus is a huge lymphatic organ just in front of the heart in the chest. In children it is very well developed but, after puberty, it tends to shrink, presumably under the influence of sex hormones.

When I saw that the lymphatic organs had so rapidly disintegrated in the rats, I naturally also examined the lymphocytes in the blood. Their number had also diminished under the influence of my tissue extracts, but while studying them I accidentally found an even more striking change in the blood picture: the almost complete disappearance of the *eosinophil cells.*

These are somewhat larger white blood cells, which have received their name because they stain very easily with a dye called *eosin.* This coloring agent is frequently used for histologic studies to make cells more visible under the microscope. The function of the eosinophils is also still debated, but they seem to be related to immunologic adaptive reactions, particularly allergy, because their number increases remarkably when a person suffers from asthma, hay fever, or allied conditions.

3. There appeared bleeding, deep *ulcers* in the lining of the stomach, and that uppermost part of the gut, just after the stomach, which we call the duodenum.

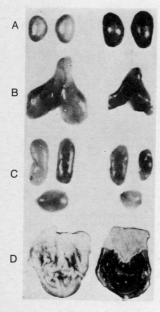

A

B

C

D

Fig. 1 The typical triad of the alarm reaction. A. Adrenals. B. Thymus. C. A group of three lymph nodes. D. Inner surface of the stomach.

The organs on the left are those of a normal rat, those on the right of one exposed to the frustrating psychologic stress of being forcefully immobilized. Note the marked enlargement and dark discoloration of the adrenals (due to congestion and discharge of fatty secretion granules), the intense shrinkage of the thymus and lymph nodes, and the numerous blood-covered stomach ulcers in the alarmed rat. *(After H. Selye, "The Story of the Adaptation Syndrome," courtesy of Acta, Inc., Montreal.)*

These three types of changes formed a definite syndrome, because they were closely interdependent in some way. When I injected only a small amount of extract, all these changes were slight; when I injected much extract, they were all very pronounced. But with no extract could I ever produce one of these three changes without the others. This interdependence of lesions is precisely what makes them a syndrome *(Fig. 1.)*

Incidentally, a syndrome such as ours, which consists of three types of changes, is usually called a *triad.*

Now, from all this I concluded that my extracts must contain some very active substance, and having been prepared from ovaries, this was first presumed to be an ovarian hormone. In apparent agreement with this view, one major manifestation of the triad was a change in an endocrine gland, the adrenal cortex, and another was the involution of the thymicolymphatic apparatus, a type of tissue known to shrink under the influence of sex hormones.

Of course, to me, the most important thing was that no ovarian hormone, or combination of ovarian hormones, known at that time ever produced adrenal enlargement, thymicolymphatic involution, and ulcers in the intestinal tract. It seemed rather obvious that we were dealing with a *new* ovarian hormone.

You may well imagine my happiness! At the age of 28, I already seemed to be on the track of a new hormone. I even had a perfect method with which to identify it in extracts, namely, the appearance of the triad just described in rats treated with this hormone. It seemed only a matter of time now before I would concentrate and isolate the new hormone in pure form.

Unfortunately, this happiness was not to last long. Not only ovarian, but placental, extracts also produced our triad. This did not worry me very much at first; after all, we knew that both the ovaries and the placenta can produce female sex hormones. I began to be somewhat confused, however, when it turned out subsequently that even pituitary extracts produced the same syndrome.

> The *pituitary* (or hypophysis) is a little endocrine gland embedded in the bones of the skull, just below the brain. It produces a number of hormones, but, as far as we knew, no ovarian hormones.

Yet, even this was not too disturbing, since mine was supposed to be a new hormone and (who knew?) perhaps the pituitary could also manufacture this one.

But I really became puzzled when I found, a little later, that extracts of kidney, spleen, or any other organ would produce the same triad. Was the causative factor some kind of general "tissue hormone" that could be produced by almost any cell?

Another inexplicable fact was that all efforts to purify the active extracts led to a diminution of their potency. The crudest preparations—the most impure ones—were invariably the most active. This did not seem to make sense.

Great Disappointment

It was then that a horrible thought occurred to me: for all I knew, this entire syndrome might be due merely to the toxicity of my extracts, to the fact that I did not purify them well enough.

In this case, of course, all my work would mean nothing. I was not on the track of a new ovarian hormone; indeed, I was not even dealing with any specific ubiquitous "tissue hormone," but merely with damage as such.

As I thought of this, my eyes happened to fall upon a bottle of Formalin on a shelf in front of my desk.

> Formalin is an extremely toxic and irritating fluid. We use it in the preparation of tissues for microscopic study, as a fixative. Just as you use fixatives in photography, so for microscopic work, we employ certain agents to *fix* the structure of cells by instantly precipitating their constituents in the natural state.

Now, I thought, if my syndrome is really due only to tissue damage, I should be able to reproduce it by injecting rats with a dilute Formalin solution. The cells in immediate contact with the Formalin would be precipitated and killed, causing considerable tissue damage. This provided a good way to formulate the question I wanted to ask: could even a toxic fluid not derived from any living tissue produce my syndrome?

I immediately undertook such experiments and, within 48 hours, when I examined the organs of my animals, the answer was only too clear. In all the rats there was even more adrenocortical enlargement, thymicolymphatic atrophy, and intestinal ulcer formation than I had ever been able to produce with any of my tissue extracts.

I do not think I had ever been more profoundly disappointed! Suddenly all my dreams of discovering a new hormone were shattered. All the time and all the materials that went into this long study were wasted.

I tried to tell myself, "You must not let this sort of thing get you down; after all, fortunately, noth-

ing has been published about the 'new hormone,' so
no confusion has been created in the minds of others and there is nothing to retract." I tried to tell
myself over and over again that such disappoint-
ments are inevitable in a scientist's life; occasionally anyone can follow a wrong track, and it is
precisely the vision necessary to recognize such
errors that characterizes the reliable investigator.
But all this gave me little solace and, indeed, I
became so depressed that for a few days I could not
do any work at all. I just sat in my laboratory,
brooding about how this misadventure might have
been avoided and wondering what was to be done
now.

Eventually I decided that, of course, the only
reasonable thing to do was to pull myself together,
admit my defeat, and return to some of the more
orthodox endocrinologic problems that had occupied my attention before I was sidetracked into
this regrettable enterprise. After all, I was young
and much of the road still lay ahead. Yet, somehow
I could not forget my triad, nor could I get hold of
myself sufficiently to do anything else in the laboratory for several days.

The ensuing period of introverted contemplation
turned out to be the decisive factor in my whole
career; it pointed the way for all my subsequent
work. But much more important than that, it
revealed vistas sufficiently alluring in their promise of adventure and fulfillment to inspire that irre-
sistible curiosity about Nature's ways which was to
be my delightful damnation ever after.

chapter 3

The Birth of the G.A.S.

The first publication on the stress syndrome.
A word about discovery.   The search for a name.

As I repetitiously continued to go over my ill-fated experiments and their possible interpretation, it suddenly struck me that one could look at them from an entirely different angle. If there was such a thing as a single nonspecific reaction of the body to damage of any kind, this might be worth study for its own sake. Indeed, working out the mechanism of this kind of stereotyped "syndrome of response to injury as such" might be much more important to medicine than the discovery of yet another sex hormone.

As I repeated to myself, "a syndrome of response to injury as such," gradually, my early classroom impressions of the clinical "syndrome of just being sick" began to reappear dimly out of my subconsciousness, where they had been buried for over a decade. Could it be that this syndrome in man (the feeling of being ill, the diffuse pains in joints and muscles, the intestinal disturbances with loss of appetite, the loss of weight) were in some manner clinical equivalents of the experimental syndrome, the triad (adrenocortical stimulation, thymicolymphatic atrophy, intestinal ulcers) that I had produced with such a variety of toxic substances in the rat?

If this were so, the general medical implications of the syndrome would be enormous! Some degree of nonspecific damage is undoubtedly superimposed upon the specific characteristics of any disease, upon the specific effects of any drug.

If this were so, everything we had learned about the characteristic manifestations of disease, about the specific actions of drugs, would be in need of revision. All the actually observed biologic effects of any agent must represent the sum of its specific actions and of this nonspecific response to damage that is superimposed upon it.

If this were so, it would mean that my first classroom impressions about the one-sidedness of medical thinking were quite justified and by no means sterile questions without practical implications. If the "damage syndrome" is superimposed upon the specific effects of all diseases and remedies, a systematic inquiry into the mechanism of this syndrome might well furnish us with a solid scientific basis for the treatment of damage as such.

If this were so, we had been examining medicine—disease and treatment—looking only for the specific, but through glasses tinted with the color of nonspecificity. Now that we had become aware of this misleading factor, we could remove the glasses and, for the first time, study the true characteristic properties of disease and treatment apart from the confusing nonspecific haze imparted by the glasses.

It had long ago been learned by sheer experience that certain curative measures were nonspecific, that is, useful to patients suffering from almost any disease. Indeed, such measures had been in use for centuries. One advises the patient, for example, to go to bed and take it easy; tells him to eat only easily digestible food and to protect himself against drafts or great variations in temperature and humidity.

Furthermore, there were all the nonspecific treatments that we had learned about in medical school, such as injection of substances foreign to the body, fever therapy, shock therapy, or bloodletting. They were unquestionably useful in certain cases. The trouble was that they often did not help, and sometimes caused much harm. One knew nothing about the mechanism of their action; using them was like taking a shot in the dark.

If we could prove that the organism had a general nonspecific reaction-pattern with which it could meet damage caused by a variety of potential disease-producers, this defensive response would lend itself to a strictly objective, truly scientific analysis. By clarifying the function of the mechanism of response through which Nature herself fights injuries of various kinds, we might learn how to improve upon this reaction whenever it is imperfect.

I was simply fascinated by these new possibilities and immediately decided to reverse my plans for the future. Instead of dropping the stress problem and returning to classic endocrinology, I was now prepared to spend the rest of my life studying it. I have never had any reason to regret this decision.

It may be worth mentioning that I often had to overcome considerable mental inhibitions in my

efforts to carry on with this plan. Nowadays it is
perhaps difficult to appreciate just how absurd my
concept seemed to most people before I had more
facts to show that it worked. For example, I
remember one senior professor whom I admired
very much and whose opinion meant a great deal to
me. I knew he was a real friend who seriously
wanted to help me with my research efforts. One
day, during these busy weeks, he asked me into his
office for a good heart-to-heart talk. He reminded
me that for months now he had attempted to convince me that I must abandon this futile line of
research. He assured me that, in his opinion, I
possessed all the essential qualifications of an
investigator and that I could undoubtedly contribute something to the generally recognized and
accepted fields of endocrinology, so why bother
with this wild-goose chase?

I met these remarks with my usual outbursts of
uncontrolled youthful enthusiasm for the new
point of view; I outlined again the immense possibilities inherent in a study of the nonspecific damage which must accompany all diseases and all but
the mildest medications.

When he saw me thus launched on yet another
enraptured description of what I had observed in
animals treated with this or that impure, toxic
material, he looked at me with desperately sad eyes
and said in obvious despair, "But, Selye, try to
realize what you are doing before it is too late! You
have now decided to spend your entire life studying
the pharmacology of dirt!"

Of course, he was right. Nobody could have

expressed it more poignantly; that is why it hurt so much that I still remember the phrase today, forty years later. Pharmacology is the science which explores the actions of specific drugs or poisons and I was going to study nothing but their undesired, contaminating, that is, nonspecific side effects. But to me, "the pharmacology of dirt" seemed the most promising subject in medicine.

Yet I could not say that I never wavered; as time went by, I often doubted the wisdom of my decision. Almost none of the recognized, experienced investigators, whose judgment one could usually trust, agreed with my views; and, after all, was it not silly and pretentious for a beginner to contradict all of them? Perhaps I had just developed a warped viewpoint. Was I, perhaps, merely wasting my time?

In such moments of doubt I derived considerable strength and courage from the fact that, right from the beginning, one of the most respected Canadian scientists, Sir Frederick Banting, was manifestly interested in my plans. At that time, he frequently visited university laboratories throughout Canada, since he acted as an adviser to the Canadian National Research Council. When in Montreal, he often dropped in quite informally at my somewhat overcrowded little laboratory. There was not much space and he usually settled down on top of the desk, listening attentively to my daydreaming about the "syndrome of being sick."

Nothing could have done me more good! He also helped to secure the first modest financial aid ($500) for this kind of research, but that was comparatively unimportant. More than anything in the world, I needed his moral support, the reassuring feeling that the discoverer of insulin, a Nobel Prize Laureate, took me seriously.

I often wonder whether I could have stuck to my guns without his encouragement.

The next point to decide was how to go about studying *the new syndrome*. Right from the start a multitude of questions arose:

1. To what extent is this syndrome *really nonspecific?*

2. Apart from those already observed, what *other manifestations* are part of it?

3. *How does it develop in time?* Is the degree of its manifestations merely proportional to the magnitude of the damage at all times, or does the syndrome—like many infectious diseases—go through distinct stages in a certain chronologic order?

4. To what extent are the manifestations of the nonspecific syndrome *influenced by the specific actions* of the agents which elicit it? All germs, poisons, and allergens have special characteristics which distinguish their effects from those of all other agents. Yet, when any substance acts upon the body, it automatically mobilizes the nonspecific mechanism also. Hence, the resulting picture would have to be a composite one, consisting of both specific and of nonspecific actions. Could these be separated?

5. What could we find out about the *mechanism*, the "dynamics" of this reaction; that is, the pathways through which the various organ changes are produced?

These and many other questions not only pre-

sented themselves quite spontaneously, but
became immediately accessible to objective scientific analysis, as soon as the concept of the "nonspecific syndrome" had crystallized. Now it was only a
matter of time to find the answers to all these
questions which could not even have been asked
before the theory of a single "stereotyped response
to damage" had taken a precise form.

I thought that our first question should be, "Just
how nonspecific is this syndrome?" Up to now, I
had elicited it only by injecting foreign substances
(tissue extracts, Formalin). Subsequent experiments showed that one can produce essentially the
same syndrome with purified hormones such as
adrenaline (a hormone of the adrenal medulla) or
with insulin (a hormone of the pancreas). One can
also produce it with physical agents, such as cold,
heat, x-rays, or mechanical trauma; one can produce it with hemorrhage, pain, or forced muscular
exercise; indeed, *I could find no noxious agent that
did not produce the syndrome.* The scope of this
approach appeared to have no limits.

At this point I first became painfully aware of the
purely linguistic difficulties arising out of new
viewpoints in medical research. Novel concepts
require new terms with which to describe them.
Yet most of us dislike neologisms, perhaps
because—especially in referring to clinical syndromes and signs—new names are so often proposed merely to give a semblance of a new discovery. Moreover a new designation, if badly chosen or
superfluous, can confuse more than clarify. However, now I clearly needed terms for two things:
first, for the nonspecific syndrome itself, and sec-

ond, for that which produced it. I could not think of any good name for either.

The First Publication on the Stress Syndrome

My first paper, in which I endeavored to show that the syndrome of stress can be studied independently of all specific changes, happened to come out on American Independence Day, July 4, in 1936 amid a nationwide shower of firecrackers. It was a brief note of only 74 lines in a single column of the British journal *Nature,* under the title, "A Syndrome Produced by Diverse Nocuous Agents."

Although previously in conversation and in lectures I had often used the term *biologic stress* in referring to what caused this syndrome, by the time the first formal paper was published—yielding to violently adverse public opinion—I had temporarily given up this term. There was too much criticism of my use of the word *stress* in reference to bodily reactions, because in everyday English it generally implied nervous strain. I did not want to obscure the real issues by such squabbles over words and hoped that the word *noxious* (especially after being refined to *nocuous* by the British editor) would be considered less obnoxious than *stress.*

In this same paper I also suggested the name *alarm reaction* for the initial response—that is, the previously mentioned triad—because I thought that this syndrome probably represented the bodily expression of a generalized call to arms of the defensive forces in the organism.

But this alarm reaction was evidently not the whole response. My very first experiments showed that upon continued exposure to any noxious agent capable of eliciting this alarm reaction (unless it killed immediately), a stage of adaptation or resistance followed. In other words, no living organism can be maintained continuously in a state of alarm. If the body is confronted with an agent so damaging that continuous exposure to it is incompatible with life, then death ensues during the alarm reaction within the first hours or days. If survival is possible at all, this alarm reaction is necessarily followed by a second phase which I called the *stage of resistance*.

The manifestations of this second stage were quite different from, and in many instances the exact opposite of, those which characterized the alarm reaction. For instance, during the alarm reaction, the cells of the adrenal cortex discharged their microscopically visible, hormone-containing granules of secretion into the blood stream. Consequently, the stores of the gland were depleted. Conversely, in the stage of resistance, the cortex accumulated an abundant reserve of secretory granules. In the alarm reaction, the blood became concentrated and there was a marked loss of body weight; but during the stage of resistance, the blood was diluted and the body weight returned toward normal. Many similar examples could be cited, but these suffice to illustrate the way one can objectively follow resistance changes in various organs.

Curiously, after still more prolonged exposure to

any of the noxious agents I used, this acquired adaptation was eventually lost. The animal entered into a third phase, the *stage of exhaustion,* the symptoms of which were, in many respects, strikingly similar to those of the initial alarm reaction. At the end of a life under stress, this was a kind of premature aging due to wear and tear, a sort of second childhood which, in some ways, resembled the first.

All these findings made it necessary to coin an additional all-embracing name for the entire syndrome. Since the latter appeared to be so evidently related to adaptation, I called the entire nonspecific response the *general adaptation syndrome,* usually abbreviated as G.A.S. This whole syndrome then evolves in time through the three stages which I have just mentioned, namely: (1) the alarm reaction (A.R.), (2) the stage of resistance (S.R.), (3) the stage of exhaustion (S.E.).

I called this syndrome *general,* because it is produced only by agents which have a general effect upon large portions of the body. I called it *adaptive* because it stimulates defense and thereby helps in the acquisition and maintenance of a stage of inurement. I called it a *syndrome* because its individual manifestations are coordinated and even partly dependent upon each other.

We have seen that the idea of stress goes back to the *pónos* of Greek medicine and that even certain nonspecific effects of drugs had long been known. The practical use of stress-producing measures of treatment had been repeatedly hailed as a panacea, each time only to be rejected a few years later as mere superstition and charlatanism. The parts of this concept were too elusive to be connected and grasped as a whole, hence it could not be analyzed and understood.

Significantly, in English, as a synonym for the word *understand* we use *grasp*, precisely because it means "to hold or grip a physical object with our hands." To *understand* is to "lay hold of with the mind." You can physically grasp something only if you manage to get hold of it between other things, for instance, your fingers, over which you have control.

Understanding is quite similar. It is not a totally new mental experience, essentially different from observation, any more than physical grasping is essentially different from touching. Understanding merely represents the solid fixation of a thing relative to the rest of our knowledge.

Throughout recorded medical history, parts of the stress concept have floated about aimlessly, like loose logs on the sea, periodically rising high on the crests of waves of popularity, then sinking low into the troughs of disgrace and oblivion. First we had to bind the loose logs (observed facts) together by solid cables (workable theories), and then secure the resulting raft (G.A.S.) by mooring it to generally accepted, solid supports (classical medicine) before we could make use of the timber.

That is what I had in mind when I spoke about the essence of discovery. To discover does not mean to *see*, but to *uncover* sufficiently that many may see and continue to see.

As regards the G.A.S., the process of grasping

and permanently attaching it to the rest of our
knowledge had progressed by this time in two
dimensions: (1) *In space*, three fixed points have
been established as comprising a coordinated
syndrome: the adrenal, the thymicolymphatic, and
the intestinal changes. These have been described
as a triad. (2) *In time*, it has been shown that the
G.A.S. goes through three distinct phases: the
alarm reaction, the stage of resistance, and the
stage of exhaustion. It thus follows a predictable
path of evolution.

This picture was woefully sketchy and incomplete. Much had been said before about *pónos*.
Much more has been written since on the many
additional changes subsequently recognized as
belonging to the G.A.S. or the *stress syndrome*, as it
is also called now. The only important thing about
our fixed points in space and time was that they
just sufficed to get a hold on stress; they were just
strong enough to prevent the concept from ever
slipping through our fingers again; they made it
amenable to a precise scientific analysis. We could
now draw a blueprint for a systematic plan of
research on stress. There will be more to say about
this blueprint later; but just to take an example,
we could now devise experiments to see whether
the effect of stress on lymphatic tissue depends
upon adrenal activity. To establish this, we only
had to verify whether the thymicolymphatic tissue
of experimental animals shrinks during stress
even after removal of the adrenals. We could not
have formulated such precise questions about the
mechanism of stress before our fixed points were
established.

A Word about Discovery

When one starts out in a research career, it is
somewhat discouraging to think that, because
through so many centuries so many outstanding
minds have explored the salient problems of medicine, presumably most of the important things
have already been discovered.

In talking to my students I hear this view
expressed again and again. Many beginners are
also convinced that to make really interesting discoveries today one would need vast sums of
money, modern laboratories equipped with all
kinds of complicated, expensive machinery, and a
large staff of highly-trained assistants. Some students are often discouraged by the thought that
the times have gone when it was possible to make
an immortal medical discovery by merely looking
at a hitherto unexplored part of the human body.

Take the adrenals, which play such a prominent
role in my own story: the most important fact
about them is that they exist. Without knowing
this, we could have discovered nothing else about
them. Well, this basic fact was revealed in 1563 by
Bartolommeo Eustacchio, physician to Cardinal
della Rovere. Because of his connections in high
places, Eustacchio managed to get permission to
perform dissections in Rome. After that it was easy:
merely by prodding about in the fat around the
upper pole of the kidneys, he could not help it—he
had to discover the adrenals. There was nothing to
it.

I think it is very wrong to look at things this way.
First, it must have taken insatiable scientific curi-

osity to overcome the prejudices of the sixteenth
century sufficiently to ask for and use permission
for the dissection of a human body. Second, it
required great perspicacity to recognize that the
inconspicuous little piece of whitish tissue, embedded in fat of almost the same color, is a separate
organ, worthy of being described. We must always
measure the importance of a discovery against the
background of the times in which it was made; and
I should think that each period offers just about
the same proportion of facilities and handicaps for
scientific investigation. We should not envy the
ancient anatomists for having been able to make a
great discovery with simple means, any more than
we should complain that our research tools are
undoubtedly very primitive in comparison with
those to be used by the investigators of coming
centuries.

Often it is not so much the existence of things
that we *do not know*, or about which we are too
uncertain, that handicaps our research, but the
existence of things we *do know* and about whose
interpretation we are quite certain—although
they may turn out to be false. Lack of equipment,
or even lack of knowledge, is much less of a handicap in original research than an overabundance of
useless materials or useless (and sometimes false)
information cluttering up our laboratories, our
files, our desks, and our brains.

You will recall that the indexes of stress upon
which the concept of the G.A.S. was based were:
adrenocortical enlargement, thymicolymphatic
involution, and intestinal ulcers. Then came the
realization that this syndrome is triphasic, with

the initial appearance of marked acute manifestations (alarm reaction), their subsequent disappearance (stage of resistance) and finally, a breakdown
in the organism, with complete loss of resistance
(stage of exhaustion). These were the facts upon
which the first note on "A Syndrome Produced by
Diverse Nocuous Agents" was based. All this is
easy to see. Actually, a pair of scissors with which
to open my rats was the only diagnostic instrument
I had used up to that time, and the production of
stress by toxic substances certainly necessitated
no complicated apparatus either.

It is true that I did use a syringe for the injection
of Formalin, and even that I had a "staff" in the
person of Mr. Kai Nielsen who, at the time, was an
untrained laboratory assistant. He helped me by
holding the rats steady for injection, but mainly by
steadying me during those busy days, through the
stabilizing effect of his always friendly, even-
minded personality.*

When the problem arose as to whether or not
stress could be produced without injecting anything, I wanted to expose animals to cold. We had
no suitable ventilated cold-room. But let me assure

*Incidentally, Mr. Nielsen worked with me for 35 years until
his retirement in 1970, and came to master a great many complex laboratory techniques. Yet, in retrospect, when everything is said and done, I feel that, in 1935, when we were both
young, as well as in 1970 when we were a little less so, his
undoubtedly enormous contribution to the study of stress was
very simple. He always was an utterly reliable, straightforward person and a warmhearted friend upon whose level-
headed judgment one could count. Let me assure you that in
the actual practice of research these characteristics of an asso-
ciate can be much more helpful than the largest staff of technical assistants.

you that here, in Canada, this presented no problem during the major part of the year, especially in
the McGill Medical Building of 1935, with its conve-
niently wind-swept flat roof.

As the years went by, I managed to acquire
every available facility that modern science can
offer in the way of the most sophisticated techniques of histology, chemistry, and pharmacology.
I have been given the means to construct one of the
best-equipped institutes of experimental medicine
and surgery in the world and have acquired a staff
which, at the peak of its activity, comprised about
100 trained assistants, technicians, and secre-
taries. Yet today, as I look back upon the years that
have elapsed since those early observations in
1935–1936, I am ashamed to say that, despite all
this help, I have never again been able to add
anything of comparable significance to those first
primitive experiments.

My advice to a novice scientist is to look for the
mere outlines of the big things with his fresh,
untrained, but still unprejudiced mind. At a more
advanced stage, one may no longer be able to see
the forest for the trees. (But by that time one will
have the money to buy fancy tools and hire assistants to exploit the details.)

There are two ways of detecting something that
no one has yet seen: one is to aim at the finest
detail by getting as close as possible with the best
available analyzing instruments; the other is
merely to look at things from a new angle where
they show hitherto unexposed facets. The former
requires money and experience; the latter presupposes neither; indeed, it is actually aided by sim-

plicity, the lack of prejudice, and the absence of those established habits of thinking which tend to come after long years of work. The G.A.S. could have been discovered during the Middle Ages, if not earlier; its recognition did not depend upon the development of any complicated pieces of apparatus, new techniques of observation, nor even upon much training, ingenuity, or intelligence, as far as that goes, but merely upon an unbiased state of mind, a fresh point of view.

The Search for a Name

As time went by, little by little, the main features of the G.A.S. had been recognized and named, but we still had no precise idea of what produced it, and even less a suitable name to describe its cause. In my first paper, I spoke of *nocuous agents*, but this term was evidently inadequate. Even such innocuous physiologic experiences as a brief period of muscular work, excitement, or a short exposure to cold proved sufficient to produce certain manifestations of an alarm reaction, such as an adrenocortical reaction. Obviously, these could not be described as strictly nocuous agents; we needed a more fitting name.

In search of one, I again stumbled upon the term *stress*, which had long been used in common English, and particularly in engineering, to denote the effects of a force acting against a resistance. For example, the changes induced in a rubber band during stretching, or in a steel spring during pressure, are due to stress. Physical stress is certainly nonspecific. In a sense, the nonspecific manifestations of the G.A.S. could be viewed as the biologic equivalents of what had been called the results of stress in inanimate matter. Perhaps one could speak of *biologic stress*.

Another advantage of this term was that, although its meaning, as applied to biology, had never been defined before, it was not strictly a neologism, even in medicine. For instance, the expressions *nervous stress* and *strain* had often been used by psychiatrists to describe mental tension. Walter B. Cannon, the eminent physiologist who introduced the term *homeostasis*, also spoke in general terms of the stresses and strains caused when an agent puts pressure on certain specific mechanisms necessary for homeostasis, that is, the maintenance of a normal, steady state in the body.

Although the term had not been used previously for any nonspecific reactions, and of course, even less for a coordinated triphasic syndrome, I saw no reason why it should not be employed in this new sense. So, during the subsequent years—despite much initial opposition—that is what I did in all my scientific papers and books.

The layman may think it ridiculous to speak so much about a name. After all, as Shakespeare said, "What's in a name? That which we call a rose/By any other name would smell as sweet." In science names have a much more profound significance, especially when they apply to novel concepts. You can discuss a rose by any name because everybody knows exactly what is meant by a rose, but you cannot discuss, and far less define, a new scientific concept, such as an atom or a molecule, without first identifying it in some way by a name. I have tried to convey the importance of this by speaking about the naming of stress before I was able to define the concept of stress in precise scientific language. That unfortunately is the order in which events actually develop in science.

One of the objections against my use of the term *stress* was that it might lead to confusion with other possible meanings of the word. For instance, some scientists were afraid that stress, in my sense, might be identified with the specific stresses and strains upon individual homeostatic mechanisms, the "built-in homeostats" (Norbert Wiener), or automatic regulators of certain actions. But Cannon had clearly shown, for example, that the specific stabilizing or *homeostatic reaction* to lack of oxygen is quite different from that with which the body meets exposure to cold; this, in turn, is virtually the reverse of that required to resist heat. These and many other highly specialized adjustments (for example, specific serologic reactions against certain microbes, the strengthening of individual muscle groups in response to frequent use) represent precisely *that part of the over-all response to an agent which we have to subtract in order to arrive at our stress syndrome*. The features of the G.A.S. (for instance, the increased production of adrenocortical hormones, the involution of the lymphatic organs, or the loss of weight) are the purely nonspecific residue that remains after this subtraction. Besides, Cannon never proposed the term *stress* as a scientific name for anything in particular; it does not even appear in the subject index of his book and, as far as I know, he used it only figuratively in one semipopular lecture.

Anyway, in practice, the possible other meanings of the word have not led to much confusion. Had I coined a totally new name by just putting letters together at random, its meaning would have been difficult to remember; it seemed preferable to use an existent term in a newly-defined connotation. After all, the words *general, adaptation, syndrome, alarm, reaction, stage, resistance,* and *exhaustion* were not new either. They had all been used before in connection with medical topics other than the general adaptation syndrome and its three stages. This likewise caused no real difficulties of understanding (although none of these terms was immediately well received either).

The initial resistance to my use of the word *stress* is an integral part of the story of stress, because here rejection of the name was largely due to a failure to grasp the new concept. Again and again, in the discussion periods following my lectures before scientific societies, someone would get up and ask why I had to speak of stress, when I actually used Formalin, cold, or x-rays. Would it not be more straightforward to say that the adrenals were stimulated by cold, when it was cold that my experimental animal was exposed to and the adrenals that were enlarged?

I tried to point out that it could not be cold itself that was necessary for adrenal stimulation, since heat or any number of other agents produced the same effect. By way of a comparison, I mentioned that a pharmacologist examining the effects of ether should not look upon adrenocortical enlargement or thymus involution as being caused by ether in the same sense as anesthesia is. Indeed, I emphasized that now, in my opinion, one would have to reexamine the whole of pharmacology to distinguish the changes merely due to stress from such specific drug actions as anesthesia or the cure of rickets.

Others pointed out that, actually, *stress is an abstraction* and does not occur as such in the pure state. In other words, it is just a purely hypothetical thing, which possesses no real independent existence. Hence, my opponents said, it is impossible to isolate stress for the objective, direct, scientific observation and measurement of its own effects, which would be indispensable for any scientific treatment of this problem. You cannot study stress; you can merely explore real and tangible things such as the effects of exposure to cold, injections of Formalin, infections, and so forth. Some people still say so today. For these reasons, I was told, even if we admitted the existence of stress, it would not lend itself to scientific study.

Of course, the concept of stress *is* an abstraction; but so is that of life, which could hardly be rejected as irrelevant to the study of biology. No one has studied life in a pure, uncontaminated form. It is always inseparably attached to something else which is more tangible and seemingly more real, such as the body of a cat, a dog, or a man; still, the whole science of physiology is built upon this abstraction.

To study the laws of gravity, the concept of weight must be separated from other characteristics of objects, even if weight, as such, does not exist. An automobile and a piece of rock both weighing 2,000 pounds are identical as regards weight, though, in most other respects, the automobile is quite unlike the stone.

Yet, during the first few years, such arguments convinced but very few people. It was only gradually, through habit rather than logic, that the term *stress*, employed in my sense, slipped into common usage, as the concept itself became a popular subject for research.

Even after that, when people began to speak of stress in my sense of the word, I was again exposed to severe criticism because of a new terminologic difficulty. It was pointed out that the word *stress* is indiscriminately applied both to the agent which produces the G.A.S. and to the condition of the organism exposed to it. Actually, some people do speak of having applied cold-stress, heat-stress, and—oh, horrors!—even infectious-stress, when referring to cold, heat, or infection employed to produce stress; but they also use the same expressions for the state of stress caused in the body by these agents.

This lack of distinction between cause and effect was, I suppose, fostered by the fact that when I introduced the word *stress* into medicine in its present meaning, my English was not yet good enough for me to distinguish between the words "stress" and "strain." It was not until several years later that the *British Medical Journal* called my attention to this fact, by the somewhat sarcastic remark that according to Selye "stress is its own cause." Actually I should have called my phenomenon the "strain reaction" and that which causes it "stress," which would parallel the use of these terms in physics. However, by the time that this

came to my attention, "biologic stress" in my sense
of the word was so generally accepted in various
languages that I could not have redefined it.
Hence, I was forced to create a neologism and
introduce the word *stressor*, for the causative
agent, into the English language, retaining *stress*
for the resulting condition.

Although these terms are now generally
accepted in biology, occasional confusions still
arise and hence I would like to state here clearly
that the concepts of stress and strain in physics
correspond, respectively, to those of stressor and
stress in biology and medicine.

A little later, yet another unforeseen complication arose, namely, that the word *stress* could not be
translated accurately into foreign languages. Of
course, as always, the Greeks had a word for it,
pónos, but apparently no modern language had an
expression like *stress*, a term which would have
suggested the new meaning. I became acutely
aware of this in 1946, when the Collège de France
honored me by an invitation to give a series of
lectures on the G.A.S. in Paris.

Now, here I was to speak in this famous research
institution where, a hundred years earlier, the
great Claude Bernard himself delivered his classic
lectures on the importance of maintaining the constancy of the *milieu intérieur* (internal environment). As I was to teach there as a representative
of a French-Canadian university, I took great
pains to deliver my lectures in good French. This
was all the more important, since it is the charming
tradition of this venerable institution of learning to
honor visiting foreign lecturers—at least on the

occasion of their inaugural address—by the presence of all the professors of the Collège de France, irrespective of their personal fields of interest. This meant that, right in the first row, in front of me, sat several of the most illustrious French men of letters. You may well imagine that my linguistic responsibilities weighed heavily upon my shoulders! Yet, I had to use at least one anglicism, the word *stress*, because I could not think of a proper French substitute for it.

After my lecture, there ensued a rather spirited debate about the correct translation of *stress* among these distinguished custodians who watch over the purity of the French language. I feel quite incompetent to give you an adequate account of their scholarly discussions, but you may be interested to learn the result.

Having eliminated as unsuitable, one by one, such terms as *dommage, agression, tension, détresse*, the unanimous conclusion was that there is no exact equivalent and hence one must necessarily be coined. Upon weighing the matter carefully, it was decided first that—for reasons I still cannot fathom—the gender of stress would have to be masculine. Then it was agreed that the best French term for it would be:

le stress.

Thus a new French word was born, and this experience did much to encourage me during subsequent lectures in Germany, Italy, Spain, and Portugal, to speak without the slightest hesitation of *der Stress, lo stress, el stress*, and *o stress*. This gave me the satisfaction of knowing that even if my scientific accomplishments should prove to be of little value, mine will be forever the glory of having enriched all these languages by at least one word.

If we are to use this concept in a strictly scientific manner, it is especially important to keep in mind that stress is an abstraction; it has no independent existence. We cannot cause stress without also producing some specific actions characteristic more particularly of the agent with which we produced it. What we actually see when something acts upon the living body is a combination of stress and the specific actions of the agent.

I should not end this section without emphasizing that, in colloquial English, such terms as "cold stress," and "interpersonal stress," have become so generally accepted that it would be difficult in practice to insist on replacing them with the cumbersome expressions, "stress produced by cold," "stress produced by interpersonal relations." As long as one clearly understands the difference between *stress* and *stressor*, I believe that such minor laxities are pardonable, just as is the occasional use of a dangling participle. To quote B. F. Skinner, "No one looks askance at the astronomer when he says that the sun rises or that the stars come out at night, for it would be ridiculous to insist that he should always say that the sun appears over the horizon as the earth turns or that the stars become visible as the atmosphere ceases to reflect sunlight. All we ask is that he can give a more precise translation if one is needed."

These considerations were important in preparing the mind for the science of stress, which we have recently tried to use even as the basis of a natural code of behavior, designed to master inter-personal and international stress. However, at this point, sketching a blueprint to investigate the mechanics of the stress syndrome was our next objective.

BOOK II

The Dissection of Stress

Summary

For scientific purposes, stress is defined as *the nonspecific response of the body to any demand*. It was first recognized by evidence of adrenal stimulation, shrinkage of lymphatic organs, gastrointestinal ulcers, and loss of body weight with characteristic alterations in the chemical composition of the body. It was later found to comprise many other changes as well that form a syndrome, a set of manifestations which appear together. This was called the *general adaptation syndrome* (G.A.S.).

In tissues more directly affected by stress, there develops a *local adaptation syndrome* (L.A.S.); for instance, there is inflammation where microbes enter the body.

The L.A.S. and the G.A.S. are closely coordinated. Chemical *alarm signals* are sent out by the directly stressed tissues, from the L.A.S. area to the centers of coordination in the *nervous system* and hence to the endocrine glands, especially the *pituitary* and the *adrenals*. These produce *adaptive hormones*, to combat wear and tear in the body. Thus the generalized response (G.A.S.) acts back upon the L.A.S. region.

Roughly speaking, the adaptive hormones fall into two groups: the *anti-inflammatory*, or *glucocorticoid hor-*

mones (ACTH, cortisone, cortisol), which inhibit excessive defensive reactions, and the *proinflammatory* and/or *mineralocorticoid hormones* (STH, aldosterone, DOC), which stimulate them.

Collectively these hormones are called *syntoxic* (from *sym* or *syn* = together, as in syndicate, symbiosis, synergy) because they facilitate coexistence with a pathogen, either by diminishing sensitivity to it or by encapsulating it within a barricade of inflammatory tissue. They are to be distinguished from the *catatoxic hormones* (*cata* = down, against, as in cataclysm, catabolism) which enhance the destruction of potential pathogens, mostly through the induction of poison-metabolizing enzymes in the liver.

The effects of all these substances can be modified, or conditioned, by other hormones (adrenalines, or the thyroid hormones), nervous reactions, diet, heredity, and tissue memories of previous exposures to stress. Derailments of this G.A.S. mechanism produce *diseases of adaptation,* that is, stress diseases.

In a nutshell, the response to stress has a tripartite mechanism, consisting of: (1) the direct effect of the stressor upon the body; (2) internal responses which stimulate tissue defense or help to destroy damaging subtances; and (3) internal responses which cause tissue surrender by inhibiting unnecessary or excessive defense. *Resistance and adaptation depend on a proper balance of these three factors.**

*This section is intended only for those who are seriously interested in the nature of normal and morbid life. Like Book IV, it is somewhat heavy, but those who would rather skip the details can do so by carefully reading this summary, which will provide the necessary continuity.

chapter 4

Blueprint for Dissection

The facts.   Abstractions and definitions.
Materials and techniques.

To understand the nature of disease is the fundamental object of medicine, for knowledge about a thing is the best way to acquire power over it. Of course, the limited capacities and the unlimited curiosity of the human brain probably will never permit man to completely solve this, or any other fundamental question. Yet, if it comes to a subject of such immense importance to mankind, even a few steps toward understanding are very rewarding. Could the stress concept help us to make some progress in this direction? We have learned that stress is an inherent element of all disease. If we manage to understand more precisely what stress really is and through what mechanisms it acts, we may perhaps bring some order into our thoughts about the nature of disease.

To understand a complex engine you have to take it apart. To understand a human body you have to dissect it. But how does one dissect an abstract concept such as stress? What is the stuff a concept is made of? Its parts are linked by imponderable ties which have no substance of their own; yet we cannot do without them if we are to handle effectively, as one coordinated thing, a mass of

ponderable and substantial but disconnected facts.
Think of the units of a navy—submarines, battleships, aircraft carriers—which, though very different in appearance and geographic position, are
nevertheless held together for effective use as one
coordinated thing. What makes this possible is one
abstraction: the concept of their nationality. This
notion would be difficult to measure; it has no
physical reality and yet it is much stronger than
the most mighty of the battleships. It dominates
the whole navy. Concepts always work through abstractions, for it is only by first abstracting from
the distinct, individual features of each factual
object that we can arrive at some common hold on
many of them, by which they can all be coordinated
from a single point.

Could the abstraction of stress furnish us with
such a common hold by which to grasp all the
individual manifestations of the G.A.S., and thus
coordinate them so as to understand the very
nature of disease?

To begin with, we must clearly realize that stress
is a condition, a state, and as such it is imponderable, but it manifests itself by measurable changes
in the organs of the body. By using these alterations as indicators of stress, we should be able to
come closer to an understanding of stress itself.
For instance, we could examine whether the various organ changes seen in patients during the
G.A.S. are closely interdependent; whether removing one or the other organ in experimental animals
will block all or part of the stress reaction; whether
treatment with certain drugs can increase or
decrease resistance to stress, and so forth.

What are the elements of stress and what procedures could we use for their analysis?

The Facts

First, there was the alarm reaction triad. The
adrenocortical enlargement and the *atrophy of the
thymicolymphatic organs* could be objectively measured in terms of the weights of these organs. The
gastrointestinal ulcers were less easy to appraise
accurately, but at least we could see whether they
were severe, mild, or absent.

Later, during the course of 1937, many other
such nonspecific changes were recognized. Among
these the most important ones were the *loss of
body weight, derangements in the regulation of
body temperature, disappearance of eosinophil cells*
from the circulating blood and a number of *chemical alterations* in the constitution of the body fluids
and tissues.

It was not clear just what part, if any, all these
changes might play in the body's *resistance to
stress*, but that was precisely what we wanted to
find out. Experimental animals and even human
beings can die from stress, and much could be
gained for practical medicine if we succeeded in
determining just what kind of change is necessary
to raise stress resistance. Of course, resistance
itself could also be used as an objective indicator of
stress. We could measure the survival rate of
experimental animals under different conditions.

Finally, perhaps one of the most important indicators of stress proved to be its effect upon *inflammation.* Normally, stress applied to a limited part of

the body causes inflammation, but the ability of
parts to respond locally in this way is impaired
when the whole body is under stress. In other
words, experiments showed that animals exposed
to some general stressor (such as a blood-borne
infection, intense nervous excitement, or extreme
muscular fatigue) failed to react with inflammation
at sites where some local stressor (for instance, a
substance to which they were allergic) was directly
applied to their body. Inflammation is also a tangible fact which can be measured, for example, in
terms of the degree of swelling, reddening, or the
histologic changes which characterize this local
response to injury. Do the general stressors act
directly upon all cells to prevent inflammation, or
through the intermediary of some hormone produced by a gland, perhaps by the enlarged adrenal?

In another dimension, in time, the *triphasic evolution* of the stress response can be used as a measurable fact. All the changes just enumerated varied during the three phases of the G.A.S. in a
characteristic and predictable manner. This varia-
tion of response during exposure to an unvarying
stressor made it possible to use the measurable
indicators of stress (structural or chemical
changes) for the appraisal of the evolution of the
G.A.S. in time.

It is rather significant that this list is so short. At
the beginning of this study in 1937, we were particularly short on facts. But the important thing is
that all these *changes are measurable* manifestations of stress, and, therefore, suitable indicators of
how the various parts of the stress machine work.

Abstractions and Definitions

It is generally agreed that a definition should be a concise explanation of the meaning of a word. According to Aristotle, it is the statement of the essence of a concept. In textbooks the definition comes first and leads you to the concept; the reverse is true in actual life. Be it ever so vague, you must first have a concept—derived from observation and symbolized by a name—before you can even try to delimit it more precisely by a definition.

If we want to present the story of stress as it actually developed, we have to proceed the same way, from observation to concept, and hence to definition. But it must be realized that, in any event, definitions applied to biologic concepts are never quite satisfactory. In the final analysis, most abstractions of biology—as that of life itself—are embraced by experience rather than by rational delimitation. We all know much better what life is than we know how to define it.

In some disciplines (for instance, in jurisprudence and in mathematics), definitions are rigid laws which make a concept what it is; in biology, definitions can only serve as concise descriptions of the way we perceive things at present. We must keep in mind that at any time our concepts may be modified by further observations. It is in this spirit that the following definitions are presented.

Definition of stress. The term *stress* has been used so loosely, and so many confusing definitions of it have been formulated, that I think it will be best to start by clearly stating *what it is not*. Contrary to some current, but vague or misleading statements:

1. *Stress is not simply nervous tension.* Stress reactions do occur in lower animals and even in plants, which have no nervous system. The general manifestations of an alarm reaction can be induced by mechanically damaging a denervated limb. Indeed, stress can be produced under deep anesthesia in patients who are unconscious, and even in cell cultures grown outside the body.

2. *Stress is not an emergency discharge of hormones from the adrenal medulla.* An adrenaline discharge is frequently seen in acute stress affecting the whole body, but it plays no conspicuous role in generalized inflammatory diseases (arthritis, tuberculosis) although they can also produce considerable stress; nor does it play any role in local stress reactions limited to directly injured regions of the body.

3. *Stress is not everything that causes a secretion by the adrenal cortex of its hormones, the corticoids.* ACTH, the adrenal-stimulating pituitary hormone, can discharge corticoids without producing any evidence of stress.

4. *Stress is not always the nonspecific result of damage.* Normal activities—a game of tennis or even a passionate kiss—can produce considerable stress without causing conspicuous damage.

5. *Stress is not the same as a deviation from homeostasis*, the steady state of the body. Any specific biologic function (the perception of sound or light, the contraction of a muscle) eventually causes marked deviations from the normal resting state in the active organs. This is undoubtedly associated with some local demand for increased vital activity, but it can cause only local stress and even this does not necessarily parallel the intensity of the specific activity.

6. *Stress is not anything that causes an alarm reaction.* It is the stressor that does that, not stress itself.

7. *Stress is not identical with the alarm reaction or the G.A.S.* as a whole. These reactions are characterized by certain measurable organ changes which are caused by stress and hence could not themselves *be* stress.

8. *Stress is not a nonspecific reaction.* The pattern of the stress reaction is very specific. It affects certain organs (for instance, the adrenal, the thymus, the gastrointestinal tract) in a highly selective manner.

9. *Stress is not a specific reaction.* The stress response is, by definition, not specific, since it can be produced by virtually any agent.

10. *Stress is not necessarily something bad.* It all depends on how you take it. The stress of exhilarating, creative, successful work is beneficial, while that of failure, humiliation, infection is detrimental. The stress reaction, just as energy consumption, may have good or bad effects.

11. *Stress cannot and should not be avoided.* Since stress is the nonspecific response of the body to any demand, everybody is always under some degree of stress. Even while quietly asleep our heart must continue to beat, our lungs to breathe, and even our brain works in the form of dreams. Stress can be avoided only by dying. The statement of "he is under stress" is just as meaningless as the expression "he is running a temperature." What we actually mean by such phrases is an *excess* of stress or of body temperature.

If we consider these points, we may easily be led to conclude that all this is so confusing and vague that stress cannot be defined. Perhaps the concept itself is just not sufficiently clear to serve as the object of scientific analysis.

But what is vague? The abortive attempts at a definition are, but surely not stress itself. It has a very clear, tangible form. Countless people have actually suffered or benefited from it. Stress is very real and concrete indeed. I think it would be correct to say that *stress is the common denominator of all adaptive reactions in the body*. This is simple and true, but perhaps still too vague.

Let us see now whether the following, more precise, definition will fit all our facts:

STRESS IS THE STATE MANIFESTED BY A SPECIFIC SYNDROME WHICH CONSISTS OF ALL THE NONSPECI-FICALLY-INDUCED CHANGES WITHIN A BIOLOGIC SYSTEM. Thus stress has its own characteristic form and composition but no particular cause. The elements of its form are the visible changes due to stress, whatever its cause. They are additive indicators which can express the sum of all the different adjustments that are going on in the body at any time.

This is essentially an "operational definition"; it tells what must be done to produce and recognize stress. A state can be recognized only by its manifestations; for instance, the state of stress by the manifestations of the stress syndrome. Therefore, you have to observe a great many living beings exposed to a variety of agents before you can see the shape of stress as such. Those changes which are specifically induced by only one or the other agent must first be rejected; if you then take what is left—that which is nonspecifically induced by many agents—you have unveiled the picture of stress itself. This picture is the G.A.S. Once this is established, you can recognize stress no matter where it turns up; indeed, you can even measure it by the intensity of the G.A.S. manifestations which it produces.*

It seems to me that this formulation was the password which opened the door to a whole new concept of medicine. Rarely, if ever, has it been possible to say this about a single sentence with more justification. It is true that some physicians who have contributed much to our understanding of stress have used this definition, only subconsciously, and without ever clearly formulating it. Yet, at the root of all research on stress, if you look for it, you find this definition. It gives unity and significance to the many individual observations on the G.A.S., the adaptive hormones, and the diseases of adaptation, which would otherwise

---

*At first I was tempted to define stress as *the rate of wear and tear* within the body at any one time, because this is the immediate nonspecific result of function and damage. Reactions which tend to repair wear and tear (e.g., corticoid secretion) are not strictly stress, but rather responses to stress. However, in practice, it is rarely (if ever) possible to distinguish clearly between damage and repair. Besides, in practice wear and tear cannot be objectively measured. Hence, this formulation—though theoretically more satisfying—could not have acted as a basis for a truly "operational" definition which we needed to give the concept of stress a solid objective foundation.

remain isolated facts. In any case, the definition of
stress is the pivot around which every part of this
volume turns. We shall have to analyze our definition carefully now in order to grasp its full meaning.

Stress is a STATE MANIFESTED BY A SYNDROME. We
would have no way of appraising the state of stress
were it not for the changes it produces. We can say
of a man, "He is under stress," but we shall have
arrived at this conclusion only by the visible
manifestations of his being under stress. The distinction between a state and the changes which
characterize this condition is just as important
in biology as it is in physics. A rubber band can
be in a state of tension, but this is recognizable
only by physical changes in the rubber. The condition of biologic stress is essentially an adjustment,
through the development of an antagonism
between an aggressor and the resistance offered to
it by the body. This quality of tension is probably
responsible for the common, but very misleading,
error of considering *biologic stress* as equivalent to
nervous tension.

Stress shows itself as a SPECIFIC *syndrome, yet
it is* NONSPECIFICALLY INDUCED. Until quite
recently in my technical papers I have often
referred to stress as "the sum of all nonspecific
changes caused by function or damage." Because
of its simplicity this definition became popular, but
it led to much confusion. Perhaps its greatest
weakness was its failure to point out that the pattern of the stress reaction (for instance, the mosaic
of changes in the adrenals, thymus, and gastrointestinal tract) is highly specific; only its causation

is nonspecific. *We must clearly distinguish between specificity in the form and in the causation of a change.*

A *nonspecifically-formed change* is one that affects all, or most, parts of a system without selectivity. It is the opposite of a *specifically-formed change* that affects only one, or at most, few units within a system. For example, pigmentation of the entire skin following total body exposure to sun rays is a nonspecifically-formed change, whereas the development of a single oval-shaped freckle on the nose is specifically-formed pigmentation.

A *nonspecifically-caused change* is one that can be produced by many or all agents. It is the opposite of a *specifically-caused change* that can be elicited by only one, or at most, by few agents. For example, simple inflammation, which can be produced by any irritant that enters the body, is nonspecifically caused, whereas the development of a calcified or iron-incrustated nodule must have a specific cause since only relatively few agents will produce it.

It is particularly important to keep in mind that *specificity is always a matter of degree.* Both among changes and among causes, there are fluent transitions between the least and the most specific. Failure to appreciate this is one of the greatest hurdles in the understanding of the stress concept, for laymen and physicians alike. The simple mechanical analogy in *Fig. 2* explains this point.

Here we have a row of ten cubes. Let the whole row represent the human body and each of the cubes one of its organs. We also have three blocks which correspond in breadth to one (A), two (B),

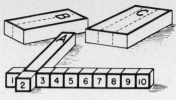

Fig. 2

and three (C) cubes. By pushing with block A, as
indicated in the drawing, I can displace a single
cube without deranging the others; this is a highly
specific action. With block B I could never displace
less than two, and with block C less than three
cubes at a time. Any intermediate type could be
constructed between the block which displaces only
a single cube and one which displaces them all. We
would need a block ten cubes wide to reliably produce a wholly nonspecific displacement of all cubes,
and even this would be a totally nonspecific change
only in this system. In a row of a thousand cubes
the displacement of ten would be a comparatively
specific change.

As regards the degree of their specificity or nonspecificity, we find the same scale among the various agents (drugs, nervous stimuli, bacteria)
which can act upon the human body.

Even the most fundamental of all biologic concepts, that of life itself, is—as we have stated
before—relative. As I sit here dictating, I feel very
much alive indeed, and yet there are parts of my
body which have already died. My hair and my
nails definitely belong to my person, but their cells
are no longer alive, in the usual sense of the word.
It would be difficult to prove that the water in my

blood is alive. I am sure that my tonsils, which were removed when I was four years old, are dead. Yet all these elements are or were parts of me.

You may argue that I chose poor examples, because the individual as a whole remains alive even if parts of him die. Perhaps we should speak of life and death only with respect to whole individuals; but where are we to draw the line between the parts and the whole? You may take a few cells from my body and make them grow on a nourishing broth in an incubator for many years; in these cells life can continue long after I have been buried. Even without such artificial experiments, through the genes in our germ cells we live on in our offspring.

So, even life itself is a relative concept.

We have explained that specificity of causation and specificity of form are two essentially different things. Yet, in practice, the two tend to run parallel. Nonspecifically-formed effects in large portions of the body are quite common; but highly selective effects upon circumscribed parts of the body are produced by comparatively few agents. For instance, wastage of body tissues is induced by starvation, infectious diseases, emotional upsets, cancer, and by many other conditions, but a truly selective and intense stimulation of the adrenal cortex can be produced only by one hormone: ACTH.

In this respect the stress response differs from most other biologic reactions, because it is nonspecifically produced and yet its form is quite specific (though modifiable by concurrently-acting additional factors). There must be some final common pathway through which the same organs can be

reached from many directions. To understand this
peculiar situation, keep in mind that stress causes
two types of changes: a *primary change*, which is
nonspecific both in its form and in its causation
(like energy consumption, it can be induced anywhere and by any kind of demand), and a *secondary change*, which has the specific pattern of the
G.A.S. The first acts as a common prompter which
can elicit the second from any part of the body.

Let us illustrate the principle of this by an example. Suppose that all possible accesses to a bank
building are connected with a police station by an
elaborate burglar alarm system. When a burglar
enters the bank, no matter what his personal characteristics are—whether he is small or tall, lean or
stout—and no matter which door or window he
opens to enter, he will set off the same alarm. This
primary change is therefore nonspecifically
induced from anywhere by anyone. The pattern of
the resulting secondary change, on the other hand,
is highly specific. It is always at a certain police
station that the burglar alarm will ring, and policemen will then rush to the bank along a specified
route according to a predetermined plan to prevent
robbery.

It is somewhat difficult, however, even in such a
simple situation, to distinguish clearly between
offense and defense, or between primary and secondary change. When the burglar opens the window to enter, this is aggression, but it is also the
trigger to set off the alarm which is part of the
predetermined defense pattern. In a complex biologic system such as the human body, it is even
more difficult to distinguish clearly between pri-

mary change, or damage, and secondary change, or defense. We recognize this difference in principle, but it is often impossible to do so in practice. Hence, it is best to consider the sum of all the changes caused by stress as one syndrome to which the secondary defensive reactions impart a specific pattern or form.

To make our analogy still more applicable to conditions of stress as they exist in the human body, we must now also bring a quantitative aspect into the alarm system. The alarm response of the body is definitely proportionate to the intensity of the aggression. That is not so with the usual burglar alarms; but, for example, a first fire alarm will bring only a limited number of men and equipment to the scene of conflagration, in comparison with a second or third alarm from the same vicinity. The defensive response is quantitatively adjusted to the number of the alarm signals.

What is here the specific and what the nonspecific part of the alarm response? In *Fig. 3*, four squares represent boxes from which fire alarms can be set off in four adjacent buildings.

All these trigger mechanisms—like the organs of the human body—are different, as indicated by the different patterns: dots, triangles, rods, and rings. The alarm may be set off by the breaking of a glass in a firebox, the activity of a thermoelectric cell, or any other device. But eventually all these mechanisms act nonspecifically through the same type of electric fire alarm which activates the same bell in the same fire station. No matter where and how the alarm is set off, the result must always be the same. Yet, despite this nonspecificity of causation, the pattern of the resulting defensive response is again highly specific and stereotyped. The bell sends men and equipment to the fire in accordance with a typical standard plan.

In our drawing, the stereotyped, that is, nonspecific, trigger mechanism was set off in the third box through its own particular activation process indicated by a discharge of the rods; this secondarily mobilized a specific pattern of defense. However, if, simultaneously, fire alarms would also go off in all three other boxes, a larger number of firemen and equipment would be sent out. Here we have a definite proportionality between the extent of the damage and the response. The analogy also shows clearly how different interventions (activation of distinct trigger mechanisms at different points)

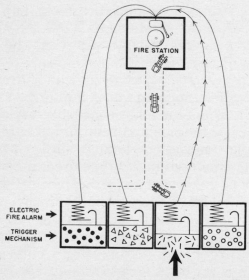

Fig. 3

can nonspecifically (always through the same signal) cause a specific pattern of response. It is only the nonspecific part (the signals) that can be summated to bring about a response proportionate to the injury.

Essentially the same situation exists in the body when the specific pattern of the stress syndrome is induced by the *sum of nonspecific signals* coming from various tissues.

There is one flaw in this analogy which I have not tried to eliminate because it is quite instructive. The signal of the bell in a real fire station is not totally nonspecific since it can indicate the site from which the alarm originated, so that help may be sent specifically there. Otherwise firemen would have to go to all locations provided with alarms. This is also the case in the human body, because stress hormones cannot be sent specifically to wherever they are most needed and, in the case of very general aggression, they may be required throughout the body.

However, now that we have made this point, we can adjust our model to fit the condition of the body more accurately. We only need to assume that the four trigger mechanisms are in different rooms of the same building, and as long as they bring the fire brigade to the burning edifice, they have accomplished their purpose.

In the triad of the alarm reaction any one change, for instance, the adrenal stimulation, is not indicative of nonspecific stress. This single change can also be reproduced by a highly specific hormone, ACTH (about which we shall say more later). When thus selectively produced, adrenal stimulation is a specific action. Only when it is induced by some stressor as an integral part of the triad—that is, simultaneously with thymicolymphatic atrophy and gastrointestinal ulcers—is it a component of the nonspecific stress syndrome.

These considerations have helped us to formulate an operational definition of stress. We find it useful for scientific purposes, but somewhat complicated to formulate or to explain. For simplicity's sake, we have recently attempted to state the essence of this concept in the following terms:

Stress is the NONSPECIFIC RESPONSE OF THE BODY TO ANY DEMAND, whether it is caused by, or results in, pleasant or unpleasant conditions. Good or bad, pleasant or unpleasant are already specific features of our response to a demand just as cold or heat are specific variants of temperature changes. Stress as such, just as temperature as such, is all-inclusive, embodying both the positive and the negative aspects of these concepts. We must, however, differentiate within the general concept of stress between the unpleasant or harmful variety, called *"distress"* (from the Latin *dis* = bad, as in dissonance, disagreement), and *"eustress"* (from the Greek *eu* = good, as in euphonia, euphoria). During both eustress and distress the body undergoes virtually the same nonspecific responses to the various positive or negative stimuli acting upon it. However, the fact that eustress causes much less damage than distress graphically demonstrates that it is "how you take it" that determines, ultimately, whether one can adapt successfully to change.

The general stress syndrome affects the whole

body; a local stress syndrome influences several units within a part; but stress always manifests itself by a syndrome, a sum of changes, not by one change. An isolated effect upon any one unit in the body is either damage or stimulation to activity; in either case, it is specific, and hence not stress.

This raises the question, *"What is a biologic unit?"* Can one organ, like the kidney or brain, be called a unit, or should we extend the meaning of this term to include any small group of cells, perhaps even individual cells and cell parts?

The definition of biologic units capable of selective reaction (*reactons*) is just as fundamental for biology as the definition of elements and subatomic particles is for chemistry and physics. We shall deal with this problem at length in Book IV. All we need to know now is that, no matter what we define as a unit of life—a whole nation, a human being, one region of man's body, or a single cell—we can speak of stress in a living system only as far as several of its constituent parts are nonspecifically affected. If a drug introduced into the general blood circulation causes changes only in the kidney, the action is specifically caused and has a specific effect within the body. Very few drugs can thus single out the kidney among all organs of the body (specificity of causation) and, of course, the kidney represents a circumscribed region within the whole individual (specificity in the type of response). On the other hand, if a drug is injected directly into the kidney and causes changes throughout the renal substance, the change is nonspecific, both as regards its form and its causation, because no part of the organ is selectively affected and such an effect can

be obtained by innumerable agents. Selective
changes in an organ—if they can be produced by
almost anything, as long as it is directly applied to
this organ—are manifestations of local stress;
whereas the changes which can be produced
throughout the body by a great variety of agents,
no matter where these are applied, constitute the
general stress syndrome.

In this distinction between local and general
stress lies the link between specificity and nonspecificity.

Throughout this analysis of our definition, we
spoke of biologic *changes*. A change, in this sense, is
any deviation from the normal resting state of the
body. But what is "normal," and what is the "resting state?"

These are again relative concepts. Clear-cut
delimitations are impossible because, in living
organisms, there are imperceptible transitions
between normal and abnormal, resting and active.

Nobody is absolutely normal; the slightest scar
or freckle is actually an abnormality. No one is ever
absolutely at rest either, while alive. Even during
sleep, your heart, your respiratory muscles, your
brain continue to work. It makes no difference that
you are not conscious of this and that these activities require no voluntary effort on your part.

Yet, in the evolution of every species (from the
simplest unicellular being to man), of every individual (from embryonic life to maturity), certain types
have formed, which we readily recognize as normal
for a given species, sex, and age. The manifold
adaptations in the evolution of each individual, of
each species, have all left their imprints and con-

tributed to the setting of these individual norms. It is normal for certain Peruvian Indians to live in the rarefied air of the Andes Mountains, but it would be highly abnormal and damaging for a man from the Netherlands to do so.

The concept of "resting" is equally relative. Only the dead can tolerate total rest. But the degree and type of activity appropriate for a six-year-old boy would be most abnormal and stressful for a seventy-year-old theoretic physicist, and vice versa.

In our mechanical analogy (page 68), the cubes were pictured as resting in a straight line during the basic condition of normalcy, before a change occurred. But if we now want to adapt this picture to what we have just learned, we may well imagine that, in the course of time, they may have gradually settled into a V-shaped groove on a constantly vibrating table. In this case, a V-shaped arrangement and vibration would be normal for them, and any enforced deviation from this state—for instance, immobilization in a straight line—would be a change.

The term stress is meaningful only when applied to a PRECISELY DEFINED BIOLOGIC SYSTEM. From all this it is obvious that if a large number of agents produce the same specific reaction pattern (say, inflammation) in one organ (say, the stomach), they act as stressors for this particular biologic system, and here their effect can be described as a local stress syndrome. But if they act only on one organ, their action is still highly specific with reference to the body as a whole.

Every conceivable agent has both specific and nonspecific actions; every individual, or part of an

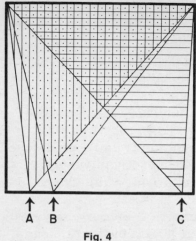

Fig. 4

individual, can be influenced specifically as well as nonspecifically. This is illustrated in *Fig. 4*.

Here the whole field represents the body, and A, B, and C represent three agents which produce specific changes (horizontal lines, vertical lines, or dots) in different sectors of the body. But only with reference to the smallest triangular sector (filled with squares and dots) can we speak of nonspecifically-induced changes, because only this sector is affected by all three agents. The changes in this sector correspond to the selective organ changes (in adrenals, thymus, stomach, etc.) of the G.A.S.

Definition of a stressor. Having thus identified the state of stress—at least as far as the limitations of biologic definitions permit—a *stressor* is naturally "that which produces stress." In view of what we have already said about the relativity of stress, it is also self-evident that any one agent is more or less a stressor in proportion to the degree of its ability to produce stress, that is, nonspecific demands and changes.

Definition of the G.A.S. Now we shall have to bring the important *element of time* into our considerations of nonspecific responses. While stress is reflected by the sum of the nonspecific changes which occur in the body at any one time, the general adaptation syndrome (or G.A.S.) encompasses all nonspecific changes as they develop throughout time during continued exposure to a stressor. One is a snapshot, the other a motion picture of the response to nonspecific demands.

We saw that a fully-developed G.A.S. consists of three stages: the alarm reaction, the stage of resistance, and the stage of exhaustion. There is stress at any moment during these stages, although its manifestations change as time goes on. Furthermore, it is not necessary for all three stages to develop before we can speak of a G.A.S. Only the most severe stress leads rapidly to the stage of exhaustion and death. Most of the physical or mental exertions, infections, and other stressors, which act upon us during a limited period, produce changes corresponding only to the first and second stages: at first they may upset and alarm us, but then we get used to them.

In the course of a normal human life, everybody goes through these first two stages many, many times. Otherwise we could never become adapted to perform all the activities and face all the demands which are man's lot.

Even exhaustion does not always need to be irreversible and complete, as long as it affects only parts of the body. For instance, running produces a stress situation, mainly in our muscles and cardiovascular system. To cope with this, we first have to limber up and get these organs ready for the task at hand; then for a while we will be at the height of efficiency in running, but eventually exhaustion will set in. This could be compared with an alarm reaction, a stage of resistance, and a stage of exhaustion, all limited primarily to the muscular and cardiovascular systems. But such an exhaustion is reversible; after a good rest we will be back to normal again.

The same is true of our eyes. When we come out of the dark and try to look into the sun, at first we see nothing. Then we adapt ourselves, but eventually our eyes become exhausted if we keep on looking into the strong light.

Everybody knows this from personal experience of the muscles and of the eyes; it is notoriously true also of various intellectual pursuits. Most human activities go through three stages: we first have to get into the swing of things, then we get pretty good at them, but finally we tire and lose our acquired efficiency.

It is less generally known that this triphasic evolution of adaptation is quite characteristic also of all bodily activities, including those that only the physician can fully appraise; for instance, of inflammation. If some virulent microbes get under the skin, they first cause what we call acute inflammation (reddening, swelling, pain), then follows

chronic inflammation (ripening of a boil or abscess),
and finally an exhaustion of tissue resistance
which permits the inflamed, purulent fluid to be
evacuated (breaking through of an abscess).

*Relationship between the G.A.S. and the
L.A.S.—the concept of adaptation energy.* The
selective exhaustion of muscles, eyes, or inflamed
tissue all represent final stages only in local adaptation syndromes (L.A.S.). Several of these may go
on simultaneously in various parts of the body; in
proportion to their intensity and extent, they can
activate the G.A.S. mechanism. Only when the
whole organism is exhausted—through senility at
the end of a normal life-span, or through the accelerated aging caused by stress—do we enter into
the terminal stage of exhaustion of the G.A.S.

It is as though we had hidden reserves of adaptability, or *adaptation energy,* in ourselves throughout the body. As soon as local stress consumes the
most readily accessible local reserves, local exhaustion sets in and activity in the strained part must
stop. This is an important protective mechanism
because, during the period of rest thus enforced,
more adaptation energy can be made available,
either from less readily accessible local stores or
from reserves in other parts of the body. Only when
all of our adaptability is used up will irreversible,
general exhaustion and death follow.

*Relationship between adaptation energy
and aging.* There seem to be close interrelations
between the G.A.S. and aging. We have already

mentioned that several local adaptation syndromes may develop consecutively or even simultaneously in the same individual. People can get used
to a number of things (cold, heavy muscular work,
worries), which at first had a very alarming effect;
yet, upon prolonged exposure, sooner or later all
resistance breaks down and exhaustion sets in. It
is as though something were lost, or used up, during the work of adaptation; but what this is, we do
not know. The term *adaptation energy* has been
coined for that which is consumed during continued adaptive work, to indicate that it is something
different from the caloric energy we receive from
food; but this is only a name, and even now—
almost thirty years after this hypothesis was first
formulated—we still have no precise concept of
what this energy might be. Further research along
these lines would seem to hold great promise, since
here we appear to touch upon the fundamentals of
fatigue and aging.

It is as though, at birth, each individual inherited a certain amount of adaptation energy, the
magnitude of which is determined by his genetic
background, his parents. He can draw upon this
capital thriftily for a long but monotonously
uneventful existence, or he can spend it lavishly in
the course of a stressful, intense, but perhaps more
colorful and exciting life. In any case, there is just
so much of it, and he must budget accordingly.

We shall have more to say about exhaustion
when we discuss the actual experiments on which
this view is based (see page 112) and its practical applications to everyday problems (Books III
and V.)

Definition of the diseases of adaptation. The last concept which we have to define is that of the "diseases of adaptation." These are the maladies in which imperfections of the G.A.S. play a major role. Many diseases are actually not so much the direct results of some external agent (an infection, an intoxication) as they are consequences of the body's inability to meet these agents by adequate adaptive reactions, that is, by a perfect G.A.S.

This is again a relative concept. No malady is only a disease of adaptation and nothing else. Nor are there any disease producers which can be so perfectly handled by the organism that maladaptation plays no part in their effects upon the body. Such agents would not produce disease. This haziness in its delimitation does not interfere with the practical utility of our concept. We must put up with the same lack of precision whenever we have to classify any other kind of disease. There is no pure heart disease, in which all other organs remain perfectly undisturbed, nor can we ever speak of a pure kidney disease or pure nervous disease in this sense.

Direct and indirect pathogens. It is essential to distinguish between direct and indirect pathogens. If we accidentally put our hand into boiling water or strong alkali, it will be damaged directly, irrespective of any vital tissue reaction to these agents.

They would damage even the hand of a dead man, who obviously could not put up any vital defense reactions.

On the other hand, if we are exposed to pollen, cat's dander or any food substance to which we happen to be allergic and to which we react with an extraordinarily intense immunologic defense response, our difficulties are not caused directly by the external agent to which we are exposed but by our own excessive adaptive mechanisms. It is such indirect pathogens that are the main causes of the so-called "stress diseases" or "diseases of adaptation," such as high blood pressure, heart attacks, peptic ulcers, migraine headaches, pains in the neck, certain types of asthma, toxicomanias, alcoholism, excessive obesity or leanness due to abnormal dietary patterns. These and many other diseases are not the direct results of any pathogen but of our defective bodily or mental reactions to the stressors encountered in daily life.

Under optimal conditions, indirect pathogens do not manifest their potential disease-producing effect because they are met by perfectly adjusted syntoxic or catatoxic biochemical or behavioral responses. Within normal limits, this results in a homeostatic response, the maintenance of the normal milieu intérieur, that is, an essentially healthy condition. However, in the event of excessive demands, usually adequate adaptive responses no longer suffice. The cybernetic mechanism (one might almost be tempted to say "thermostat") has to be set at a higher level to maintain equilibrium in the face of such very excessive demands.

During evolution, immunologic reactions, which lead to the destruction of microbes and other foreign tissues, undoubtedly developed as useful defensive mechanisms against potentially dangerous foreign materials. When the attack against the "foreign" agent is unnecessary or even harmful, as in the case of many allergens, heart transplants, etc., man can improve upon the wisdom of Nature by suppressing this hostility.

On the other hand, when the aggressor is dangerous, the defensive reaction should not be suppressed but, if possible, increased beyond the normal level. This can be achieved, for example, by catatoxic substances which carry the chemical message to the tissues to destroy the invaders even more vigorously than would normally be the case.

The concept of heterostasis. Natural homeostatic mechanisms are usually sufficient to maintain a normal state of resistance. When faced with unusually heavy demands, however, ordinary homeostasis is not enough. The "thermostat of defense" must be raised to a higher level. For this process, I proposed the term *heterostasis* (from the Greek *heteros* = other) as the establishment of a new steady state by treatment with agents which stimulate the physiologic adaptive mechanisms through the development of normally dormant defensive tissue reactions. Both in homeostasis and in heterostasis, the milieu intérieur participates actively.

In homeostatic defense, the potential pathogen (which threatens the fixity of the milieu intérieur) automatically activates usually adequate catatoxic or syntoxic mechanisms; when these do not suffice, such natural catatoxic or syntoxic agents can also be administered readymade by the physician. Heterostasis depends upon treatment with artificial remedies which have no direct curative action, but which can precipitate the production of unusually high amounts of the body's own natural catatoxic or syntoxic agents so as to achieve fixity of the milieu intérieur despite abnormally high demands that could not be met without outside help *(Fig. 5)*.

We can stimulate the production of natural protective agents by treatment with chemicals that augment the induction of catatoxic or syntoxic enzymes, or by immunization with bacterial products (e.g., vaccination) which increase the manufacture by the body of serologic antibodies to combat infections.

The most salient difference between homeostasis and heterostasis is that the former maintains a normal steady state by physiologic means, whereas the latter "resets the thermostat" of resistance to a heightened defensive capacity by artificial interventions from the outside.

Heterostasis differs essentially from treatment with drugs (e.g., antibiotics, antacids, antidotes, pain killers) which act directly and specifically rather than by strengthening the body's own natu-

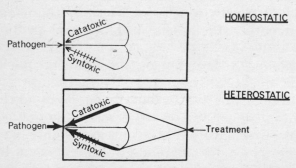

Fig. 5 Comparison of homeostatic and heterostatic defense mechanisms.

ral nonspecific defenses. In treatment with drugs, the milieu intérieur is passive.

In the preceding passages I have had to lead you through a rather detailed analysis of abstractions, but these concepts are quite indispensable for the understanding of stress as it affects us in everyday life. They had never been precisely formulated before and it is only through them that stress could be explored in the laboratory.

Materials and Techniques

Experimental animals. If we want to learn something about any aspect of life, we first need a sample of its pattern as expressed in the body of an animal or man. The structural organization of living beings can often be studied by dissection after death, but vital processes can only be explored during life.

Since it is not justified to perform dangerous operations on man, experimental animals are quite indispensable for such studies. This involves what is often called *vivisection*. Literally, the term means "cutting into a living animal," and it implies to many laymen that this is done without anesthesia and involves unnecessary suffering. This misconception is most unfortunate, since it has led many well-meaning people to attack animal experimentation—the very basis of medical research—on grounds of cruelty. The *Encyclopaedia Britannica* concludes an extensive article on the arguments for and against vivisection with the statement that "either view to be respected must be based upon extensive and accurate knowledge, accurate statement and sincerity. Unfortunately, these are not always manifested by protagonists." It is not my purpose to go deeply into the ethical aspects of animal experimentation, although I hope that this book will give the reader the understanding necessary to form a personal opinion. All I should like to say on the authority of a life-long association with animal experiments and animal experimenters is this:

1. Almost every major step of progress in medicine has been based, at least partly, on animal experiments. Without these Pasteur and his contemporaries could not have discovered the role of microbes in infectious diseases, nor would it have been possible to develop vaccines, sera, or antibiotics against them. Without operating on animals, Ivan Petrovich Pavlov could not have developed his concept of the "conditioned reflexes," which is still a basic pillar of our knowledge about the nervous system. Banting could not have discovered insulin without making dogs diabetic (by removing their pancreas glands) to test the antidiabetic action of his first extracts. And finally, imagine the unnecessary cruelty to man and loss of human life which would result if every surgeon were to acquire his skill by trying new operations, such as heart or kidney transplants, first on patients!

It is, in fact, against the law in the United States, Canada, and many other countries to use new drugs on man before they have been tested on experimental animals. Such testing implies, among other things, the determination of the fatal dose, a procedure which will necessarily lead to the death of many animals. Yet, few antivivisectionists would consider it more ethical to stop medical research altogether and thereby expose countless human beings to unnecessary suffering.

2. I have never met a professional investigator who was not concerned about the question of cruelty to animals and did not attempt to avoid it. Those who claim that animal experiments are never painful simply distort the truth; but every effort is made to diminish pain to the absolutely unavoidable minimum. It is important for the public to realize that, even if an experimental surgeon were a sadist and wanted to cause pain on purpose, he would nevertheless have to anesthetize his animals for major surgery because delicate operations cannot be performed if the animal struggles.

3. Legislators who pass laws which prohibit or curtail the use of experimental animals for research, or for the teaching of medical students, do so either because of sincere moral considerations or under the pressure of political exigencies. Whatever their motives, they are either uninformed or they have reconciled their consciences to the fact that they necessarily inflict untold cruelties upon their fellow men and seriously interfere with one of the noblest and most human aspirations of man, the desire to understand himself.

The better one understands the nature of life, disease, and suffering, the more one becomes incapable of brutality. This thought was not the least important among the motives which led me to write a book on the nature of disease for those who are not professionally concerned with medicine. In

our Institute last year, we used about 1400 rats a
week for research, but not one of them was exposed
to unnecessary pain because of carelessness.

Surgical techniques. Most of our experiments are performed on rats or mice. These animals have a comparatively undeveloped brain and
hence presumably (we cannot be really sure of this)
feel less anguish and pain than a cat or a dog.
Rodents also have the advantage of being small,
inexpensive, and singularly resistant to infections,
which makes them especially suitable for large-
scale experimentation.

In a standard experiment a rat is anesthetized
with ether, or some other anesthetic, until it is
completely unconscious and unable to move or feel
pain. Then the experimenter can expose a gland
and remove it to learn how the rat will react to
stress without this organ. Similarly the experimental surgeon can transect a sensory nerve if, for his
studies, he wants to render a certain region of the
body insensitive to pain. He can diminish the blood
flow through an artery by putting a constricting
loop of thread around it, and so forth. After the
operation, the animal wakes up and is then ready
for observation.

In most of these instances, the surgical intervention produces a type of deficiency which could spontaneously arise in man. By causing such a selective
disturbance, we can appraise the participation of
the individual organs in the stress mechanism.

Chemical techniques. There is much we can
learn only through the application of chemical

methods. For instance, if we want to study the actions of corticoids, we can get large quantities of beef adrenals from the slaughterhouse and extract the hormones from these glands. As explained, making an extract means chopping up the glands into fine particles and putting the resulting mush into water or some other fluid in which the hormones are soluble. From this crude extract various fractions can be precipitated out by adding chemicals which make either the hormones or the contaminants insoluble. This process of purification is continued until a hormone is separated from everything else that was in the gland, and emerges in absolutely pure, usually crystalline, form.

Purification is an especially important step, because only pure substances can be analyzed by the chemist, who wants to determine their molecular structure, that is, exactly how the individual atoms are arranged within the hormone molecule. After this is accomplished, it usually becomes possible sooner or later to make the natural substance in the laboratory, from its elements or from other simple compounds which are more readily available than glands. This is what we call *synthesis* or putting together.

It is particularly useful to learn how to synthesize hormones, because most of them are valuable remedies which must be made available in quantity for all patients who need them. Such bulk production from animal glands is always costly, and often impossible, because all the slaughterhouses in the world could not furnish enough raw material.

There are, of course, many other problems of

experimental medicine which can be solved only by
the techniques of biochemistry. The changes,
which occur during stress or after treatment with
hormones, in the chemical make-up of body fluids
and tissues furnish innumerable examples of this.

Morphologic techniques. *Morphology* literally means "the science of shape" (from Greek
morphē, shape, form, plus *-logy,* science of). The
gross anatomic knowledge gained from merely dissecting and inspecting organs falls into this category; so does the information furnished by the histologic (from Greek *histos,* tissue) structure or
cellular pattern of tissues, as revealed through the
microscope. By merely looking at them through a
microscope we can learn much about the function
of certain organs. For example, the resting adrenal
is laden with small fat droplets—readily visible
under the microscope—which contain the fat-
soluble hormones; the active gland discharges its
reserves into the blood and, therefore, contains
few or no such droplets.

*Complex laboratory and clinical tech-
niques.* Experimental surgery, chemistry, and
morphology furnish us with the basic tools for medical research. It is customary to consider separately the information yielded by *pharmacologic,
bacteriologic,* and other experimental techniques
or by *clinical* study. Yet, in essence, all these techniques are combinations of surgery, chemistry, and
morphology.

Suppose we want to find out whether an excess of
adrenal hormones spills over into the urine of a

patient under stress. We make an extract from his urine and, after suitable purification, inject it into animals previously subjected to adrenalectomy (from Greek *ectomē*, excision, cutting out). The test animals, of course, have to be adrenalectomized to avoid any uncontrollable complications due to the secretion of hormones by their own adrenals. In such adrenal-deficient animals, the thymus is always very big because they have no adrenal hormones which could cause thymus involution. If we now inject the extract, the degree of the resulting thymus involution tells us how much adrenal hormone there was in our extract. This pharmacologic method is called a *bioassay* (short for biologic assay), because you test or measure something by its biologic activity.

In essence, this procedure is a combination of chemistry (extraction), surgery (adrenalectomy), and morphology (change in thymus size).

Most of the changes caused by spontaneous diseases in man or by experimental interventions (treatment with bacteria, allergens, etc.) in animals are revealed through combinations of the three fundamental techniques which we have just outlined.

Techniques for the coordination of knowledge. The volume of medical literature has assumed such gigantic proportions that the mere registration and coordination of the accumulating medical knowledge has become a major task of contemporary research. As Vannevar Bush so aptly said to the American Philosophical Society (*The Atlantic*, August, 1955), if we fail in this task, "science may become bogged down in its own product, inhibited like a colony of bacteria, by its own exudations."

Because of my long-standing interest in stress, I have accumulated over the years the world's largest collection of publications dealing with this subject. Since 1950, between 2,500 and 7,700 publications on stress have appeared each year. Of course all these papers first have to be obtained, read, and carefully indexed before they can be useful.*

No one who has not done this kind of work himself can realize what it means to go through a collection which by now consists of about 110,000 scientific papers on stress and catalogue their substance so that it may be easy to find when needed. You cannot even fully digest and enjoy all the information contained in this mass of literature because time does not permit you to do more than skim through the pages with a sharp eye trained to pick out meaningful facts.

Naturally, among the thousands of publications on stress, there were many which I have read carefully and with great interest; indeed, some served as a basis for my own experiments. But stress and the adaptive hormones which participate in stress have inspired so many investigations that no one person could really have studied them all. And, yet,

*To cope with this task we have developed a *Symbolic Shorthand System (SSS) for Physiology and Medicine* (H. Selye in collaboration with G. Ember, Montreal: IMCE, Université de Montréal, Fourth ed., 1964). Here the concepts of medicine are represented by symbols which correspond essentially to the equations of algebra, the formulas of chemistry, or the notes of music. To give the reader some idea of how the system works we have made partial use of it in the INDEX (page 499).

it would have been quite impossible to keep the subject together and build it into a science without constructing such an international instrument of information and correlation as our documentation service.

It is wasteful to repeat experiments which have already been done elsewhere; it is futile to use obsolete techniques when better ones are available. We cannot see major gaps unless a picture of our knowledge is put together. Hence, this information center became as essential a tool for organized stress research as the experimental animals or the surgical, chemical, and microscopic techniques which we employ in the laboratory.

chapter 5

Dissecting a Biologic Mechanism

Interrelations in the endocrine system. Basic mechanisms of stress reactions. The essence of the stress response.

Interrelations in the Endocrine System

Suppose you are faced with the problem of having to figure out the system of wiring in a complex electric network, in which a battery supplies five light bulbs with current; the task would be easy but all the wires are hidden in the wall and you can reach them only around the sockets.

In a case like this, after having identified the position of the battery and the five bulbs, the simplest procedure would be to interrupt the current by disconnecting the wires at each of the possible relay points. This would show us which of the lights go out and which still remain lighted after cutting a certain connection. As a countercheck, we might then—after disconnecting the main battery—supply current at various points by providing an auxiliary source of electricity, to see which of the wires supplies which of the bulbs.

This is illustrated in *Fig. 6*.

Here, if we could only see the position of the
battery and of the five bulbs (numbered 1 to 5), it
would be quite impossible to know how they are
connected. But we could easily figure it out by a
few simple experiments. For instance, if we interrupted the current by disconnecting bulb 1, all the
lamps, except No. 3, would go out. This means that
Nos. 2, 4, and 5 are supplied through a system
which must go through point 1, while No. 3 has an
independent electric supply directly from the battery.

On the other hand, after turning off the battery
and putting on an auxiliary source of electricity
just below point 1, it will become evident that bulbs
2, 3, 4, and 5 go on. From this we may conclude that
lamp No. 3 has a dual supply of electricity, one
coming from somewhere above, the other from
below point 1. Now it will only be a matter of pa-

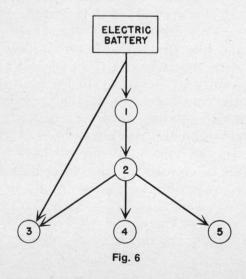

Fig. 6

tience to demonstrate, with further experiments of the same kind, that the three wires leaving point 2 go to bulbs 3, 4, and 5. Thus eventually the whole plan of the circuit can easily be determined.

Essentially the same procedure is used by medical investigators when they want to disentangle interrelations in a complex living system, such as the body of an animal or man.

The situation is very similar in the case of living organs regulated by hormones, the chemical messengers produced by endocrine glands. The principal difference is that the hormones are not carried each through its own separate channel, the way the nerves transmit their impulses through individual fibers or the electric current through separate wires.

Hormones are soluble chemicals poured out by the glands into the blood in which they travel together to all parts of the body. But each hormone carries instructions in a code which only certain organs can read. Therefore, these blood-borne messengers can influence limited parts of the body just as selectively as can nerves which are physically connected to a specific muscle. Each organ responds only to certain hormones which act either directly or through some other endocrine gland (a relay station).

Here the system is more comparable with radio or television networks, in which the emitting station sends its waves indiscriminately in every direction, but only certain sets are tuned to a particular wavelength. This is what permits the selective reception of certain programs to the exclusion of all others. The comparison can even be carried

further, in that some sets will receive a program
from the original sender, and others will get it
relayed through some local station, just as the hormones of a gland can act upon tissues directly or
after first relaying their message through another
gland.

Therefore, in the study of endocrinology (the science of the endocrine glands and their hormones)
we can use the same process of elimination to
determine the order in which the glands influence
each other. This is illustrated in the next figure by
an example taken from the field of stress research.
Here we see the effect of a stressor, or stress-producing agent, upon the hypothalamus, the pituitary gland, the adrenals, the stomach, the lymphatic tissues, and the white blood cells.

The *hypothalamus* is a coordinating brain region
and the *pituitary* (or hypophysis) is a small endocrine gland embedded in the bones at the base of
the skull just underneath the brain. The *adrenals*
are endocrines which lie above the kidneys, one on
each side. The *lymphatic tissues* are important
defensive organs consisting of small cells, similar
to the white blood cells. The lymph nodes in the
groins and armpits, the tonsils in the throat, and
the thymus in the chest belong to this system.
Among the *white blood cells*, some come from the
lymphatic organs, others from the bone marrow.
These cells are also important in defense, especially against infections.

During stress we noticed changes in all these
tissues, but we did not know how—through what
pathways—they were produced. As far as we could

tell, when we began this work, the thymus might
have produced some hormone which stimulates the
adrenals. But this possibility was soon ruled out.
After surgically removing the thymus (point 4 in
Fig. 7.) of rats, their adrenals (point 2) still became
enlarged and overactive during stress. Conversely,
however, after the adrenals were removed, the thymus no longer showed the changes characteristic
of the stress reaction. Finally, we found that injections of adrenal extracts rich in corticoid hormones
(which were not yet available in pure form at that
time) produced typical stress changes in the thymus, even after adrenalectomy. Obviously the
pathway went from adrenal to thymus and not
from thymus to adrenal.

Now the question arose, "How does the adrenal
know when there is stress and, therefore, a need
for large amounts of corticoid hormone?" In other
words, what is the immediately preceding link in

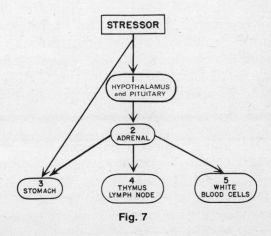

Fig. 7

this sequence of events? After unsuccessfully trying various other possibilities, we removed the pituitary and found that, after interruption of the biologic chain reaction at this point (point 1), exposure to stress now no longer stimulated the adrenal glands (point 2). On the other hand—even without stress, and even in the absence of the pituitary—injection of a pituitary hormone, ACTH (described on page 109), caused typical stress changes in the adrenal. It became enlarged and produced a great excess of its own hormones. Evidently, the adrenal was a relay station between point 1 and certain points farther down the chain.

The role of the hypothalamus as a bridge between the brain and the endocrine system was recognized much later. It was mainly through the work of Dr. A. V. Schally and my former graduate student Dr. Roger Guillemin, that we have learned about the releasing factors (such as CRF, described on page 140) which are discharged from the hypothalamus into the blood supplying the pituitary, causing the latter to produce its own hormones.

It is easy to see how—using this sketch as a blueprint for the dissection of stress—the whole complex endocrine network of the G.A.S. became amenable to scientific analysis. We merely had to interrupt the network by the removal of a gland and then correct the resulting defect by the injection of the gland's special hormone.

This kind of work is still in progress and will have to continue for quite some time. We, like hundreds of other investigators, are busy trying to disentangle the many still mysterious complexities of the stress machinery.

Basic Mechanisms of Stress Reactions

Interactions between specific and nonspecific events. Every conceivable agent which can act upon the human body, from without or from within, does certain things more than others. Those which it does more are relatively specific or characteristic for it, as compared to those which it does less. The latter, the nonspecific actions, may therefore be viewed as incidental side-effects. But they are incidental only from the standpoint of classical medicine, which is always interested in the specific causes of disease and the specific cures with which to combat them. Stress research is primarily concerned with these nonspecific actions. Whatever our point of view, we must keep in mind that, in actual practice, it is impossible to separate the specific from the nonspecific effects.

In each of the drawings in *Fig. 8*, the solid arrow represents the stressor and the other the specific— from our point of view incidental—actions of three agents.

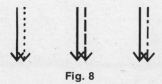

Fig. 8

Obviously, the end result of exposure to any of the agents represented by these double arrows could not be the same, even though their stressor effects are identical. The two types of actions of the same agent can influence one another. In the language of stress research, we say that the nonspecific effects are *conditioned* (modified) by the specific effects of each agent. Indeed, the specific actions of agents can, even totally, block certain nonspecific effects whenever the two happen to be diametrical opposites. Thus inevitable modifying and masking by specific actions was one of the main reasons why it took so long to draw a clear picture of stress as such.

Of course this state of affairs is encountered whenever we try to make any generalization. For instance, one of the typical features of the G.A.S. is its characteristic blood sugar curve. However, if stress is produced by the injection of insulin (the antidiabetic hormone of the pancreas), the typical blood sugar response will be obscured because the specific action of insulin is to lower the blood sugar at all times. It would be false to conclude that the blood sugar is no indicator of stress, or that insulin cannot produce a G.A.S. The stressor effect of insulin can still be recognized because, like all other stressors, at excessive dose levels, the hormone causes adrenocortical stimulation, thymus involution, and so forth. This lesson has been learned by examining many effects of many agents.

Various agents can produce the same specific syndrome. In *Fig. 9* we see four squares symbolizing potential target areas for stimuli. They might represent whole organs, tissues, or even individual cells. Each of these squares is subdivided into a top part containing alarm signals (arrows) and a bottom part which is constructed to give specific reactions upon stimulation.

Each time a specific agent acts upon any one

target, two things happen: there is a specific response (graphically represented here by the discharge of the distinct action-patterns from the lower part of the square), and a nonspecific response (represented by the discharge of the always-identical little arrows from the top part of the square).

For instance, light acting upon the eye causes vision, a diuretic induces the kidney to produce urine, a nerve impulse makes a muscle contract. These are specific responses. But, at the same time, the cells of all these organs can also send out some nonspecific alarm signals which merely indicate demands for activity. That the eye, kidney, or muscle each reacts differently and specifically to stimulation is a self-evident fact. But how can we concretely prove the nonspecific response? The chemical nature of the alarm signals has still not been definitely determined; yet, their existence has been proven beyond doubt.

When, in experimental animals or man, organs are induced to function intensely (for instance, if a large part of the musculature is forced to work), or

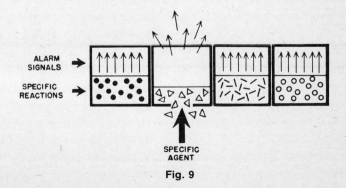

ALARM SIGNALS

SPECIFIC REACTIONS

SPECIFIC AGENT

Fig. 9

when tissues are damaged (for example, if the surface of the skin is burned), there is positive evidence of an increased secretion of ACTH, the adrenal-stimulating pituitary hormone. This substance, in turn, stimulates the hormone secretion of the adrenal cortex; consequently, the cortical hormone content of the blood rises. Evidently, somehow the directly affected organ must have sent out a message notifying the pituitary-adrenal system of an increased cortical hormone, or "corticoid," requirement.

At first it was thought that such messages could only travel through nerves. This is not the case. It has been possible to show, for instance, in a deeply anesthetized rat, that if one hind limb is completely separated from the body (except for its blood vessels) mechanical injury or scalding of that limb can still produce adrenocortical stimulation. Here, there was no nervous connection between the directly stimulated part and the rest of the body. Obviously, here, the alarm signals could not have been nervous stimuli; they must have traveled from the limb to the adrenal through the bloodstream. Presumably, these messengers are chemical compounds, *fatigue substances*, produced as metabolic by-products during activity or damage. It is equally possible, however, that the "first mediator," which carries the stress message from the directly affected area to the hypothalamus-pituitary system, is the lack of a vitally important body constituent which is consumed whenever any demand is made upon an organ. In this sense it would be a "negative by-product" of energy consumption. Finally, whatever the nature of this messenger may be, we have seen that while it is not

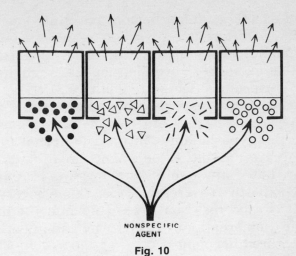

NONSPECIFIC
AGENT

Fig. 10

necessarily dependent upon the integrity of nervous pathways, there can be no doubt that nervous
stimulation itself can also produce a general stress
response. This happens, for example, when we
stimulate the sensory nerve stumps of an ampu-
tated extremity from which evidently neither positive nor negative chemical signals could reach the
body.

Experience has also shown that a specific agent
acting only on one organ usually causes less of a
stress response than a nonspecific agent acting on
many parts of the body. Why?

The explanation of this fact can again be visualized by our analogy of the four squares, as shown in
Fig. 10.

If a nonspecific agent acts simultaneously upon
all four targets, each of them will respond in its
own characteristic way (a muscle with contraction,
a nerve with conduction, and so on). But, of course,

these responses cannot be additive, since each target has a different pattern of response. On the other hand, every tissue will also discharge its alarm signals; these are identical throughout and their nonspecific effects are additive.

The hormonal response to the discharge of these alarm signals is a useful adaptive response, in which the hypothalamus-pituitary-adrenal system plays a cardinal role. Experiments on animals have shown that if any one of these organs is removed before exposure to stressors, resistance is very low. Yet, it can be restored toward normal if suitable substitution treatment is given by the injection of the required hormones.

In all these respects the mechanism of the stress response is very reminiscent of the events during a fire alarm, which we used as an analogy in the preceding chapter.

In *Fig. 11* a specific agent acts upon the third

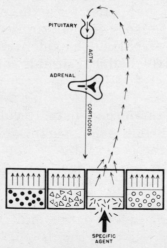

Fig. 11

square. The target reacts with its own characteristic pattern of response (downward discharge of the rods); but this specific activity automatically discharges alarm signals which travel to the hypothalamus and hence to the pituitary. The signals are nonspecific, no matter which target they come from; they just say, "Stress." But, from here on, the pattern of response is quite specific.

In the preceding chapters I spoke at length of the adrenal cortex, but the pituitary was barely mentioned. This gland is embedded in bones at the base of the skull, just beneath the hypothalamus, and regulates the production of corticoids through its adrenocorticotrophic hormone, or ACTH. It does not matter that the adrenals are placed above the kidneys at a great distance from the pituitary, because hormones are carried equally to all organs through the blood. When the pituitary produces ACTH, this trophic (from Greek *trephein*, to nourish) hormone incites the cells of the adrenal cortex to transform available raw materials into corticoids. These are then also discharged into the blood so that they can act throughout the body wherever they are needed.

The selective secretion of ACTH and corticoids under the influence of the alarm signals is a specific form of response. Its ultimate purpose appears to be the increased blood level of corticoids, which can then act back upon the directly stimulated target, to steady its work and to put out the fire of excessive activity.

If we compare the two preceding drawings, it is easy to see that the more nonspecific the eliciting agent (the less its effect is limited to individual targets), the greater its ability to elicit an intense stress syndrome. Even maximal specific stimulation of any one small target can only produce systemic stress corresponding in its intensity to the limited quantity of alarm signals this one activated unit can emit. On the other hand, if a large number of target areas is affected by a nonspecific agent which acts simultaneously in many places, the quantity of the alarm signals discharged can become enormous. Here—as in our analogy of the multiple fire alarms—there is a direct proportionality between the number of signals and the extent of the resulting defensive measures.

This hypothesis is by no means definitely proven as yet, but no other interpretation fits our experimental observations better. We have seen, for instance, that if one rat is exposed to intense sound, another to severe cold, and yet another to scalding of a paw, there is a moderate adrenal enlargement in each of them. There is a definite limit to the adrenal stimulation that can be produced by any one agent, say scalding a small area, no matter how severely. On the other hand, if a rat is exposed to sound, cold, and scalding simultaneously, the resulting adrenal enlargement will be much greater than that produced by any one of these stressors. Obviously these three distinct agents must have had some common effect through which their actions upon the adrenal could be added.

Stimulation of a small area which sends messages to many targets, however, acts as a very nonspecific stressor, affecting all these areas directly. For example, intense pain caused by stimulation of one point in a sensory nerve can be the cause of intense general stress, not through its direct effect upon the limited point of a nerve, but through the spreading of its effect through the innumerable branches of the nervous system.

It is apparently the discharge of alarm signals that makes stress the common denominator of the most diverse reactions to all kinds of agents.

The triphasic course of the stress response. If we follow the development of the G.A.S. in time, we can see that it goes through a typical triphasic course. To illustrate this I pointed out (in Chapter 2) that if an animal is continuously exposed to some stressor (say, cold), the adrenal cortex first discharges all its microscopic fat granules which contain the cortical hormones (alarm reaction), then it becomes laden with an unusually large number of fat droplets (stage of resistance) and finally it loses them again (stage of exhaustion). As far as we can see, the same triphasic course is followed by most, if not all, of the manifestations of the G.A.S.

Fig. 12 illustrates this graphically, using general resistance to injury as an indicator.

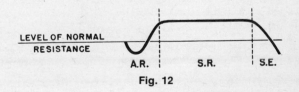

LEVEL OF NORMAL RESISTANCE

A.R.   S.R.   S.E.

Fig. 12

In the acute phase of the alarm reaction (A.R.), general resistance, to the particular stressor with which the G.A.S. had been elicited, falls way below normal. Then, as adaptation is acquired, in the stage of resistance (S.R.), the capacity to resist rises considerably above normal. But eventually, in the stage of exhaustion (S.E.), resistance drops below normal again.

To test these observations, we exposed large numbers of rats to various stressors over long periods of time and tested the resistance of sample groups among these animals at repeated intervals. For instance, in one experiment we placed a hundred rats in a refrigerated room where the temperature was near freezing. Thanks to their fur coats, they could stand this quite well, although during the first 48 hours they developed the typical manifestations of the alarm reaction. This was proved by killing ten animals at the end of the second day; all of them had large, fat-free adrenals, small thymuses, and stomach ulcers.

At this same time—after 48 hours of exposure—twenty other rats were also removed from the cold-room to test their resistance to low temperatures. They were now placed in a still colder chamber, together with normal rats which up to then had lived at room temperature. It turned out that the rats which had already developed an alarm reaction due to moderate cold were even less than normally resistant to excessive cold.

Five weeks later another sample of rats was taken from the cold-room. By that time they had fully adapted themselves to life at low temperature and were in the stage of resistance of the G.A.S. When these animals were placed in the still more refrigerated chamber, they survived temperatures which nonpretreated animals could never withstand. Evidently their resistance had risen above the normal level.

Yet, after several months of life in the cold, this acquired resistance was lost again, and the stage of exhaustion set in. Then the animals were not even capable of further surviving in the comparatively moderate cold of the refrigerated chamber in which they had spent so much time in a state of perfect well-being, ever since the initiation of the experiment.

The three waves in the curve (see page 111) (down, up, and down again) represent a summary of many such observations, because this type of experiment was repeated with various other stressors (forced muscular work, drugs, infections) and the result was always the same.

Adaptability can be well trained to serve a special purpose, but eventually it runs out; its amount is finite.

This was not what I had expected. I should have thought that once an animal has learned to live in the cold, it could go on resisting low temperatures indefinitely. Why shouldn't it, as long as it received enough food to create the internal heat necessary for the maintenance of a normal body temperature? Naturally, in order to get used to cold, the organism must learn how to produce an excess of heat by the combustion of food. For additional safety the body must also learn to prevent unnecessary loss of heat. It does this through a generalized constriction of the blood vessels in the skin which interferes with the cooling of the blood on the surface. But once all this has been learned and the animal has become well adjusted to life at low temperatures, one would expect that nothing but lack of food (caloric energy) would stand in the way

of continued resistance to cold. Observation shows
that this is not the case.

Similar experiments have then revealed that the
same loss of acquired adaptation also occurs in
animals forced to perform intense muscular exercise, or in those given toxic drugs and other stressors over long periods of time. These were the
actual observations which led to the concept of
"adaptation energy" (see page 81).

*The defense is twofold: overpower or coex-
ist.* There are two principal ways of defending
yourself against aggression: ignore (or run away
from) the aggressor, or advance and attack him. All
these techniques are also used by the defensive
forces of our tissues against foes inside the body.

If an agent is an indirect pathogen, not damaging in itself but only through the defense reactions
it elicits, it is best to ignore it since in that way it
will cause no harm. The syntoxic hormones (e.g.,
corticoids) help tissue in this effort to coexist without unnecessary inflammatory or immunologic
defense reactions. However, such peaceful attitudes are not always desirable. In these cases, we
use catatoxic defense reactions. For example,
chemicals which cannot be ignored must be
destroyed. This can be done by catatoxic hormones
which induce enzymes in the liver that chemically
disintegrate the offending agents, as we have previously explained. Similarly, there are serologic
mechanisms which can defend us against invading
microbes. When a germ gets into the blood stream
it can be killed by these purely aggressive, chemical substances which we call *antibodies*. There is

no element of retreat, no flight in this response, for the lethal microbe cannot be ignored. Conversely, if I accidentally put my hand on a hotplate, my muscles will immediately pull the burned hand back. This happens whether I want it to or not, because it is an involuntary reflex of flight. There is nothing aggressive about this; I make no effort to destroy the source of my injury, but merely draw away from it. Here again I could not avoid damage by merely disregarding the scalding heat.

To my mind, it is one of the most characteristic features of the G.A.S. that its various defensive mechanisms are always based on combinations of these two types of response: attack, or passive tolerance or retreat. It is often an interplay of antagonistic responses—that is, responses designed to activate opposing forces. I rather think that it is the subconscious realization of this fact that gave the word *stress* its connotation of "tension" in everyday English. In physics, tension is the result of two balancing forces, and that is very much what antagonistic, nervous, or hormonal tensions create during stress in the human body. Of course, advance and retreat cannot occur simultaneously and at the same place, but the *forces* of advance and those of retreat can both be mobilized concurrently at any one place.

Let me illustrate this again by a simple, mechanical analogy, one which incidentally represents a procedure of defense actually used by the human body.

The black rods in *Fig. 13* represent the two large bones in the arm; the two white spindles correspond to the bending (flexor) and stretching (exten-

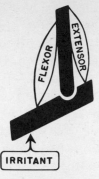

Fig. 13

sor) muscles. It is evident from this drawing how
contraction of the flexor will bend, and how contraction of the extensor will stretch, the arm. If
both these antagonistic muscles contract simultaneously with the same force, the arm does not move
but becomes tense and hence more steady.

When an irritant touches my wrist I can retreat
from it by contracting the flexor muscle (flight); I
can push it away by contracting the extensor muscle (advance); or I can steady myself against it by
contracting both (tension).

So, we see that actually the two antagonistic
mechanisms give us three possibilities of reaction:
retreat, advance, or steadiness, all of which can
have their uses; and we must choose among them,
depending upon the circumstances. Only in the
rare instance where you really succeed in totally
disregarding a potential source of trouble, without
even having to force yourself, do you avoid tension.

Survival depends largely upon a correct blending
of attack, retreat, and standing one's ground. To

obtain the best results these three types of reaction must be perfectly coordinated, not only in time but also in space, so as to adjust our reactions to the changing demands of the situation at various times, in various parts of the body. When faced with an aggressor, it is by achieving this coordination with minimal distress that an organ, an individual, or even an entire nation can successfully defend itself. For the present we will concern ourselves with the somatic basis of the mechanism of stress resistance, but in Book V we will go much deeper into the psychosomatic and psychosocial aspects of these same laws when applied to interpersonal relations in everyday life.

The principal coordinating systems of the body are the nervous and the hormonal systems. In both of these we have pairs of antagonists. As far as the fight for survival is concerned, we might call them the *pro-* and the *antidefense factors*. The former carry the message to act or to advance, the latter to relax or to retreat.

As regards the *nervous system* this had been known for a long time. The voluntary muscles of our limbs are innervated by antagonistic nerve fibers; so are the many involuntary muscles which innervate the stomach, intestines, blood vessels, and other internal organs.

How do nerves act this way? Interestingly, in the final analysis even they act through hormones. At the minute end-points of each nerve branch, hormone-like chemical substances are discharged, and it is these which influence the tissues, for instance, the muscles to cause contraction.

The *adrenalines* (adrenaline itself and its close

relative, noradrenaline)—technically called catecholamines—represent one type of such a nerve
hormone.

The noradrenaline produced by nerves resembles
adrenaline, the hormone secreted by the *adrenal
medulla*. Up to now, I have spoken almost solely
about the outer part, or cortex, of the adrenal,
because it was here that we saw the most striking
changes during the alarm reaction. Yet, the central portion, the medulla of the gland, is also important; the adrenalines which it secretes likewise
have important functions to fulfill during stress.

One wonders why the body makes such substances, once in a gland and once in nerves. Their
effects are very similar, but when adrenalines are
secreted into the blood by the glandular cells of the
adrenal medulla, the hormones are necessarily distributed equally to all parts of the body; this
assures widespread effects, but it can give no selectivity of action. On the other hand, when these
substances are liberated at nerve-endings, a high
concentration of them can be produced in certain
circumscribed territories of the body, so that their
effects may become very selective. In other words,
the hormones secreted by the adrenal medulla can
best achieve a generalized, uniform effect throughout the body, whereas those locally produced by
individual nerves are most effective in causing pronounced changes in one place without disturbing
the rest of the body. It depends upon circumstances, which of the two types of reaction is preferable, the generalized or the selective.

The nerve hormone which acts as an antagonist
of the adrenalines is called *acetylcholine*. As far as

we know, it is not produced and secreted into the general blood stream by any endocrine gland; it is liberated only at nerve-endings.

The *adrenal cortex* makes a large number of hormones. Some of these are sex hormones, quite similar to those produced by the sex glands (ovaries, testes). They have little or nothing to do with the mechanism of stress, but they may cause severe sexual derangements. For instance, most of the bearded women who exhibit themselves in circuses, are suffering from an excessive production of male hormones by their adrenals. Three- to four-year-old girls may develop the sexual characteristics of adult women merely as a result of excessive adrenal female hormone production.

These facts are mentioned only to complete the picture, but it is the so-called vital or life-maintaining hormones of the adrenal cortex that concern our discussion of stress, for when these are lacking there is no adaptability to change—and lack of adaptability spells death.

At first it was thought that the adrenal cortex produced only one kind of vital hormone; this was called *cortine.* But further research showed that there are at least two types of such hormones. It was at that time—some thirty years ago—that I proposed the term *corticoid hormones,* as a collective name for this group.

The outstanding effect of one type of corticoid is to inhibit inflammation. Inflammation is a defense reaction of the tissues; so this type of hormone can be regarded as an antidefense hormone, in that it prevents a defensive reaction. There are several such hormones. I called them *anti-inflammatory*

corticoids. To this group belong cortisone and cortisol COL), which have become generally well-known
because of their conspicuous beneficial effects in
rheumatoid arthritis, allergic inflammation,
inflammation of the eyes, and other inflammatory
diseases. With them we can also prevent other
defensive reactions, for example, those that
develop immunity to foreign substances and
microbes. Such immunity is most useful in resisting smallpox or poliomyelitis but, unfortunately,
the body cannot always distinguish between harmful and useful foreign bodies; hence it also rejects
grafts of tissues which come from foreign donors
(as in the case of heart or kidney transplants).

The opposite kind were quite naturally designated as the *proinflammatory corticoids*. These are
less well-known by the general public, because we
are just beginning to learn something about their
role in clinical medicine. Aldosterone and desoxycorticosterone are two such proinflammatory hormones.

To follow our argument, it is not essential to burden your memory with all these complex names.
Remember only that many corticoids have been
discovered: some of them are anti-inflammatory
and generally antiaggressive (syntoxic), others
proinflammatory and generally aggressive (catatoxic). Although, for the sake of simplicity, we
group them this way, we must constantly bear in
mind that these terms are merely symbols; they do
not tell the whole story. First, it is only under certain conditions that the two types of corticoids
inhibit or stimulate inflammation. Second, they do
many other things besides acting on inflammation.

For instance, the anti-inflammatory corticoids can also raise the blood sugar; hence I suggested that biochemists could call them *glucocorticoids* (from *glucose*). On the other hand, one of the most outstanding chemical effects of proinflammatory corticoids is to influence mineral metabolism; they are *mineralocorticoids* in that they cause a retention of sodium and an excretion of potassium.

It is somewhat confusing to have several names for the same group of compounds, but this is necessary, even in designating things encountered in everyday life. For instance, the same region may be called *wheat country* or *oil country*, depending upon whether one is interested in the products of the surface, or of the depths, of the land. Incidentally, in additon to acting on inflammation, immunity, sugar and mineral metabolism, the corticoids have many other effects—for instance, upon the pigmentation of the skin, emotional reactions, and blood pressure—just as any geographic region has many characteristics apart from producing wheat or oil.

Finally, it must be kept in mind that although the anti- and proinflammatory corticoids do, under certain conditions, diametrically oppose each other's effects on inflammation, this is not always so; nor are these hormones necessarily antagonistic as regards their other actions. In some respects they may actually be synergistic, that is, they may work together and mutually increase each other's effects.

Any agent which acts upon the body produces dual effects. Some are specific, others nonspecific. In this discussion we are not concerned with specific actions, so we shall say no more about them here. The nonspecific component acts three ways:

1. Directly, on whatever tissue the agent happens to touch (target area). For instance, microbes on a splinter of wood which gets under our skin can destroy cells in their immediate surroundings by the direct effect of bacterial poisons.

2. Indirectly, by mobilizing the antireactive part of the antagonistic defense system, which is actually a chemical message to retreat from, or at least ignore, the aggressor (syntoxic).

3. Indirectly, by mobilizing the other part of this same system which is prodefensive, that is, a message to encapsulate (proinflammatory) and, if possible, to destroy the aggressor (catatoxic).

Incidentally, both the anti-inflammatory and the proinflammatory effects are considered to be syntoxic, since they promote coexistence with a potential pathogen, either by ignoring it or by surrounding it with an inflammatory barricade which separates it from the rest of the body. On the other hand, enhanced degradation of toxic substances by the induction of hepatic enzymes is a catatoxic effect, as is the formation of immunologic antibodies that actively attack and destroy microbes and other foreign matter.

It is easy to see how a whole human being, or even part of one—for instance, an arm—could either attack or retreat from an aggressor. But how could these descriptions be applicable to tissue reactions? We shall try to show this by using inflammation and drug detoxication as examples; but first we shall have to become more familiar with the principle of *conditioning*, which I have barely mentioned up to now.

The importance of conditioning factors. Suppose you are given some strawberries to eat—would your reaction depend only upon the quality of the fruit? Certainly not. It would depend upon many other conditions. If you like strawberries and have not had any for a long time, you would welcome them with enthusiasm. If strawberries were all you had had to eat for weeks, they would probably disgust you. If you should happen to be allergic to strawberries, they would even make you sick.

The reactions of our tissues to various agents are dependent upon very similar conditioning factors. Generally speaking, we distinguish two types of these: the internal and the external. The *internal conditioning factors* are those which have become part of the body. Heredity and past experiences have some trace, some "tissue memories," which influence the way we react to things. For instance, cold is less damaging to a polar bear than it is to a tropical fish whose whole genetic evolution was oriented toward life in a warm climate. But, in any one animal, the reaction to cold will also largely depend upon whether this particular individual has previously been living in a cold or a hot atmosphere. Remember that the same cold which initially produced an alarm reaction in our rats and decreased resistance to more cold, eventually produced a stage of resistance with an increased cold tolerance. Thus, both inherited genetic factors and previous exposure of an individual can create internal conditions which alter resistance from within.

On the other hand, whatever acts upon us from without can also influence our response to a simultaneously-acting agent, even if it causes no permanent change in our body. The food we take, the climate we live in are such *external conditioning factors*.

Our discussion of physiologic reactions to stressors would be very incomplete and misleading if we failed to make the importance of conditioning quite clear. Take the case of conditioning by food substances. The same amount of proinflammatory (mineralocorticoid) hormone which causes marked kidney damage and hypertension in a rat kept on a high salt intake has no such effect on a salt-free diet. It is especially noteworthy that stress itself can act as a conditioning factor for the adaptive hormones produced during stress. For instance, the same amount of cortisone which markedly inhibits inflammation in a patient who has just undergone a major surgical operation will be relatively ineffective in a perfectly healthy person.

At first we thought that this was merely due to increased corticoid production by the patient's own adrenals. Of course, the effect of the internally-formed corticoids is added to that of the injected cortisone. But this is not the whole story. Such conditioning by stress (or, in the previous example, by salt) occurs even in adrenalectomized animals in which no corticoids could possibly be produced. Here we must be dealing with some direct interaction between the conditioning factors (the dietary salt, the stress of surgery) and the corticoids.

Stress apparently acts in two ways: directly and indirectly. For instance, to inhibit inflammation, it increases both the production of, and tissue sensitivity to, anti-inflammatory corticoids. *Fig. 14* shows how:

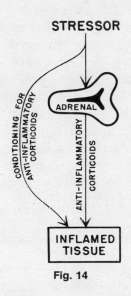

Fig. 14

The Essence of the Stress Response

What we have said up to now is already sufficient to give us a fairly correct picture of the basic mechanisms involved in all types of stress reactions. They can be visualized in *Fig. 15.*

Again we note that the agent produces both specific and nonspecific actions through which it influences the whole body (here represented as a square). But *Fig. 15* also shows that the agent does not act on the whole body evenly; it usually hits some part, the direct target area, more than other regions.

For example, if I accidentally swallow some corrosive fluid, my whole body suffers to some extent, but no part of it will be as much affected as the tissues between my lips and stomach, which came into direct contact with the poison. These represent the target area in this case. Yet, organs far removed from this region are also affected; for instance, the adrenals are stimulated to produce an excess of proinflammatory and/or anti-inflammatory corticoids; there are nervous and emotional reactions and various biochemical changes which influence metabolism. As a result of all this, virtually every tissue in the body is eventually affected to some extent.

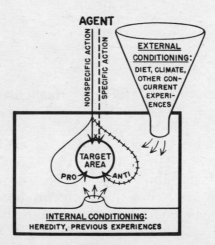

Fig. 15

Fig. 15 also reminds us that the whole development of the reaction largely depends on conditioning factors. These can be invariables which act upon us from within: our hereditary predispositions and previous experiences (internal conditioning), as well as variables which influence our body simultaneously with the agent from without (external conditioning). All these are integral elements of the response during stress; they all contribute something to the picture of the G.A.S.

This general view of the stress mechanism now permits us to consider in more detail the application of our concept to a special problem.

chapter 6

Stress and Inflammation

Forms of inflammation. The structure of
inflammation. The purpose of inflammation.
The regulation of inflammation: relations
between the L.A.S. and the G.A.S.

Forms of Inflammation

Inflammation has been defined as "a local reaction to injury." It may occur almost anywhere in the body and it can take many forms; yet it is always the same kind of reaction. When fully developed it is always characterized by swelling, reddening, heat, and pain.

If a particle of dust gets under your eyelid, there will be some pain, with reddening and swelling of the membranes around the irritated spot; the eyes become hot, and tears form, which usually succeed in washing the offensive particle away. But while the irritation lasts, it is actually an inflammation of the outer eye-membrane, the conjuctiva; we call it *conjunctivitis.*

If a child develops a sore throat, what usually happens is that certain microbes proliferate in his tonsils and cause local swelling, reddening, heat, and pain. This is an inflammation of the tonsils; we call it *tonsillitis.*

A patient may come down suddenly with violent

pain in his abdomen because microbes have gotten
out of control in one small part of his intestine, the
appendix, and caused swelling, heat, reddening,
and pain there; this is *appendicitis*. If the wall of
the appendix can no longer resist aggression by the
microbes, it perforates. Then the bacteria attack
the whole of the fine membrane which covers the
outer surface of our intestines: the peritoneum.
The resulting inflammation, if not treated, is
usually fatal; we call it *general peritonitis*.

The disorders which I have just mentioned are
very different, indeed; yet all of them are forms of
inflammation. In medicine it became customary to
add the suffix *-itis* after the name of the *organ*
affected, to indicate that an inflammation had
developed in it. This fundamental process of
defense plays a leading part in a great variety of
disease conditions. Inflammation of the liver is
hepatitis, of the kidney, *nephritis*, of the joints,
arthritis, of the nerves, *neuritis*.

Viruses (living beings even smaller than bacteria), which cause paralyzing inflammatory changes
in certain portions of the central nervous system,
elicit *poliomyelitis*. Some larger microbes tend to
irritate the inner surface of the heart and produce
endocarditis. Ingestion of irritating foods can
cause an inflammation of the stomach, that is, *gas-
tritis;* and exposure of the skin to allergens or x-
rays may lead to *dermatitis*.

Even the mending of a wound, if you have cut
your hand, will depend on inflammation, and so will
the healing of a tuberculous focus in the lung. Hay
fever, an inflammation of the nasal mucosa, develops in certain persons because something in their

bodily structure has made them especially sensi-. tive to certain plant-pollens in the air. The innocuous sting of a mosquito, just as an almost fatal exposure to the atomic bomb, is met by the body with what we call inflammation.

From all this it is evident that virtually any agent can cause inflammation in virtually any part of the body, and the resulting conditions present the most varied aspects. Yet when you examine the affected organs under the microscope, the cellular changes in them are very similar in every case.

The Structure of Inflammation

We have said, "Inflammation is a local reaction to injury." If so, it must be something active; it is not merely the passive result of injury, but a positive reaction against it. By calling it a *reaction*, we also imply that it has a purpose; apparently its object is to inactivate the aggressor and mend whatever damage has been caused.

But what is its structure? What does inflammation look like? In going through our long—though still quite incomplete—list of the inflammatory diseases, we have repeatedly pointed out that there is reddening, heat, swelling, and pain. This is the classic syndrome of inflammation.

The reddening and heat are due to a dilatation of the blood vessels in the inflamed area. The swelling is caused partly by the leakage of fluids and cells from the dilated blood vessels into the surrounding solid tissues, and partly by an intense proliferation of the fibrous connective tissue, whose cells rapidly multiply in response to irritation. The pain is due to an irritation of the sensory nerve-endings which are caught in and invaded by this inflammatory process.

These cardinal signs have long been known to physicians. They were first clearly described in the Third Book of the famous *Treatise on Medicine*, which Aurelius Cornelius Celsus, the great Roman physician, wrote just a few years before the birth of Christ. This volume contains what is probably the most quoted sentence in medical writing: "Indeed, the signs of inflammation are four, redness and swelling, with heat and pain." To this was later added: "and interference with function," because the swelling and the pain always diminish the functional efficiency of inflamed organs.

In the schematic drawing *(Fig. 16)*, we see on the left side the microscopic appearance of a small, normal connective tissue territory. There are spindle-shaped connective tissue cells and, between them, connective tissue fibers which surround a branching, small blood vessel. In the latter we notice both red and white blood cells. Connective tissue is the material which cements all our other tissues together. Here we have described its microscopic features, but with your naked eyes you have already seen it. Whenever some abrasion or a cut takes a bit of skin away, the sticky, pinkish material you see beneath is connective tissue.

After exposure to air and contact with various irritating substances that we may use to dress the wound, its surface usually becomes granular, and sometimes whitish pus forms on it. That is the naked eye appearance of inflamed connective tissue. The granules are due to proliferation of connective tissue cells and fibers. The whitish pus is essentially a mass of white blood cells which have penetrated to the surface—through the vessel walls and the connective tissue—toward the source of irritation.

On the right side of *Fig. 16*, we see a microscopic picture of such inflamed tissue. It is actually the same region which has been shown on the left as an example of normal tissue, but now an irritant has acted upon it. The blood vessel became dilated and engorged with blood cells. Many of these, especially the white cells, emigrated into the connective tissue around the vessel, traveling particularly in the direction of the irritant. The connective tissue cells and fibers proliferated to form a thick, impenetrable barricade of the inflammatory tissue which prevented the spread of the irritant into the blood.

An important thing which cannot be shown in *Fig. 16* is that, from the blood and from the connective tissue, chemical substances are also secreted toward the irritant: they enmesh and surround it, preventing it from spreading and tending to

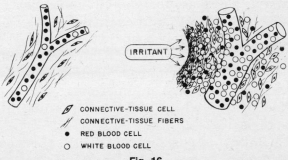

IRRITANT

🖋 CONNECTIVE-TISSUE CELL
∥ CONNECTIVE-TISSUE FIBERS
● RED BLOOD CELL
○ WHITE BLOOD CELL

Fig. 16

neutralize its poisons and to kill any bacteria that it may contain.

The Purpose of Inflammation

Judged by its structure, inflammation is undoubtedly an active defense reaction: it represents fight, not flight. It also comprises an element of repair, in that any wound, any tissue defect caused by an injury, is filled out and mended by the rapidly proliferating connective tissue cells and fibers. As the fibers mature, they tend to contract; this further helps to abolish the defect.

Once we have thus understood the structure of inflammation, it appears to be self-evident that this reaction is useful for the maintenance of health. This is often true, but not always. If the irritant is really dangerous—say, the deadly microbe of tuberculosis which, if allowed to multiply and invade the blood vessels, would spread throughout the body—then inflammation certainly is useful. It can prevent the irritant from invading farther, by putting a strong barricade of connective tissue around it. If microbes are thus restrained, there is not enough food for them to multiply indefinitely, and eventually they become bogged down by their own exudations. Furthermore, many of the surviving bacteria are killed by the antibacterial chemicals formed by inflammatory tissue, and other microbes are actually engulfed by the white blood cells, which literally eat bacteria.

But what could possibly be the use of responding with inflammation to something like a harmless

plant-pollen, which cannot multiply or invade anyway, and which is not damaging to tissue? Yet
some sensitive persons react to such plant-pollens
with the intense inflammation of certain mucous
membranes which we call *hay fever*. You may say,
perhaps Nature knows best; perhaps inflammation
has a protective value even here. After all, who
could tell whether the nasal tissues of a sensitive
person would not be destroyed by such plant-pollens if there were no inflammation? The same may
be suspected of any other substance to which we
happen to be allergic. This is not so and we can
prove it. If a hay fever-sensitive person is first
given large doses of the syntoxic, anti-inflammatory cortisone, contact with plant-pollens will not
cause inflammation in his nose; still, under these
conditions the nasal structures are not damaged.
Indeed a person so protected by cortisone could not
even know that he had been exposed to the pollens
which normally would produce most distressing
symptoms in him. In other words, we might say
that here inflammation is no protection against
disease: it *is* the disease.

To summarize, we may say that inflammation is
undoubtedly a reaction to injury. If the injury is
serious, and especially if it threatens life because
the causative agent could spread into the blood and
throughout the body, then this reaction is useful
for the maintenance of health. It essentially consists of putting a strong barricade around the
invaded territory, thereby clearly demarcating the
sick from the healthy. The diseased part may have
to be sacrificed; the destructive cells and fluids of
inflammation enter the quarantined area to kill

the invader, but usually they also kill the invaded tissues. The pus evacuated from a boil contains the dead bodies of both the microbes and the tissue cells. Other disadvantages are the swelling, pain, and interference with function, which the proliferating inflammatory tissue necessarily produces. This is still a small price to pay for the preservation of life. But if the invader is harmless, there is no point in reacting at all. In this case inflammation does not help, it only hurts. The same is true not only of inflammation but also of all other excessive reactions to indirect pathogens.

In a sense, inflammation is intermediate between syntoxic and catatoxic responses. The encapsulation of a potential pathogen, or its enmeshment in a restraining tissue mass, is syntoxic since it merely permits coexistence with an aggressor by separating it from the rest of the body. However, when this separation is followed by aggression, through inflammatory cells and enzymes, a true catatoxic element is added since these latter responses are designed to destroy the enemy, not merely to ignore it.

If we compare inflammation with the defensive reactions of a whole human being, or even of a whole nation, we find striking similarities in the over-all pattern everywhere. By recognizing these we may gain more insight into the mechanism, and even the philosophy, of defense in general, insight which penetrates far beyond the confines of medicine.

When an alarm is sounded to announce the approach of the enemy, the threatened nation may immediately stop its peaceful activities to mobilize for war; it may place all available manpower under arms, put up barricades of all sorts—or it may do nothing at all. Which course is better depends largely upon the aggressor. If the foe is well-armed and dangerous, it may be preferable to fight. But if the approach of a small band of marauders happened to set off the alarm, a nationwide mobilization of defenses would only hurt the population by unnecessarily interfering with its normal activities.

In all these examples of reactions—whether we deal with the problems of a few cells, with those of a whole man, or of an entire nation—defense may bring salvation or it may bring self-inflicted injuries. Whether to fight or not to fight depends upon circumstances; and, on the whole, cells are more judicious than people, and individuals wiser than the leadership of nations, in making this choice. Yet all biologic groups from the microscopic to the geographic are singularly short-sighted when it comes to this alternative. It is, as it were, a difficult selection to make *from within,* for tissues, men, and nations alike. These situations are best appraised by looking at the disturbed unit *from without,* whence you can see its position within a larger context. This is especially true whenever the result depends largely upon possible help from without.

We shall have more to say about such psychosocial implications of these biologic response forms in Book V. Here we merely wanted to prepare the reader to observe the singular similarity of adap-

tive reactions to demands on the somatic and mental levels.

The Regulation of Inflammation: Relations between the L.A.S. and the G.A.S.

What regulates inflammatory defense from within
the body? How can we help to regulate it from
without?

I shall use as an example mainly the role of the
endocrines—especially that of the adrenals and of
the pituitary—because it is with these that I am
best acquainted through personal investigations.
Also, it so happens that we have learned more
about the role of hormones in the regulation of
inflammation than about that of nerves and other
factors.

It is easy to see how, by discharging ACTH into
the blood, the pituitary can inform the adrenal that
a situation of local stress exists somewhere in the
body; but how does the pituitary "know" there is
stress? This question about the nature of the "first
mediator" of the stress message has still not been
fully answered.

ACTH induces the adrenals to produce mainly
anti-inflammatory corticoids (such as cortisol and
cortisone); hence this chemical messenger of the
pituitary can only inhibit inflammatory reactions
to injury. What happens when stimulation of
inflammation is needed? Intensive work along
these lines is still in progress today in many laboratories and clinics throughout the world. But we
have learned enough about the problem to draw at
least a preliminary sketch (see *Fig. 17*) of stress

and inflammation as a part of the G.A.S. blueprint.*

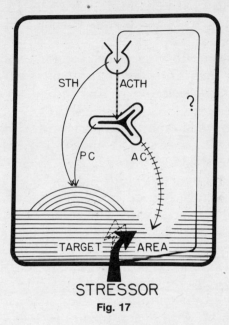

STRESSOR
Fig. 17

Here we shall not consider internal and external
conditioning, nor the specific actions of agents.
These have already been discussed on pages 123-
124 and may now be taken for granted. The whole
square field represents the body. The funnel-

*If I may be permitted a small aside before I confront you with
this sketch, let me point out that it is taken—without the
slightest change—from *The Story of the Adaptation Syndrome*
published in 1952. It is rather satisfactory to me that now, 24
years later, it is still possible to present all the fundamental
facts for the understanding of this problem in essentially the
same manner. Although in the meantime numerous additional
facts have come to light, those noted almost a quarter of a
century ago still appear to be valid.

shaped structure at the top is the hypothalamus on the floor of the brain; the round body just beneath it is the pituitary. In the middle we see the Y-shaped cross section of one adrenal with its light cortex and dark medulla.

The *stressor* (for instance, a colony of microbes) acts upon the *target area* (any part of the body) both directly (thick arrow) and indirectly by way of the pituitary and adrenals.

To begin with, some alarm signal (labeled by a question mark) travels from the directly injured target area to the pituitary. This *first mediator* of the stress response undoubtedly exists, but, as we have said before, we do not know what it is. Perhaps it is not even always the same signal. In some instances, it may be a chemical substance formed in the directly affected tissue, in others a nervous impulse elicited by pain or excitement. It often appears to travel first to the brain, and then through the hypothalamus to the pituitary, notifying this gland that a condition of stress exists, so that more ACTH is needed.

The message to release ACTH is transmitted from the hypothalamic nerve cells to pituitary gland cells by a substance called CRF, for corticotrophin releasing factor (corticotrophin is a synonym for ACTH).

The subsequent increase in ACTH secretion stimulates the adrenal cortex to make more anti-inflammatory corticoids (ACs). The adrenal can also produce proinflammatory corticoids (PCs); but this is regulated by a variety of complex factors, among which ACTH plays only a minor role as compared to renal blood pressure regulators and electrolytes.

By changing the proportion between pro- and anti-inflammatory stimuli, the body can regulate the ability of tissues to undergo inflammation in response to local injury. This change in reactivity can be accomplished in various ways:

1. Any increase in ACTH secretion necessarily shifts the balance in favor of an inhibition of inflammation because this hormone stimulates mainly the production of ACs.

2. As I have said, we still do not know much about what stimulates the adrenals to produce an excess of PCs, but it has been established with certainty that the blood concentration of these hormones also fluctuates, and quite independently of the AC content of the blood. Evidently the production of both types of corticoids can be independently regulated.

3. In order to change the proportion between pro- and anti-inflammatory stimuli in the body, it is not even necessary that the proportion between PCs and ACs be changed. We found, for example, that if both types of corticoids are very plentiful in the blood (we call this *hormonal tension*) the ACs always win the contest. This is so, no matter how much PC is simultaneously present.

4. Yet another way of changing the inflammability of tissues is through a pituitary substance which blocks certain effects of ACTH. This compound is known as the *growth hormone*, because it stimulates the growth of the body as a whole. Most of the giants you can see in circuses are "pituitary

giants," whose growth was stimulated by an abnormal excess of growth hormone. The international scientific name of this substance, *somatotrophic hormone*, is derived from the Greek *soma*, body, plus *trophic*, nourishing, and I have recommended for it the symbol STH (in analogy to ACTH).

Specialists are still divided in their views on the possible effects of STH upon the adrenals. Some think that STH stimulates proinflammatory corticoid production, just as ACTH enhances the secretion of anti-inflammatory corticoids; but this is still uncertain and of minor importance, for, in any event, STH can unquestionably increase the activity of proinflammatory corticoids and thereby shift the hormone balance toward the left side of *Fig. 17*. This is accomplished by the direct effects of STH upon connective tissue.

The local response of any directly injured territory to nonspecific stressors, the *local adaptation syndrome* (L.A.S.), is mainly characterized by tissue death and reactive inflammation. It is clear, from what we have just learned, that this L.A.S. is powerfully influenced by the G.A.S. It is largely— though by no means entirely—dependent upon the balance between proinflammatory and anti-inflammatory hormones secreted by the endocrine glands in reply to alarm signals set off by the stressor itself.

In *Fig. 17* the results of enhancing inflammation are depicted on the left side. Here strong barriers of inflamed connective tissue are shown. They develop under the combined influence of: (1) local irritation by the stressor, and (2) stimulation of defense against the stressor by STH and proinflammatory corticoids. These barriers prevent the spread of the irritant toward the interior of the body. Conversely, on the right side of the diagram, we see the results of an anti-inflammatory hormone predominance. This manifests itself as an atrophy of connective tissue elements, a prevention of their inflammatory proliferation, and thus essentially an opening of the way for invasion by the aggressor.

It will depend largely upon the nature of the aggressor which of the two responses is more useful for the maintenance of health.

chapter 7

Synoptic View of the Whole Stress Mechanism

Inflammation is undoubtedly one of the most important features of the response to localized stress situations during the L.A.S. But the endocrine regulators of general stress reactions—for instance, the pituitary and the adrenals—also participate in the control of localized inflammation; hence there are close interactions between the L.A.S. and the G.A.S. A primarily local stress, if sufficiently severe, can produce a G.A.S., and general stress influences the L.A.S.

But what happens when a stressor does not act selectively upon any one target organ to produce inflammation? What happens, for instance, when nervous tension (worry, fear, pain), total irradiation of the body with x-rays, or a sudden change in atmospheric pressure, initiates a G.A.S.? None of these agents enters the body through any one limited portal and consequently none of them produces a well-defined L.A.S. Besides, even when there are more or less well-defined direct target areas which react with inflammation, what happens to the other internal organs besides the pituitary and the adrenals? In short, what does the picture of the whole G.A.S. look like? Inflammation is, at the most, a limited part of the whole picture.

Virtually every organ and every chemical constituent of the human body is involved in the general stress reaction. We should now try to draw a sketch of the whole G.A.S. Of course such an ambitious general map will have to be quite incomplete. In a book of this kind we could not even describe all parts of the human body. Besides, the participation of every organ in the G.A.S. has not yet been fully explored. Still, we badly need a sketch of this kind right now. We must have it, just as an explorer must at least have some idea of where the gaps, the unknown regions, are before he can begin to chart them. In medicine, as in geography, or in any other field, we must form some picture of what is known—and even of what can reasonably be suspected—in order to show where further investigation is most likely to be worth the effort.

To draw such a broad picture of the G.A.S., the scientist must start by forgetting all the little problems of detail which happen to occupy him in his daily laboratory work; only then will the well-established fundamental facts stand out clearly.

Now I must ask the reader not to give up in despair as he goes through these following pages, because, even if we limit ourselves to the most important facts, we are faced with such a multitude of apparently disconnected observations that their complexity appears to be insurmountable. However, since I want to tell this story as it confronted us, I must start by presenting the picture as it first appeared, full of well-established individual data with apparently no connections between them. The best way to learn about this fascinating mechanism is first to take stock of the facts and then to try to coordinate them, arriving in the end at the synoptic picture on page 151. In any event, the facts enumerated below are all well-established and important; hence, they have a value of their own and we should know about them even if at present we cannot yet be certain of the connections between them.

What are the most important landmarks which necessarily must be in the picture? The *kidney*, for instance, will certainly have to be included, because it plays a central part in maintaining the steady equilibrium of the body during the G.A.S. It regulates the chemical composition of the blood and tissues by selectively eliminating certain chemicals from the body. The kidney can also adjust blood pressure which is essential for the normal life of all tissues—by regulating the production of renal pressor substances, "RPS" (renin, angiotensin). Renin can act back upon the adrenal cortex to stimulate its secretion of aldosterone, the most potent natural mineralocorticoid, which also raises the blood pressure through a complicated mechanism largely dependent upon salt balance. These facts have been clarified mainly through the work of two groups of clinical investigators, directed respectively by Drs. J. H. Laragh of New York and J. Genest of Montreal.

The renal mechanism of *blood pressure regulation* is complicated and still only partially understood; but we have learned many important facts about it, mainly through animal experiments performed by three distinguished scholars: H. Goldblatt and I. Page of Cleveland, and E. Braun-

Menendez of Buenos Aires. We have learned, for
instance, that when the renal arteries are partially
constricted, the kidney produces an excess of renal
pressor substances. It is also known—chiefly
thanks to Arthur Grollman of Dallas—that the
blood pressure also rises if we remove both kidneys
from an experimental animal. Here we have a curious paradox: both too much and too little renal
activity can result in high blood pressure and over-
load the circulation with fluid that cannot be eliminated.

We have seen that in general PCs and ACs antagonize each other; yet large amounts of both these
hormones can raise the blood pressure and cause
renal damage.

The first experiments that demonstrated the
existence of what we called "mineralocorticoid
hypertension" were performed in our laboratories
at McGill University in 1943. We showed that the
only mineralocorticoid then available, desoxycorticosterone (DOC), when given in large amounts to
rats, produces a kidney disease of the kind which
also occurs spontaneously in man and is called
nephrosclerosis. No matter whether this disease is
produced in animals by overdosage with such corticoids, or whether it develops spontaneously in man,
nephrosclerosis is accompanied by a marked rise in
blood pressure.

At the same time hardening, rigidity, and inflammatory changes develop in the walls of the arteries
throughout the body. These changes, *arteritis* or
arteriosclerosis, belong to the group of diseases
commonly seen in the aged, presumably as one of
the irreversible results of lifelong stress.

We have already had occasion to speak of the antagonistic effect of PCs and ACs upon connective tissue responses, particularly *inflammation.* We have likewise mentioned that during stress the *lymphatic cells* in the thymus, the lymph nodes, and the circulating blood disintegrate. At the same time the *eosinophil cells* tend to disappear from the circulation.

All this would somehow have to be fitted into an over-all picture of the G.A.S.

But this is not all. The work of Walter B. Cannon and his school at Harvard University had taught us, long ago, that during acute emergencies the adrenal medulla and certain nerves secrete an excess of *adrenalines.* The significance of *noradrenaline* became evident in this respect much later, chiefly through the investigations of Ulf von Euler of Stockholm.

The whole important concept of *neurohumoral transmission* of nerve impulses had been clarified by the classic investigations carried out by Sir Henry Dale in England and Otto Loewi in Austria. These were the men who first showed that both noradrenaline and acetylcholine are produced at nerve-endings, and that it is through these two fundamentally antagonistic nerve hormones that the brain and the nerves exert their manifold actions.*

---

*Incidentally, the work of Dale, Loewi and von Euler was considered to be of sufficient importance to earn each of them a Nobel prize. I think most of us agree that Cannon would have deserved the same honor, but presumably he died before the enormous importance of his contribution was generally recognized.

The *thyroid*—a gland which lies just before the windpipe in the neck—is also often affected during stress; through special hormones which intensely stimulate the metabolism of every tissue, this organ can influence all organs in the body.

The *liver* is a sort of central chemical laboratory of the organism. It participates in most of the biochemical adjustments to stress. Firstly, by providing energy-yielding materials to satisfy the increased demands, it regulates the concentration of sugar, protein, and other important tissue foods in the blood. It can also check an excess of corticoids by destroying the surplus when the adrenals make too much. Finally, it plays a decisive role in the detoxication of various environmental pollutants, or poisonous substances that arise in the body. This activity is largely stimulated by the catatoxic hormones that induce drug-metabolizing liver enzymes.

The *white blood cells* (particularly the thymicolymphatic cells and eosinophils) regulate *serologic immune reactions* and *allergic hypersensitivity responses* to various foreign substances.

Obviously all these tissues have important parts to play during the G.A.S. A general outline of the stress response will not only have to include brain and nerves, pituitary, adrenal, kidney, blood vessels, connective tissue, thyroid, liver, and white blood cells, but will also have to indicate the manifold interrelations between them.

This is attempted in the following synoptic drawing, but I present this "atlas of stress" with great reservations because, despite the enormous mass of available data, the picture is still very incomplete. Besides, it lists only structures, hardly mentioning the many chemical changes characteristic of stress which are not clearly dependent upon any one organ.

In *Fig. 18*, the whole field again represents the entire body. The *conditioning factors* (heredity, previous exposures, diet, etc.) are symbolized by the dotted frame within which all reactions must

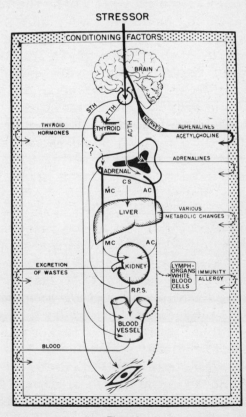

Fig. 18

develop. The main regulators of the stress syndrome (brain, nerves, pituitary, thyroid, adrenals,
liver, kidney, blood vessels, connective tissue cells,
white blood cells) are each represented by special
symbols. The interactions between these main regulators are shown in the usual way by connecting
arrows. Many arrows do not go specifically to any
one organ, but are drawn through the frame, point-
ing back into the body as a whole. The exact pathways through which they act will be the subjects of
future research; meanwhile we know only that
they can influence the response selectively at various points. It is this possibility of a *selective conditioning* that explains why every person reacts
somewhat differently to stress, depending upon his
inherited and acquired characteristics.

Since this general diagram attempts to illustrate
the fundamental pattern of all stress situations,
the *stressor* is not shown as acting upon any one
target area in particular. We merely indicate that,
wherever it happened to act first, it eventually
produced generalized stress reactions in the whole
body. This generalization of the response can be
accomplished by way of the two great coordinating
systems: the endocrine and the nervous.

In the nervous mediation of stress reactions, an
important part is played by the *reticular formation.* This is phylogenetically a very old part of the
central nervous system (CNS), well-developed even
in the lowest vertebrates in which it represents the
bulk of the CNS. In higher vertebrates, it is particularly developed in the spinal cord, brain stem, and
thalamus, consisting of closely-intermingled gray
and white substances. Its main function appears to

be one of correlation among various parts of the nervous system and it thus undoubtedly plays an extraordinarily important role in adaptation to the most diverse stressors.

Acting through the *nerves*, stressors produce *adrenalines* and *acetylcholine* which can influence the G.A.S. mechanism selectively at any point, without having to go through the endocrine gland system. These two types of nerve hormones generally antagonize each other. For instance, in an inflamed area, the adrenalines can produce circumscribed blood vessel constriction which interferes with inflammation; whereas acetylcholine has an inverse effect. The movements of the intestinal tract and many other physiologic functions are also antagonistically influenced by nerves through the production of adrenalines or acetylcholine.

A few nerve filaments go directly to the *adrenal medulla*, which is not stimulated by any hormone but by nervous stimuli which cause it to produce adrenalines. These hormones of the adrenal medulla act just like the adrenaline-producing nerve-endings; in fact, the adrenalines made by the gland are chemically similar to those secreted by nerves. The main difference is that the former are secreted into the circulating blood and, therefore, cannot act selectively anywhere, whereas nerves can produce adrenalines in limited tissue regions without disturbing the rest of the body.

At the same time the other great pathway, the endocrine, is activated through the *hypothalamus*, which sends an order (CRF) to the *pituitary* for the secretion of ACTH. Here we are in well-known territory. As we have seen before, ACTH stimulates the *adrenal cortex* to produce predominantly anti-inflammatory glucocorticoids (GC). These, in turn, repress the thymicolymphatic organs and certain *white blood cells* (lymphoid cells, eosinophils) which are necessary both for immunity and for allergic hypersensitivity reactions. Consequently, such immune and allergic responses are inhibited by the cortisone-like hormones. In addition, the GCs provide glucose, a readily-available source of energy, for various defense phenomena. Indeed, because ACs act predominantly upon glucose metabolism, they are often referred to as glucocorticoids, or GCs. Similarly, the proinflammatory corticoids (PCs) which exert their major action upon mineral metabolism, are also called mineralocorticoids, or MCs (as explained on pages 121-122). These two sets of terms (AC-PC and GC-MC) are virtually interchangeable and we shall use only the terms GC and MC from here on.

The GCs also influence the *connective tissue* (represented at the bottom of the picture by a single, spindle-shaped connective tissue cell, surrounded by connective tissue fibers) to inhibit inflammation no matter how produced. (Inhibition is shown here by cross-hatched arrows.)

The *liver*, as we have said, is perhaps the most important chemical plant in the body. Substances brought to it by the blood can be stored here for later use or transformed into other substances to meet requirements. Under the influence of certain chemicals, e.g., catatoxic steroids, the liver can also inactivate poisonous substances, and even hormones. For instance, while the corticoids go through the circulation of the liver, a large proportion of them is destroyed or transformed into other types of corticoids. Consequently, the liver can change the corticoid content of the blood, even when the adrenals produce these hormones at a constant rate.

The GCs also act upon the *kidney* and—at least under certain circumstances (for instance, when MCs are also plentiful)—they can even produce permanent histologic changes in it. Curiously, as regards their known actions upon the kidney, the GCs and MCs are not antagonistic, although in most other respects they do counteract each other. Among the renal changes produced by the corticoids are certain inflammatory arterial lesions which tend to constrict the blood vessels of the kidney. A change then results, very similar to that which Goldblatt had produced mechanically by putting a constricting clamp around the main renal artery. The principal difference is that the hormones, through their chemical actions, put such constrictions upon many minute arteries inside the kidney. We may reasonably assume that such a vessel constriction, no matter how elicited, increases the production of *renal pressor substances* (RPS). These, in turn, constrict the blood vessels throughout the body and thereby increase the peripheral resistance against which the heart pumps. It is precisely this pumping against great resistance that then raises the blood pressure.

This effect is especially pronounced if, through renal failure, fluid retention increases vascular filling. As shown in our drawing, RPS (particularly angiotensin) act back upon the adrenal cortex to increase MC secretion. Thereby a vicious circle may

result, which eventually leads to severe hypertension.

In any event, the renal changes produced by
corticoids—like those elicited by a mechanical constriction of the main renal artery—can produce
inflammatory, arteritic, and arteriosclerosis-like
changes in the *blood vessels* throughout the body.
Since ACs generally inhibit inflammation, we were
not surprised to find that they also prevent this
arteritis, at least under certain conditions. I say
"under certain conditions" because—as the drawing clearly shows—their ability to do so depends
upon the proportion between their kidney-
mediated and direct actions. If the kidney is hyper-
sensitized by MCs a concurrent excess of ACs may
cause renal lesions, and, through these, a rise in
blood pressure so pronounced that the arteritis is
actually aggravated, although the direct effect of
ACs is to inhibit it (cross-hatched arrow).

Now, to the left side of the picture. We have
reason to suspect that the STH secreted by the
pituitary can act upon the adrenal cortex to stimulate MC production, but this is still uncertain
(hence the question mark). In any event, through
its direct effect upon connective tissue cells, STH
certainly helps MCs to stimulate inflammation. In
most other respects STH is also an ally of the MCs,
due to its direct (not adrenal-mediated) actions.
Curiously, it does not appear to act this way
directly on the kidney. STH imitates the kidney-
damaging action of MCs in intact animals, but not
after adrenalectomy. This is one of the main reasons why we also have to consider the possibility of
an indirect STH action which is relayed through

the adrenals. We still do not know with certainty what the normal stimulator of MC production might be. As we have said, these are called *mineralocorticoids*, because, apart from acting on inflammation, they also influence mineral metabolism. Probably certain minerals in the blood (sodium and potassium) can act back on the adrenal to regulate the production of mineralocorticoids in accordance with requirements.

Finally, the graph shows that during stress the production of TTH, or thyrotrophic hormone, is also important. As the name indicates, this pituitary substance stimulates the thyroid. The thyroid hormones are among the most potent accelerators of chemical reactions in the body: they stimulate metabolism as a whole.

This then is the general atlas of the stress reaction as far as I can make it out at present. It comprises the most important known pathways through which our bodily reactions are regulated during the G.A.S. But now we are tempted to ask, "Just what is adaptation?"

The events depicted here are nonspecifically produced. They occur when our muscles have to adapt themselves to hard work, when our nerves must be used to coordinate activities for an exacting new task, when our connective tissue has to fight an invasion by bacteria; they occur under any condition necessitating adjustment. Yet adaptation to different agents certainly poses different problems to different organs. What is the relationship between these distinct adaptive activities and the stereotyped G.A.S.?

chapter 8

The Nature of Adaptation

Adaptation is always a concentration of effort at the site of demand. Implications of the spatial concept of adaptation.

Webster's Dictionary defines biologic adaptation as:

> Modification of an animal or plant (or of its parts or organs) fitting it more perfectly for existence under the conditions of its environment.

In the foreword of *Stress* (Acta Inc., Montreal, 1950), I wrote, in a somewhat more philosophic vein, and without attempting a definition, that:

> Adaptability is probably the most distinctive characteristic of life.
>
> In maintaining the independence and individuality of natural units, none of the great forces of inanimate matter are as successful as that alertness and adaptability to change which we designate as life—and the loss of which is death. Indeed there is perhaps even a certain parallelism between the degree of aliveness and the extent of adaptability in every animal—in every man.

Webster's comments were dictated by pure intellect, whereas mine were perhaps more influenced by my emotional attachment to a phenomenon which I have learned to admire during our lifelong association. But both these descriptions merely try to say what adaptation is like, not what its mechanism consists of.

To find out more about how adaptation occurs, compare the way you perform a task before and after having done it often. You will notice first of all that almost invariably you have gradually learned to do it better as time went by. The degree of adaptation you can acquire varies from case to case, but there are very few things in life which you cannot learn to do at least a little better with practice.

What is the most characteristic difference between the way we do something before and after we have learned to do it well? To me, it is that at first we invariably put many more mechanisms to work on our problem than later. This is so with virtually any task I can think of.

If I have to lift a heavy weight with my right hand, at first I have to pull, not only with the muscles of my arm, but also with my shoulders. I may even have to bend my knees and then stretch them suddenly to give the weight enough momentum. If I lift the weight several times, my heart will have to beat more rapidly in order to get enough blood into the working muscles; my respiration will be accelerated so as to oxygenate this blood sufficiently for the liberation of enough energy for the chemical reactions which take place in the muscles. However, after adequate training, the whole response will become much more localized to the particular muscle-group which is really essential for the performance of the required work. The muscles of the right arm gradually become large and strong, so that the work may be adequately performed by them without having to strain any other part of the body.

Now, take an altogether different situation: suppose I suddenly have to resist great cold. At first I shiver, wave my arms, and run around, because only intense muscular activity can increase the internal heat production rapidly enough to maintain the normal body temperature under these conditions. But if I spend much time in the cold every day for months, gradually my thyroid will produce more of its metabolism-stimulating hormones to increase internal heat production even without excess muscular work. At the same time my skin vessels will learn to contract so as to minimize heat losses from the surface. Gradually I shall have learned to resist low surrounding temperatures by using only a few of the particular mechanisms which can best be trained to cope with this situation.

The same is true of mental reactions. When we are first confronted with a complex mathematical problem, we attempt to solve it in different ways. We check our results repeatedly to see whether, using various approaches, we will always arrive at the same conclusion. This process may be quite exhausting, but if similar problems come up again and again, eventually we learn always to use the simplest formula which will give us the correct answer with a minimum of effort.

The same gradual simplification by the concentration of effort occurs even in such fundamental tissue reactions as inflammation. When irritating germs penetrate through the skin into connective tissue, they first cause an acute inflammation with considerable swelling, reddening, and pain. The reaction will tend to spread and to involve a comparatively large adjacent region of tissue; indeed, there may even be fever and a general blood poisoning because the microbes cannot be adequately confined and many of them enter the blood. The characteristic adaptation in this case is the development of a strong connective tissue barricade which limits the damage to the minimum by restricting the microbes and their poisons to the point of invasion.

Inflammation can also be produced by excessive function in an organ not adapted to intensive activity. For example, excessive work can cause inflammation in and around muscles, due to local irritation by the metabolic products of activity. This is what causes the muscle stiffness and pain when we perform physical work to which our musculature is not adapted. Inflammation is a sort of nonspecific auxiliary mechanism of adaptation everywhere; it helps to close all doors and to clean up the debris in any overactive compartment of the body.

All this suggests that *an essential feature of adaptation is the confinement of stress to the smallest area capable of meeting the requirements of a situation.*

Now that we have found a general, that is nonspecific, feature of adaptation, we can explore the relationships between the specific problems facing the body and its fundamental reaction pattern (the G.A.S.) during adjustment to anything.

Adaptation Is Always a Concentration of Effort at the Site of Demand

In *Fig. 19* the heavy black line on top represents adrenocortical activity during the three stages of the G.A.S. As the alarm reaction develops, corticoid activity rises sharply; during the stage of resistance it falls to a level only slightly above normal; finally, in the stage of exhaustion, it rises again to, or even above, the maximum level reached during the alarm reaction. These are facts which can be

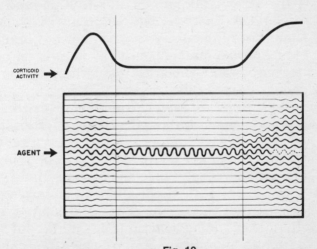

CORTICOID ACTIVITY →

AGENT →

Fig. 19

Alarm Reaction
Auxiliary mechanisms are mobilized to maintain life so that the reaction spreads to large territories. No organ system is as yet specially developed to cope with the task at hand.

Stage of Resistance
Adaptation is acquired due to optimum development of the most appropriate specific channel of defense. Spatial concentration of the reaction makes corticoid production unnecessary.

Stage of Exhaustion
The reaction spreads again due to wear and tear in the most appropriate channel. Corticoid production rises, but can maintain life only until auxiliary channels are exhausted.

verified by actual determinations of corticoids in the blood, or by studying the bodily changes which are characteristic of increased corticoid activity (for instance, disappearance of blood eosinophils, involution of the lymphatic organs, or the generalized loss of body weight). All these signs are pronounced only during the alarm reaction and the stage of exhaustion.

In the lower part of *Fig. 19* each of the horizontal lines symbolizes the activity of a particular organ or tissue. When an agent acts upon the point indicated by the arrow, it demands maximum adaptive work here, and overactivity will begin at this point. But without training, this one point cannot immediately respond adequately, so that activity must spread to the neighborhood to meet the situation. If the agent is a microbe, not only the cells in its immediate vicinity but even those at some distance from it will become inflamed. Indeed, often no extent of local reaction can prevent some microbes from entering the general circulation; then, to prevent catastrophe, the whole body will have to respond with fever and the production of serologic antibodies against the germs. This is accompanied by a well-marked alarm reaction: adrenal enlargement, lymphatic involution, and all the other characteristics of generalized stress.

But, as irritation at the original point of attack continues, gradually the local adaptive responses can develop sufficiently to cope with the situation. The growth of connective tissue around the microbes will be able to hold them in check, and adaptation becomes limited to the smallest area that must necessarily be involved. Since now only a small tissue territory is irritated, the number of alarm signals going forward to the hypothalamus and the pituitary diminishes; hence adrenocortical activity will no longer be maximally mobilized. The whole reaction has been concentrated to one point.

However, if irritation continues over a very long time, the directly-affected cells eventually break down from "fatigue," wear and tear, or, if you wish, from exhaustion of all local stores of *adaptation energy*. Then, during the stage of exhaustion, the reaction spreads again because wear and tear have led to the disintegration of the most appropriate channel of defense. Now the reaction must again extend to neighboring areas. In our example, the inflammatory barricade breaks down; the germs invade the surroundings; and eventually, through the blood, they spread to all parts of the body. At this time, when many tissues become involved and resume sending out their alarm signals, the pituitary and the adrenal cortex are again activated. But, after the auxiliary channels have also become exhausted, recovery is no longer possible and death follows.

In essence, the adaptive hormones of the pituitary-adrenal system appear to be most necessary for survival whenever large tissue regions are under stress. By their maintaining life during the alarm reaction, the body gains the time necessary for the development of specific local adaptive phenomena in the directly-affected region. During the subsequent stage of resistance, this region can cope with the task without the help of adaptive hormones. Finally, they help with the acquisition of adaptation by alternative channels and thereby prolong survival, but only until even the auxiliary mechanisms are worn out; after that there is no further line of defense and death must necessarily ensue.

Implications of the Spatial Concept of Adaptation

It is curious to note such a close interdependence between adaptation and the spatial extension of the body's response to an agent; but the realization of this relationship helped us to form a clearer picture of four hitherto quite inexplicable facts:

1. It had long been established empirically that the more extensive the tissue damage, the more does it stimulate the production of ACTH and of corticoids. This fact agrees with the hypothesis that, within a given time interval, each cell can only discharge a limited number of alarm signals; consequently, past a certain level, it is more the extent than the intensity of tissue damage that stimulates ACTH and corticoid production.

2. It had also been shown that an adrenalectomized individual tolerates very intense injury or actual death of a few cells much better than mild injury, or even malfunction of many cells. This explains why, for the purpose of self-preservation during stress, the body must produce corticoids in proportion to the anatomic extent of the involved region.

3. The standard response to tissue injury anywhere in the body is inflammation. Damage or uncustomary function, no matter how produced, can cause inflammation in any part of the body.

Thus inflammation is a specific reaction pattern of nonspecific causation, that is, a manifestation of local stress wherever it occurs. It is of fundamental biologic significance, therefore, that whenever stress spreads to large portions of the body, it automatically evokes a general hormonal stress reaction which tends to diminish excessive inflammation. When only limited territories are attacked, inflammation is useful; it prevents the spread of the causative agent (for example, of germs or allergens). On the other hand, when disease has already become generalized anyway, it is in the best interest of the body not to put up defensive inflammatory barricades. This is so because: (1) the more the damage has spread, the less can be accomplished by barricades; (2) inflamed organs do not function well; and (3) inflamed tissue produces toxic substances (enzymes, tissue decomposition products) which may endanger life when the reaction is very extensive. It is most fortunate therefore that our body possesses a fire alarm system which automatically puts out the flame of inflammation as soon as its spread is too extensive and actually threatens life.

4. Finally, we have learned (in Book I) that stress (bloodletting, shock therapies, and so forth) can have a therapeutic value, especially in certain chronic diseases. We have vaguely hinted that it looks as though, during chronic exposure to certain irritants, our adaptive mechanisms would "get into a groove," and that stress would help us to snap out of it. Our last diagram attempts to outline a more precise picture of what actually happens in such cases. Apparently, sometimes when the body uses

one organ system preferentially to cope with a threatening situation, disease can result, either from the disproportionate, excessive development of this particular system or from its eventual breakdown due to wear and tear. Here it is desirable to activate possible collateral channels, thereby giving the preferential one a rest.

In this discussion on the nature of adaptation— as in all our previous considerations—we have tried to point out clearly what is theory and what is fact. It is important not to confuse the two. Yet it is not enough to recognize facts; we must also try to formulate ideas about the way the body behaves in health and disease. Only such theoretic concepts can guide us logically to new facts.

I have attempted to define the essence and to dissect the mechanism of successful adaptation. But no biologic reaction is always perfect; the stress response is no exception. When it fails to cope adequately with a potential disease-producing situation, the body develops what I have called *diseases of adaptation*. We shall now consider how these arise and how they can be prevented.

BOOK III

The Diseases of Adaptation

Summary

First we shall consider the signs of danger, the warnings by which either the physician or you yourself can monitor your stress status. Then we shall turn to the actual diseases of adaptation.

There is an element of adaptation in every disease; but, in some maladies, the direct effects of the disease producers, in others the body's own defensive adaptive reactions, are more prominent. Only in the latter case do we commonly speak of *diseases of adaptation*. Usually adaptation consists of a balanced blend of defense and submission. Some diseases are due to an excess of defensive, others to an overabundance of submissive, bodily reactions.

It has been possible to simulate a number of renal and cardiovascular diseases in animals by giving them an excess of DOC. This called attention to the possible *role of excessive or insufficient corticoid production in the development of various diseases* which had never been thought to be related to hormones.

The rest of this section is devoted to a critical discussion of maladaptation as a factor in: *high blood pressure, diseases of the heart and of the blood vessels, diseases of the kidney, eclampsia, rheumatic and rheumatoid arthritis, inflammatory diseases of the skin and eyes, infec-*

tions, allergic and hypersensitivity diseases, nervous and mental diseases, sexual derangements, digestive diseases, metabolic diseases, cancer, and diseases of resistance in general.

In discussing these maladies I shall briefly describe the design of the laboratory experiments which helped me to appraise the maladaptation factor in each case. This will permit the correlation of the experimental diseases produced in animals with the corresponding clinical conditions as they occur in man, so that the reader may see for himself *how the laboratory analysis of a malady can guide the physician in his efforts to treat it.* This will act as a preparation for Book V where we shall try to show that through a better understanding of the underlying mechanisms we can also learn to face stress more efficiently in our daily life. Only by intelligent adjustment of our conduct to the biologic rules is it possible to achieve full enjoyment of eustress without distress.

chapter 9

The Signs of Danger

Medical symptoms.   Self-observable signs.

How can a person know that he is experiencing
undue stress before he suffers evident damage,
with obvious diseases of adaptation such as a nervous breakdown, peptic ulcers, or a heart attack? A
certain amount of stress is needed to tune you up
for action and keep you on your toes. This is especially true of eustress, which is enjoyable in itself
and actually gives purpose to life. On the other
hand, we must learn the limits of our endurance
before we exceed them dangerously.

As we have so often said, certain signs and reactions are common to stress as such, be it healthy or
unhealthy. All these are also, therefore, characteristic of distress which must be avoided as much as
possible.

Medical Symptoms

Among the most generally used and reliable measures of stress are the blood levels of *adrenalines*,
corticoids, ACTH and a drop in *blood eosinophils*.
The latter is a consequence of increased GC secretion and can easily be determined, even by the
general practitioner in the consulting room. *CRF*,
the chemical factor primarily responsible for the

discharge of ACTH and subsequently of adrenal corticoids, rapidly disappears from the blood. Hence, its measurement is extremely difficult and uncertain.

On the other hand, the blood *creatine/creatinine* ratio, the elevation in certain blood lipid substances, such as *cholesterol* and *free fatty acids*, are comparatively simple to estimate, although they do require a chemical laboratory. Rises in *STH*, *glucagon*, *insulin* and *prolactin* are not only more difficult to determine, but also less reliable indicators of stress reactions in man.

The measurement of the electrical activity of the brain by the *electroencephalogram (EEG)* gives useful indications, but also requires special machinery.

A rise in *blood pressure* can be determined even without medical training, if you learn the use of a relatively simple apparatus. Nowadays, in many public places (such as supermarkets and department stores) you can have this tested as a courtesy service. However, unless hypertension is constant and severe, it has little diagnostic significance since daily blood pressure variations can depend merely upon minor fluctuations associated with normal responses to ordinary life events.

The electrical conductivity of the skin known as *galvanic skin resistance (GSR)* is primarily an indicator of sweat secretion, but special instruments can detect its variations during stress, even if it is not of sufficient intensity to result in evident sweat droplet formation.

It is useful to know that these are fairly reliable

indicators of any kind of stress (both eustress and distress), but they can be accurately determined and interpreted only by experts.

Self-observable Signs

On the other hand, there are much more immediately useful signs of stress which the average person can follow throughout his working day. For example a man quietly sitting in his living room was eating his dinner while watching TV. Suddenly the newscaster announces the crash of a plane on its way from Santiago to Buenos Aires. There were no survivors. The passenger list included the name of J. Browne. Now the man knew that his father, John Browne, intended to travel on the same route at about this time, and of course he believed him dead. However, a few hours later, the name was spelled out as Joseph Brown. Our TV watcher felt just as overjoyed to learn that the victim was not his father, as he had felt shocked by sorrow at first. Yet, in both instances he immediately stopped eating, got up from the chair and walked about the room in agitation (though he did not want to go anywhere); his heartbeat was accelerated, his blood pressure rose and he began to perspire. These manifestations—inability to eat or keep still, accelerated pulse rate, increased blood pressure (which you can even feel by the thumping of your heart) and sweat secretion—are all characteristic both of eustress and of distress, as our example shows. Actually, to a large extent, all these easily-detectable manifestations of stress are the results of deranged hormone secretion or nervous activity. These mechanisms cannot be checked by all of us, but the end results are manifest and they suffice.

There are a number of other indexes of stress, particularly of the more dangerous distress, which are not such immediately evident, constant consequences of an acute impact as those in our typical example, but which we could be well advised to monitor throughout our lifetime. Depending upon our conditioning, we all respond differently to general demands. But on the whole, I think that each of us tends to respond particularly with one set of signs, caused by the malfunction of whatever happens to be the most vulnerable part in our machinery, and when they appear, it's time to stop or change your activity—that is, find a diversion.

1. General *irritability, hyperexcitation, or depression*. This is associated with unusual aggressiveness or passive indolence, depending upon our constitution. It often manifests itself under what is sometimes called "the prima donna complex," personality traits associated with singers and actors, but also with scientists, politicians, military commanders, highly successful businessmen, and other "heroes" who are virtually always the center of attention. It is certainly objectionable to capitalize unduly on being extraordinary in any respect. As far as possible one should try to master the offensive aspects of the stress of being prominent and always "in the public eye," but on the other hand, no one can be expected to accomplish unusual things without being unusual.

2. *Pounding of the heart,* an indicator of high blood pressure (often due to stress).

3. *Dryness of the throat and mouth.*

4. *Impulsive behavior, emotional instability.*

5. *The overpowering urge to cry or run and hide.*

6. *Inability to concentrate,* flight of thoughts and general disorientation.

7. *Feelings of unreality, weakness, or dizziness.*

8. Predilection to become *fatigued,* and loss of the "joie de vivre."

9. *"Floating anxiety,"* that is to say, we are afraid although we do not know exactly what we are afraid of.

10. Emotional *tension and alertness,* feeling of being "keyed up."

11. *Trembling, nervous ticks.*

12. *Tendency to be easily startled* by small sounds, etc.

13. *High-pitched, nervous laughter.*

14. *Stuttering and other speech difficulties* which are frequently stress-induced.

15. *Bruxism,* or grinding of the teeth.

16. *Insomnia,* which is usually a consequence of being "keyed up."

17. *Hypermotility.* This is technically called "hyperkinesia," an increased tendency to move about without any reason, an inability to just take a physically relaxed attitude, sitting quietly in a chair or lying on a sofa.

18. *Sweating.* This becomes evident only under considerable stress by inspection of the skin, but is readily detectable by the GSR, as explained previously.

19. *The frequent need to urinate.*

20. *Diarrhea, indigestion, queasiness in the stomach, and sometimes even vomiting.* All signs of disturbed gastrointestinal function which eventually may lead to such severe diseases of adaptation as peptic ulcers, ulcerative colitis, the "irritable colon," with which we shall deal later.

21. *Migraine headaches.*

22. *Premenstrual tension or missed menstrual cycles,* both of which are frequently indicators of severe stress in women.

23. *Pain in the neck or lower back.* In conversational English, the expression "this is nauseating," "he gives me ulcers," "this business is an awful headache," or "he gives me a pain in the neck" are not merely colorful expressions, but based on actual experience. For example, the pain in the neck or back is usually due to increases in muscular tension that can be objectively measured by physicians with the electromyogram (EMG).

24. *Loss of or excessive appetite.* This shows itself soon in alterations of body weight, namely excessive leanness or obesity. Some people lose their appetite during stress because of gastrointestinal malfunction, whereas others eat excessively, as a kind of diversion, to deviate their attention from the stressor situation. Besides, a well-filled stomach and intestine shift a great deal of blood to the abdomen, resulting in a relative decrease in brain circulation which tranquilizes by decreasing mental alertness.

25. *Increased smoking.*

26. *Increased use of legally prescribed drugs,* such as tranquilizers or amphetamines.

27. *Alcohol and drug addiction.* Like the phe-

nomenon of overeating, increased and excessive
alcohol consumption or the use of various psychotropic drugs is a common manifestation of exposure to stressors beyond our natural endurance.
Here again, we are actually dealing with flight
reactions, known as diversion or deviation, to
which we resort presumably because they help us
to forget the cause of our distress and tend to
temporarily replace it by the eustress of psychic
elation, or at least tranquilization.

    28. *Nightmares.*

    29. *Neurotic behavior.*

    30. *Psychoses.*

    31. *Accident proneness.* Under great stress
(eustress or distress) we are more likely to have
accidents at work or while driving a car. This is also
a very important reason why pilots and air traffic
controllers must be carefully checked for their
stress status.

Many questionnaires have been devised in order
to help a person to appraise his own stress situation. There are also various mechanical instruments—known as "stress meters" or "stress poly-
graphs"—which measure even such characteristics
as cannot be directly appraised by the layman; however they can register only a few indicators which
are usually, but not always, characteristic of stress.
Of course, the more signs and symptoms are measured, the more reliable the general picture becomes; yet even the best of these procedures avoid
the crucial difference between eustress and distress. Moreover, beyond this distinction there lies
a still more significant fact which not only psychologists have realized: it is our ability to cope with

the demands made by the events in our lives, not the quality or intensity of the events, that counts. And this brings us back to our key phrase, namely, that what matters is not so much what happens to us, but the way we take it.

chapter 10

Diseases of the Kidney, the Heart, and the Blood Vessels

The chickens: disease caused by corticoids.
Pituitary hormones can produce renal and
cardiovascular diseases.   The role of the
adrenals in the spontaneous renal and
cardiovascular diseases of man.   Metacorticoid
hypertension.   Eclampsia.   The sudden heart
attack.

Some diseases have specific causes, the direct actions of certain particular, disease-producing agents, such as microbes, poisons, or physical injuries. Many more diseases are not caused by any one thing in particular; they result from the body's own response to some unusual situation.

It is not always immediately obvious that, in the final analysis, our diseases are so often due to our own responses. For instance, if a man is hit over the head with the club of a policeman and suffers permanent brain damage from the injury, it is obvious that his disease was caused by the club. But, if you come to think of it, the blow was not the real first cause; it was but one link in the sequence of a chain reaction that eventually led to brain

injury. What actually happened may have been
that the officer asked the man not to loiter, whereupon the latter reacted by violently insulting and
assailing the policeman, who in turn hit him over
the head with the club. So, in fact, the principal,
immediate cause of the man's injury was his own
unwarranted, aggressive behavior.

The parts of the body work in a similar way. We
have seen, for instance, that if a dirty splinter
of wood gets under your skin, the tissues around it
swell up and become inflamed. You develop a boil or
an abscess. This is a useful, healthy response,
because the tissues forming the wall of this boil
represent a barricade which prevents any further
spread throughout the body of microbes or poisons
that may have been introduced with the splinter.
But sometimes the body's reactions are excessive
and quite out of proportion to the fundamentally
innocuous irritation to which it was exposed. Here,
an excessive response, say, in the shape of inflammation, may actually be the main cause of what we
experience as disease. Since we had learned that
inflammation, in turn, is regulated by adaptive
hormones, the question arose whether excessive or
deficient hormonal responses to injuries might
play a part in the development of various diseases.
Could, for instance, the excessive production of a
proinflammatory hormone, in response to some
mild local irritation, result in the production of a
disproportionately intensive inflammation, which
hurts more than it helps? Could such an adaptive
endocrine response become so intense that the
resulting hormone excess would damage organs in
distant parts of the body, far from the original site

of injury, in parts which could not have been affected by any direct action of the external disease-producing agent?

We have already learned to distinguish between direct and indirect pathogens (page 83); the latter were precisely defined as those in which normally useful bodily responses are excessive or perverse, so that mechanisms which have evolved to create resistance actually become the decisive ingredients of a disease. In other words, these maladies are actually caused by maladaptation itself; they are "diseases of adaptation."

The Chickens: Disease Caused by Corticoids

Frankly, I cannot remember just why I suddenly decided to work with newly-hatched chicks, when the problem of the diseases of adaptation arose in 1940. For me it was certainly an unusual thing to do: we did not keep any chickens in the lab; I had never experimented with them before; and I knew nothing about how to raise them. But the oddest thing about it is that I had no conceivable reason for selecting chicks in preference to any of the usual laboratory animals, such as mice, rats, guinea pigs, or rabbits. Yet the choice was certainly lucky. It turned out that the next thing I wanted to do had to be done on newly-hatched chicks; it could have been done on none of our usual experimental animals, and not even on older fowl.

The problem we faced may be stated like this: if the adrenal must produce an excess of corticoids to maintain life during stress, it is quite probable that the resulting hormone excess in itself may have dangerous consequences. It is a well-known fact that flooding the body with any hormone produces disease. When the thyroid secretes too much of its hormones, metabolism is unduly accelerated. When the pituitary manufactures huge amounts of STH, the result is gigantism. When the adrenal medulla discharges an excess of its adrenalines, the pulse quickens and the blood pressure rises dangerously. It was quite natural to ask, therefore, "What would happen if the adrenal secreted an excess of corticoids?" It obviously does so during stress. But this question could not be answered by just examining a patient in stress; in him it would be impossible to distinguish between the effects of the corticoids and those of stress itself.

There is a curious disease called the *adrenogenital syndrome,* which had been traced long ago to an overactivity of the adrenal cortex. In this malady there is an excessive, and often premature, development of the sex organs, but these morbid changes are due to overproduction of adrenocortical sex hormones. Typical corticoids, such as MCs and GCs, could not be responsible for this disease because they do not affect sex. We had to discover the syndrome caused by flooding the body with these adrenal hormones.

If an electric heater maintains the temperature of a room, we can compensate for excessive cold by using more current. But this is possible only within certain limits. As more and more current is used, there comes a point when the wires burn out; then the whole heating mechanism breaks down, and, significantly, its failure is the direct result of efficient heat regulation. This kind of breakdown can occur in most compensatory mechanisms. It seemed unlikely that, in the adjustment to stress, the secretion of corticoids would be an exception.

Naturally, the thing to do was to give enormous amounts of corticoids to normal experimental animals and just see what happened. But, in 1941 when we reached this point in our work, only one corticoid, DOC (one of the MC hormones), was available in adequate amounts for such experiments, and even it was very scarce and expensive. Besides, most of the common experimental animals are singularly resistant to DOC. If one just injects this hormone into the usual laboratory animals nothing obvious happens; and, of course, at that time nobody knew how to sensitize or condition the body for this substance. Curiously, even now, after some thirty-five years of research, I have found no animal which would be more sensitive to DOC (without special conditioning) than the newly-hatched chick. This is why it was fortunate that, by sheer accident, I happened to use young chicks for my first experiments.

Since the demonstration of the role played by corticoids in the causation of renal disease has opened interesting new avenues to medical research, it may be amusing to learn how the first relevant experiments were actually carried out in practice.

To start with, I bought 24 three-day-old, white Leghorn chicks. After consultation with people who knew something about how to raise pullets, Mr. Nielsen—whom I have already introduced to you (page 43)—constructed a large wooden box for them in an attic under the roof. He equipped this

box with electric bulbs because we had learned
that young chicks cannot maintain their body temperature unless they are kept warm. Soon we also
found out, much to our dismay, that they would not
eat the usual rat food, so we got them a special diet,
commercially prepared (and sold under the self-
explanatory name of Chick-Startina) to start
chicks off in life. I mention these details only
because it still puzzles me just why I went to all
this trouble when there was nothing to indicate
that young chicks were the only kind of animals in
which our experiment would work.

When we were satisfied that our birds were well
taken care of, we divided them into two groups:
twelve received daily injections of DOC, and the
other twelve acted as untreated controls. During
the first ten days I could see no difference between
the two groups. Then all the DOC-treated chicks
began to drink much more water than the controls,
and gradually they developed a kind of dropsy.
Their bodies became enormously swollen with
fluid accumulations under the skin and they began
to breathe with difficulty, gasping for air, just like
certain cardiac patients.

On the twentieth day, we killed both the DOC-
treated and the control pullets to examine their
internal organs. Upon dissection it was striking
that, under the influence of the hormone, large
amounts of fluid had also accumulated in their
body cavities, and especially within the sac that
surrounds the heart (the pericardium). The heart
itself was much enlarged and the walls of the blood
vessels had become thick and rigid; they looked

very much like those of patients suffering from high blood pressure.

The most pronounced changes occurred in the kidneys, which were swollen and had an irregular, discolored surface. Upon histologic examination, they showed lesions which had been described in man more than a hundred years earlier. In 1827 at Guy's Hospital in London, Richard Bright discovered such renal changes in patients with enlargement of the heart and dropsy. Ever since then the condition has been known to physicians as *Bright's disease.* In this malady, the heart becomes big and strong, presumably because it must pump the blood under high pressure to get it through the narrow and hardened arteries.

Bright had noticed another important sign which he considered characteristic of this disease: the presence of protein in the urine. In chicks the urine and the intestinal contents are eliminated together through one opening, so that even normally their excretions are rich in proteinacious matter which comes from the gut. But, on histologic sectioning, it could be clearly seen that in our DOC-treated pullets, the fine renal tubules, which carry the urine within the kidney, were also filled with protein precipitates. This was not so in the untreated chicks.

It is difficult to determine the blood pressure in birds accurately, but in several instances we succeeded in showing that under the influence of DOC it rose to very high levels.

Clearly, here we had reproduced all the six major features of Bright's disease in an experimental ani-

mal: (1) characteristic structural changes in the
kidneys; (2) enlargement of the heart muscle; (3)
thickening and hardening of the arteries; (4) high
blood pressure; (5) generalized dropsy; and (6) elimination of protein into the urine.

Now, before going further, we shall have to say
more about kidney diseases. In man there are
three common types: nephrosis, nephritis, and
nephrosclerosis. Some physicians regard these as
essentially distinct maladies, but this is improba-
ble because there are many transitions between
them; presumably they are all closely interrelated.
Nephritis usually develops into nephrosclerosis as
time goes by; this corresponds to Bright's disease.
The former is a simple inflammation; the latter is a
kind of scar formation due to the healing of chronic
renal inflammation. Nephrosis is considered to be a
degenerative disease. But it is not always possible
to distinguish the inflammatory from the degenerative changes, and nephrosis may develop into
nephritis; hence there are no sharp borderlines
between these diseases. In any event, the derangement produced by DOC in our chicks exhibited elements of all three renal diseases, although in its
final stages, it corresponded most closely to nephrosclerosis. I must mention these details to avoid a
distortion of my description by oversimplification;
but actually the important point in this experiment
was the demonstration that an equivalent of clinical
kidney disease can be produced by overdosage with a
corticoid hormone.

I published these first observations on the hormonal production of renal disease during 1942 in
the *Canadian Medical Association Journal,* con-

cluding my article with the sentence: *"Hence it is perhaps not too far-fetched to suspect adrenocortical involvement as a causative agent in nephrosclerotic hypertension."*

This paper started a great controversy in medical literature. Hypertensive kidney disease is one of the most common fatal maladies of man; and since nothing was known about its cause, naturally any clue had to be carefully analyzed. Physicians were particularly reluctant to accept my view, because, in the whole of endocrinology, there was no precedent of any such inflammatory or degenerative disease caused by hormones. At that time the textbooks on hormones were virtually limited to the discussion of the primary diseases of the endocrines, i.e., maladies which originate within a hormone-secreting gland. In principle, we distinguish two types of such diseases: those caused by the destruction of an endocrine gland (for instance, by cancer or a localized atrophy), and those which result from a primary overgrowth of an endocrine gland (for instance, hypertrophy or tumor formation). These are the derangements which cause such typical endocrine conditions as diabetes, gigantism, sexual anomalies, and hyperthyroid goiters. The production of nephrosclerosis by DOC seemed to fall into an altogether different category. No wonder the idea of "adrenocortical participation in nephrosclerotic hypertension" was received with great skepticism.

The first question which now arose was whether an experimental Bright's disease could be produced by corticoids only in chicks or also in mammals. The structure of the kidney is similar in man and in other mammals, but in birds it is quite different. Naturally we wanted to repeat our experiments on mammals. In this we failed. When DOC was injected into rats, guinea pigs, dogs, or cats, no obvious changes were noted in the kidneys or the heart or the blood vessels. It seemed for a while as though we had just accidentally stumbled upon some peculiar hypersensitivity for corticoids, characteristic only of newly-hatched chicks: a mere laboratory curiosity which could have no bearing upon the causation of human diseases.

It was at this time that the idea of some special "conditioning" for corticoids began to take shape. Could we identify the factor which renders chicks particularly sensitive to an excess of corticoids? Would this same factor participate significantly in the development of corticoid overdosage diseases in man?

Medical experience had shown long ago that patients suffering from Bright's disease cannot stand much salt. Perhaps the kidney of the baby chick resembles the diseased human kidney in having a low salt tolerance. Would ordinary kitchen salt (sodium chloride) be the factor we were looking for? If we could prove that with salt, chicks can be further sensitized to the kidney-damaging action of DOC, this would be yet another important fact suggesting a relationship between the experimental and the clinical forms of Bright's disease. Besides, using sodium chloride as a sensitizing procedure, it might even become possible to show—at least under certain conditions—that corticoids can produce renal and cardiovascular disease in mammals.

With this in mind, we proceeded to give newly-hatched chicks dilute solutions of sodium chloride as a drinking fluid; half of them, the controls, received no hormone treatment; the other half were given injections of DOC. It turned out that surprisingly small doses of DOC can produce Bright's disease in birds kept on dilute sodium chloride solutions which caused no damage in themselves.

We had proved that the experimental DOC disease also resembled clinical Bright's disease in that both were aggravated by salt supplements.

(An interesting by-product of this work grew out of the observation that, on more concentrated solutions of sodium chloride, baby chicks develop a kind of Bright's disease, even without any hormone treatment. This malady is well-known to farmers and veterinarians as a "spontaneous" disease of pullets. It had been given many names—such as *avian Bright's disease*, *pullet disease* or *blue comb disease*—but nothing definite was known about its cause. Usually it occurs in epidemics, so that most people believed it to be contagious. Our observations on its causation by salt were subsequently confirmed by veterinarians in various countries. It had been shown that avian Bright's disease tends to occur whenever the food of pullets contains too much sodium. This would explain the epidemic character of the malady, although salt is probably not the sole causative factor. Now that the importance of sodium chloride has been clarified, it

has often been possible to get rid of the condition
in hatcheries by simply reducing the salt content of
the food and water.)

What we had learned so far suggested that perhaps DOC could produce renal damage even in
mammals if they were kept on a high sodium diet.
This approach proved to be fruitful. In rats forced
to drink 1 per cent sodium chloride instead of
water, DOC did produce nephrosclerosis and hypertension. Yet very large doses of hormone had to be
injected for many weeks, and even so the changes
were rather mild.

We then argued that the immature pullet may
not have a sufficient safety margin of renal function
to adjust itself well to overdosage with salt and
corticoids. If so, perhaps we could further augment
the DOC sensitivity even in mammals by simply
taking out one of their kidneys and throwing the
entire load on the other.

In the next experimental series we removed the
right kidney in a group of rats which were then
forced to drink 1 per cent sodium chloride while
receiving DOC. Here the hormone produced
extremely marked and rapidly fatal nephrosis and
nephrosclerosis-like changes in the kidney,
enlargement of the heart, hardening and inflammation (arteritis) of the blood vessels, as well as a
pronounced rise in blood pressure. Most of these
rats died from coronary lesions and cardiac
infarcts, or brain hemorrhages ("strokes") similar
to those common in hypertensive patients.

Thus, we finally succeeded in developing an
experimental technique of conditioning which consistently permitted the production, by a corticoid

hormone, of Bright's disease in a mammalian species.

This was an important turning point in the analysis of these diseases. Within the next few months
it could be shown that, after suitable conditioning
(removal of one kidney and administration of salt
supplements), DOC also produces similar renal and
cardiovascular changes in other mammals, such as
the mouse, guinea pig, cat, dog, and even in the
monkey, the closest relative of man among the
laboratory animals *(Fig. 20)*.

These observations left no room for doubt; it was
quite clear now that, at least under certain circumstances, corticoids could produce inflammatory or
degenerative diseases even in mammals, the class
of animals to which man himself belongs.

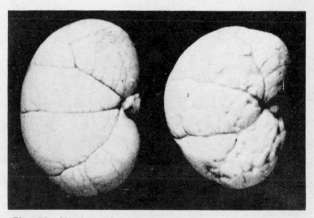

Fig. 20 Nephrosclerosis produced by DOC in a cat.
Compare the smooth surface, marked only by the normal
blood vessels, in the kidney of the untreated control cat
(left), with the granular, shrivelled-up surface of the kidney in the DOC-treated animal. *(After H. Selye, "Textbook
of Endocrinology," courtesy of Acta, Inc., Montreal.)*

Pituitary Hormones Can Produce Renal and Cardiovascular Diseases

As I have explained before, corticoids are made by the adrenals under the influence of certain pituitary hormones. It was reasonable to suppose, therefore, that, through their effect upon the adrenals, pituitary extracts would act like DOC. But, contrary to expectations, large amounts of ACTH (the most powerful adrenal-stimulating pituitary hormone) did not do this. Even rats specially sensitized, by removal of one kidney and administration of salt supplements, failed to develop renal or cardiovascular changes comparable to those we had produced with DOC. Apparently, ACTH stimulates the adrenals to produce large amounts of GCs (COL type), but not of MCs (DOC type).

On the other hand, pituitary extracts rich in STH did reproduce (in suitably sensitized rats) a syndrome virtually identical with that seen after DOC treatment. Interestingly, these same extracts were quite ineffective in this respect after adrenalectomy. This finding seems to agree with the view that STH acts upon the kidney and the cardiovascular system by stimulating the production, or by increasing the activity, of DOC-like hormones in adrenal tissue. We are still not certain that this explanation is correct: up to now it has been impossible to show beyond doubt, by chemical means, that the DOC content of the blood increases after administration of STH.

But no matter what the mechanism of the STH action, one thing is certain: STH can damage the kidney and the cardiovascular system only in the presence of the adrenals.

As we have explained (page 155) and illustrated, angiotensin (an RPS) has been found to be an active stimulator of aldosterone secretion, and the latter represents an even more potent MC than DOC. Perhaps STH may stimulate the production or activity of renin by the kidney, but only in the presence of adrenal tissue. All these are questions yet to be explored if we are to disentangle the complex mechanism of what I have called "mineralocorticoid hypertension." But in order to solve such questions, they must first be formulated.

To summarize the essence of what we have learned from this particular experimental series, we may say that: (1) the pituitary produces substances which can lead to renal and cardiovascular disease; (2) STH (or some substance which is inseparable from it) is responsible for this effect; and (3) the production of renal and cardiovascular disease by STH preparations depends upon the presence of living adrenal tissue in the body.

The Role of the Adrenals in the Spontaneous Renal and Cardiovascular Diseases of Man

All this still did not really prove that corticoids (or STH) actually do play a part in the causation of human diseases resembling those imitated by DOC in animals. Besides, our experimentation was not in accordance with an almost routine time-honored pattern for this kind of study; usually, when we want to establish the cause of a disease, we proceed quite differently. If we suspect that some agent (a microbe, poison, or hormone) is the cause of a disease, it must be shown that: (1) when the disease is present the agent is demonstrable in the body; (2)

when the agent disappears, the disease disappears.
Only after establishing all this has it been possible,
in some cases, to furnish the ultimate proof by
actually reproducing the disease in experimental
animals through the administration of the causative agent.

For instance, let us take the case of tuberculosis.
This disease had first vaguely been ascribed to a
variety of causes: bad food, hereditary predisposition, overwork, life in crowded quarters, and so
forth. In fact many physicians doubted that tuberculosis always had the same cause. Then, when
suspicion fell upon a certain germ as the possible
specific cause of tuberculosis, research to prove
this theory progressed in accordance with the classic pattern. First, it was shown that the *tubercle
bacillus* is present in all patients who suffer from
tuberculosis; indeed, it is usually most plentiful in
those parts which are most severely affected. Second, it was demonstrated that when the bacilli
disappear the disease also disappears. Only after
all this did bacteriologists finally succeed in reproducing the disease at will, by injecting guinea pigs
with tubercle bacilli. The success of this last crucial
experiment was then generally accepted as irrefut-
able proof of the bacterial theory.

In our studies on Bright's disease, we happened
to start with this final step; we first reproduced a
simile of the disease with DOC in animals and then
tried to progress in reverse. As I shall explain presently, the next thing to be shown was that removal
of the causative agent (the adrenal) leads to
improvement. What is usually the first indication
of such a cause-and-effect relationship—namely,
that an excess of the suspected (DOC-like) agent is

present in the body during the disease—was the last point to be attacked in this study. Before we had accidentally produced the malady in animals with DOC, there was no reason to suspect that corticoids were particularly plentiful in patients who suffer from similar diseases; nor was it known whether withdrawal of DOC-like hormones (by adrenalectomy) would be of curative value here.

Of course, it may seem that once you have caused a disease with a certain agent you have proved beyond doubt that the disease is caused by that agent. This type of argument can be misleading. It was quite conceivable, for instance, that the spontaneous renal and cardiovascular diseases of man have nothing to do with corticoids, even if DOC reproduces similar maladies in animals. After all, several roads may lead to the same destination: exercise quickens the heart rate, but, of course, this does not mean that the rapid pulse of a bedridden, feverish patient is due to excessive exercise. Such an analogy is not quite appropriate, however, because many factors can quicken the pulse, whereas the particular renal and cardiovascular diseases which we had produced with DOC are rather specific.

In any event, as we shall see, much more evidence has come forth in support of our view that cortical hormones do play a part in the development of certain renal and cardiovascular diseases of man. In discussing these clinical data we must realize that observations on human beings can seldom be made with the precision of animal experiments. The physician's first concern is to help his patient; the acquisition of knowledge about disease is a secondary consideration. This tends to inter-

fere with the interpretation of findings. If we want
to know whether the adrenals are indispensable for
a biologic reaction in animals, we can just remove
these glands—changing nothing else—and see
whether or not the response still occurs. In man
this is, of course, not possible. If the biologic reaction is a disease and we are convinced that adrenalectomy would be the best cure, we can remove the
adrenals; but the patient must also receive every
other treatment that may benefit him, even if this
obscures the interpretation of the results.

Despite these inherent limitations of clinical
investigation, a great deal of evidence has now
accumulated in support of the view that the adrenals participate in the development of various
renal and cardiovascular diseases. This evidence is
provided by two types of techniques: surgical and
chemical. The surgeon can remove the source of
the offending hormones (by adrenalectomy or
hypophysectomy) and the chemist can demonstrate an excess of them in the blood and urine of
patients with kidney or heart disease.

To prove this it was necessary to remove the
adrenals, which are the source of DOC-like material. Adrenalectomy is a very serious operation.
For one thing, a patient who has no adrenals must
take pills or injections of corticoids for the rest of
his life. If he runs out of corticoids—even if only for
a few days—he dies. As long as adequate corticoid
treatment is available, such patients may live an
essentially normal and happy life; but it is, of
course, very disturbing to be utterly dependent on
a drug. There is always the possibility that, on
some trip, at some time, corticoids may become
quite unavailable; and, for the adrenalectomized

patient, that spells death. Yet his situation is not really so much worse than that of a severe diabetic who is equally dependent on insulin. Indeed, if you come to think of it, all of us constantly require food, water, and air, but fortunately very few people are ever stranded in places where any of these vital necessities are unavailable for dangerously long periods.

Besides, often you have no choice. In patients with severe malignant hypertension there comes a point when, under ordinary conditions, death becomes inevitable because no established method of treatment is of any avail. The same is true of certain types of rapidly-progressing arterial inflammation. The physician who, in the absence of any precedent, first recommends a hazardous operation in such cases must have a great deal of vision and courage. Yet such decisions must be made whenever medicine attempts to develop a drastic new cure for a dangerous ailment.

Ephraim McDowell made a momentous decision of this kind on December 13, 1809, when he undertook to remove the ovaries of a woman at his private home in Danville, Kentucky. The patient suffered from an ovarian tumor which weighed fifteen pounds; if allowed to go on growing it would undoubtedly have killed her. Yet up to that time no such growth had ever been removed. Perhaps the operation just could not be done. The townspeople were horrified when they learned that their doctor wanted to open a live woman's abdomen and cut out her ovaries. They marched on McDowell's house, ready to hang him, thinking that he must be dangerously insane or criminally irresponsible. But finally mob violence was averted and, against all expectations, the operation succeeded; indeed, the patient lived to be eighty years old, and McDowell had the satisfaction of having initiated an entirely new era in surgery.

The basic idea of removing ovarian tumors was a sound one; still, it was largely a matter of chance that this particular patient survived. Anesthesia had not yet been discovered; nothing was known about the need for sterility of instruments; and the Kentucky pioneer's surgical technique was hair-raisingly crude. But the point is that nothing but this operation could have saved that woman in 1809, and she was saved.

The situation was not nearly as bad when the first total adrenalectomies and hypophysectomies were performed for hypertensive disease. By that time such operations had already been carried out for incurable cancer, yet it took considerable daring and insight to recommend them for hypertension, when the patient's future did not seem to be quite as hopeless. Medicine certainly owes an everlasting debt to those great physicians and surgeons who were not afraid to face the criticism which is always leveled at everything radically new.

In the *Annals of Internal Medicine* (of 1952), Dr. G. W. Thorn and his associates, at Harvard Medical School, described an impressive case to show what can be accomplished by removal of the adrenals in severe hypertension with renal dissease. W. C., a 34-year-old laborer, was known to have had hypertension for ten years. Three months before his admission to the hospital, this man developed swelling of the legs and marked fluid accumulations in his abdomen. At night he was often troubled by spells during which he could not breathe. Upon medical examination, it turned out that his blood pressure was greatly elevated; his heart was enlarged; and, as a result of cardiac failure, he had developed much dropsy. His difficulties of respiration were caused by water accumulation in his lungs. Both adrenals were removed and the patient was maintained mainly on cortisone. After the operation the dropsy disappeared, breathing became normal, and the blood pressure fell essentially within the normal range. This patient who had been totally incapacitated, was able to return to work soon after the removal of his adrenals; and reexamination one year later showed him still "very active and capable of working." From this and similar cases the Harvard group concluded that:

"It would appear, therefore, that bilateral complete adrenalectomy is justified as an experimental approach in man in an effort to determine the possible role of the adrenal cortex in patients with severe hypertensive vascular disease, including those with renal or cardiac impairment.

"In those patients whose blood pressure has fallen in response to adrenalectomy it has been possible to restore the blood pressure toward the original hypertensive levels with desoxycorticosterone [DOC]. . . ."

Later Professor J. Govaerts of Brussels demonstrated that complete adrenalectomy can also restore health in patients who suffer from a mutilating type of juvenile arteritis, which histologically resembles that produced in rats by DOC.

Almost at the same time, in Stockholm, Professors

H. Olivecrona and D. R. Luft successfully performed complete hypophysectomies in people for diabetic hypertension.

Depending upon the character and severity of the disease, the improvement may be quite slight in some cases and extremely striking in others; but the work of all these pioneer clinical investigators definitely showed that cardiovascular disease can be treated by removing the adrenals or the pituitary.

Fortunately, progress along these lines has been astonishingly rapid, and nowadays most cases of hypertensive disease can be controlled by drugs, without any surgery. The most effective and commonly used among these act by inhibiting MCs or adrenalines. They are often used in combination with diuretics which help excretion of sodium, and tranquilizers which diminish the production of the offensive stress hormones. Depending upon the type of hypertension to be treated, these drugs are used singly or in certain combinations. However, we cannot enter into a detailed discussion of practical questions related to such treatments which, in any event, could only be established by experienced specialists after careful examination of each case.

If you suspect that a patient has been poisoned, you only need to demonstrate the poison in his body to prove your point. This is not so with diseases due to DOC-like hormones. The normal body always contains MCs and their activity may become excessive, even when they are not produced in excess, because conditioning factors can render them particularly effective. For instance, a derangement in salt metabolism or a disturbance in renal function can condition the human body for DOC, just as the administration of sodium chloride and the removal of one kidney did in our animal experiments.

Nevertheless, using the latest, highly sensitive techniques, an actual increase in DOC-like material has now been demonstrated with certainty in several renal and cardiovascular diseases of man.

It has been shown, for instance, that in *nephrosis* (a renal disease accompanied by much dropsy and resembling the initial stages of DOC intoxication in animals) the urinary excretion of aldosterone (a highly potent DOC-like hormone) is way above normal. It is especially significant that, when the condition of these patients improves, either spontaneously or under the influence of some treatment, aldosterone elimination in the urine also diminishes. There appears to be a correlation between the severity of nephrosis and the excretion of aldosterone. The same has been demonstrated (by Doctors Luetscher and Venning) for certain types of *cardiac failure* which tend to cause dropsy.

Of course, the convincing value of all these observations is greatly weakened by the fact that it is often impossible to ascertain whether an increased MC production is the cause or the result of the disease.

Professor Jerome W. Conn of Ann Arbor made a very remarkable observation in 1955 which has shed light upon this problem. A 34-year-old housewife came to see him because for the past seven years she had suffered from hypertension, kidney trouble, and muscular weakness. She also had various other disturbances, similar to those that can be produced in animals by an excess of DOC—for example, a thirst compelling her to drink so much water that she had to get up several times during the night to void urine. Patients with similar symptoms have repeatedly been observed before, but no physician ever had the astuteness to think of a relationship between their complaints and the experimental syndrome produced with DOC over-dosage. Doctor Conn immediately considered the possibility that his patient might have an adrenal hypertrophy or tumor, which would produce an excessive amount of some DOC-like hormone, such as aldosterone. Analysis of the urine showed that this woman did, in fact, eliminate an extraordinarily large amount of aldosterone and, on this evidence, he recommended an operation to inspect the adrenals. The surgeon found, and immediately removed, a large adrenocortical tumor, whereupon the patient recovered her health.

Doctor Conn named this condition *aldosteronism* and concluded from his observation that in the future "patients exhibiting such clinical and laboratory manifestations be subjected to adrenal surgery." Many additional cases have since been observed by other physicians, and there can be little doubt that here the excess production of DOC-like material by the adrenals is the cause of a syndrome now known as "Conn's disease."

Until quite recently we have had no satisfactory method for the determination of aldosterone and other DOC-like compounds in the fluids and tissues of the body; this is one of the reasons why, up to now, so few investigators have searched for them in patients with ordinary *hypertension*, particularly the malignant type. There can be no doubt, however, that here the production of DOC-like material is also often increased. Of course, we cannot expect to find a significant hormone excess in every patient who suffers from hypertension. First, some cases of hypertension are due to derangements which have nothing to do with corticoids; second—though this may seem paradoxical—when a disease manifests itself, its cause is not necessarily present in the body. This has been demonstrated particularly as regards the so-called metacorticoid hypertension.

Metacorticoid Hypertension

All the clinicians agree that antimineralocorticoid treatment (or even the now obsolete adrenalectomy) for hypertension is most effective when the kidneys are not yet severely damaged by the disease. Apparently an advanced nephrosclerosis can maintain an abnormally high blood pressure even in the absence of the adrenals.

This noteworthy fact checks perfectly with earlier animal experiments performed by two of my former pupils, Professor Sydney Friedman of Vancouver, and Doctor Leal Prado of São Paulo, as well as by the late Doctor D. M. Green of Los Angeles. These three investigators found—at about the same time and yet quite independently of each other—that, in rats which have become hypertensive as a result of DOC treatment, the blood pressure returns to normal as long as hormone administration is discontinued early; on the other hand, if DOC treatment is stopped only after the kidney

has been seriously damaged, the blood pressure
continues to rise, even when no more hormone is
given.

I called this *metacorticoid* (from Greek *meta*,
after) *hypertension*, because here the disease progresses after a transient corticoid overdosage.

Unfortunately, once this stage has been reached,
the disease appears to become irreversible; at least
our experiments so far have given us no clue to a
possible treatment.

Eclampsia

A young woman, who comes from a perfectly
healthy family and never had any serious illness in
her life, may—when she expects a baby—suddenly
come down with one of the most fulminating hypertensive diseases: eclampsia. Often there is nothing
to foreshadow this complication and the patient
feels perfectly well during the first two-thirds of
pregnancy. Then, without any warning, she has
convulsions, her face becomes congested, she foams
at the mouth, and often badly bites her tongue.
During these spells she may even die, but as a rule
the convulsions are followed by more or less prolonged periods of unconsciousness (coma), from
which the patient recovers. These convulsive
attacks may become more and more frequent as
pregnancy progresses, and then the condition is
sometimes mistaken for epilepsy.

It is this sudden onset that earned the disease its
name (from Greek *ek*, out, plus *lampein*, to flash).
It has also been called the *disease of theories*
because it has stimulated so much speculation.
Doctor C. H. Davis's standard three-volume trea-

tise, *Gynecology and Obstetrics*, discusses fifteen theories of eclampsia, only to conclude: "We are wholly ignorant as to the cause of this disease." In any event, the malady belongs to the general group of the toxemias of pregnancy, which also includes the milder *preeclampsia* (minus convulsions or coma), the vomiting of pregnancy, and various types of renal and hypertensive diseases.

Actually eclampsia itself is also a hypertensive disease which affects the kidney and the blood vessels. It is characterized by frequent sudden, intense rises in blood pressure, the excretion of albumin in the urine, and morbid changes in the blood vessels which may lead to hemorrhages in the brain, liver and other organs.

The safest treatment is to accelerate delivery because, as soon as mother and baby are separated, all the symptoms and signs disappear. But if premature termination of the pregnancy is impossible, there is not much that can be done, either for the mother or for the baby. It is instructive, however, to examine what sheer experience has taught physicians about the treatment of this disease. Even before the possible participation of corticoids in the development of eclampsia was suspected, it was found that the best thing to do (apart from combating the convulsions with sedatives and complete rest) was to give much fluid or ammonium chloride, which stimulated the excretion of urine and particularly of sodium. It had also become known that, on the other hand, foods rich in sodium chloride tended to aggravate this disease.

The beneficial effect of washing out sodium, the damaging action of sodium chloride intake, and the character of the morbid changes in the kidney and blood vessels are all singularly reminiscent of the DOC-overdosage syndrome which we had produced in rats. I may add that even convulsive spells, similar to those of eclampsia or epilepsy, had been noted quite frequently in our rats treated with excessive amounts of DOC. All this strongly suggested some relationship between eclampsia and the adrenocortical hormones. But we needed more proof.

Soon additional evidence of such a relationship was brought to light by the interesting studies of my former student, Dr. Georges Masson, who worked on this subject in cooperation with Drs. I. H. Page and A. C. Corcoran at the Cleveland Clinic. These investigators found that, after pretreatment with DOC, a few injections of a blood pressure-raising kidney extract (RPS) can produce a syndrome which imitates eclampsia even more closely than the one produced by DOC alone.

Particularly illuminating relevant observations have been published by Dr. Russell R. de Alvarez. He found that DOC is definitely contraindicated in women with preeclampsia because it tends to aggravate their disease, somewhat as sodium does. Moreover, it has been demonstrated in several clinics that some women suffering from eclampsia excrete excessive amounts of aldosterone.

All these findings still do not prove definitely that the adrenal plays a decisive role in the production of eclampsia, but they do make it rather probable. In any event, we have learned enough by now about this "disease of theories" to know that the role of corticoids deserves to be systematically investigated, and that treatment based on this concept offers definite promise.

It is still largely a matter of debate which of the *diseases of adaptation* are due to an actual over-production of, or hypersensitivity to, adaptive hormones. But this is a point of secondary importance. The most significant practical outcome of our experiments was to demonstrate that *hormones participate in the development of numerous nonendocrine diseases,* that is, of maladies which are not primarily due to derangements originating in the endocrine glands themselves. Prior to these studies, we had no reason to suspect that such conditions as nephrosis or cardiovascular disease are in any way dependent upon the pituitary-adrenal axis, and that they might be effectively treated on the basis of this dependence.

The Sudden Heart Attack

Our work on mineralocorticoid hypertension and the associated cardiovascular diseases strongly suggested to us that stress, the hormones produced during stress, or both of these, could play an important role in the sudden, often fatal heart attacks that may appear even in relatively young and middle-aged people under the influence of some sudden mental or physical exertion. Reports of such attacks appear in the newspapers almost daily and nearly everyone of us can remember dramatic instances of this kind occurring in his family or among his friends. These attacks are called "coronary accidents," because until quite recently, it was thought that they are always caused by an *obstruction of one of the "coronary" or heart arteries by a blood clot.* This is true in many, but cer-

tainly not in all cases. Experts differ in their estimates of the percentage of sudden heart attacks
due to mechanical obstruction of the circulation by
a clot, as compared to those caused by metabolic
derangements in the biochemistry of the heart
muscle or derangement of the heart rhythm under
increased demand.

Whatever their cause, these heart accidents are
due to the actual death or, as we say, "necrosis" of
a portion in the heart muscle; if it happens to be an
indispensable portion, the accident is fatal. The
heart attacks caused either by occlusion of the circulation or metabolic defects leading to cardiac
necrosis must be distinguished from those induced
by functional derangements of the heart rhythm
with irregular fibrillation or arrest of the heart
beat (for example, under the influence of intense
fear, joy, or other stressors), although both may end
in sudden death.

Our work on mineralocorticoid hypertension was
instrumental in the formulation of the idea that all
the "diseases of adaptation" are actually "pluricausal" or "multifactorial" in that stress alone
causes disease only in predisposed persons. Since,
as we have said, it is always the weakest part in
any machine that breaks under heavy demand,
even the location of the breakdown caused by
stress is determined by a predisposing weakness of
one or the other organ in our body.

It has long been common knowledge among physicians that the so-called "coronary heart attacks"
primarily affect "coronary candidates," people who
are particularly prone to react this way. Among

the predisposing factors detected simply by experience were for example: pre-existent arteriosclerosis of the heart vessels due to aging, high blood pressure, excessive obesity, lack of muscular exercise, high blood cholesterol, a pushy, aggressive, overactive personality, and heredity. Heart attacks run in families to some extent, and heredity can predispose a person to develop any or all of the features just mentioned as typical of the "coronary candidate." Yet, all these factors only cause the danger of a heart attack, and do not in themselves precipitate it. The final, decisive eliciting factor is usually stress.

Many physicians questioned the fact that heart accidents can be induced chemically by stress, even *without occlusion of coronary arteries* (I am afraid this is true of some doctors even today) because, until recently, this interpretation rested exclusively on the evaluation of statistics on a very diversified human population, and this is never as convincing as a repeatable experiment on a homogeneous group of animals, kept under strictly controlled conditions.

During the early 1950s, we undertook some laboratory work on purebred rats with the hope of developing a model of stress-induced myocardial necrosis. Of course, necrosis, similar to that seen in men who die from occlusion of heart vessels, had been produced much earlier in animals by actually tying off cardiac arteries, or by giving certain specific drugs which are extremely toxic for the heart muscle and kill through chemical means. However, encouraged by our work on mineralocorticoid hypertension and the associated cardiac lesions, we experimented with various hormones and sodium salts until we could find a combination of GCs, MCs, and sodium salt which, given to healthy normal young rats, caused no visible cardiac damage, but made them into "coronary candidates." Hence, when subsequently exposed to virtually any type of stressor (frustration, forced muscular exercise, traumatic injury), they invariably died with obvious signs of cardiac failure. The latter could be confirmed at autopsy by naked eye and microscopic inspection of their muscles, showing extensive necrosis without preceding coronary occlusion.

This indeed proved to be a very helpful experimental model since it gave us and many investigators in other laboratories a chance to test the possible value of drugs which, for theoretic reasons, could be suspected of protecting against stress-induced heart accidents. Antimineralocorticoids, antiadrenalines, and drugs facilitating the excretion of sodium or the retention of potassium (which in this, as in many other respects, counteracts sodium) are now among those most efficiently and most commonly used in clinical medicine.

As a minor contribution, our model also helped to establish beyond doubt many facts that were suspected before on the basis of statistical evidence, but never generally accepted. For example, high-sodium, high-fat diets predispose our animals to hypertension and cardiac disease; and adrenaline (known to be secreted in excess during acute stress) is one of the most potent eliciting factors in rats made into "coronary candidates" by our procedure.* †

There is good evidence that sudden death may also be precipitated by acute emotional stress which causes severe functional *derangements of the cardiac rhythm without necrosis.* Not long ago, Dr. George L. Engel of Rochester, New York, collected a large number of case reports indicating that *sudden death* may occur under the influence of "psychological stress." These he classified into eight categories: (1) on the impact of the collapse or death of a close person; (2) during acute grief; (3) on threat of loss of a close person; (4) during mourning or on an anniversary; (5) on loss of status or self-esteem; (6) personal danger or threat of injury; (7) after the danger is over; (8) reunion, triumph, or happy ending.

Sudden death may also occur in animals under the influence of psychologic stress, for example when threatened by other animals or captured by

*Most people, including myself, find it difficult to follow the doctor's advice of eating salt-free, or at least very low salt foods, because they are extremely tasteless. My solution to this (being highly active, ambitious, and 68 years old, all of which are predisposing factors) is to fill my salt shaker with potassium chloride instead of the usual kitchen salt (sodium chloride). I assure you both have virtually the same taste. Some people can tell the difference—or at least they think so—when they first use potassium chloride, but after a while, I can tell you from personal experience that this ceases to be a problem.

†For the technical aspects of this work on experimental cardiac necroses and their clinical implications I refer the specialized reader to my publications, *The Chemical Prevention of Cardiac Necroses* (Ronald Press, New York, 1958), *The Pluricausal Cardiopathies* (Charles C Thomas, Springfield, 1961) the two-volume documented treatise *Experimental Cardiovascular Diseases* (Springer, Heidelberg, Berlin, New York, 1970), and *Stress in Health and Disease* (Butterworths, Reading, Mass., 1976).

man. Although the mechanism of this dramatic
sudden death is not clearly understood, it is most
probably due to abnormalities of cardiac rhythm
induced by nervous stimuli. Dr. Michael Bernreiter
of Kansas City described a series of similar case
reports which he attributed to physical or emotional stress resulting in an acute alarm reaction.
It is highly probable that sudden death caused by
the "evil eye" and by various mystic procedures
practiced by medicine men is due to a similar
mechanism.

chapter 11

Inflammatory Diseases

The inflammatory pouch test. The anti-inflammatory hormones. The proinflammatory hormones. Effect of general stress on a local disease condition. Focal infection can cause generalized disease. The experimental arthritis tests. Rheumatic and rheumatoid diseases of man. Inflammatory diseases of the skin and the eyes. Infectious diseases. Allergic and hypersensitivity diseases.

In our dissection of stress we have devoted an entire chapter to inflammation (page 129), because this is the most striking aspect of the L.A.S., the local adaptive response of tissue at the site of injury. We have seen that the principal purpose of inflammation is to put a strong barricade of activated connective tissue around a territory invaded, or least damaged, by some pathogen, thereby sharply *demarcating the sick from the healthy.*

If the invader is dangerous and threatens life because it could spread into the blood and throughout the body, then—and only then—is this reaction useful.

The whole diseased part may have to be sacrificed, because when the destructive cells and fluids of inflammation surround and quarantine an area

to choke and kill the invader, they often also kill
the invaded tissues. We have seen that the pus
evacuated from a boil usually contains the dead
bodies both of the microbes and of the body's own
tissue cells. Besides, inflammation causes swelling,
pain, and interference with the function of the
affected parts. All this is a small price to pay,
however, when this reaction is our only means of
maintaining health or even life: that is why inflammation is essentially a useful adaptive response to
injury.

But, as we have said, *if the invader is harmless*,
there is no point in reacting at all. An allergic
inflammation is a sign of morbid hypersensitivity.
Here it is actually the defensive inflammation
itself that we experience as disease. In such cases
we are not being injured, we injure ourselves. Here
the reactions of our tissues are quite comparable to
those mental overreactions (worry, anger) to inoffensive insults, which do not help but merely hurt.

The *principal problems* posed by the inflammatory diseases are: first, to determine how inflammation can be influenced (for instance, by hormones); and then to establish whether it should be
enhanced, left alone, or inhibited. We have already
seen that the body can make proinflammatory and
anti-inflammatory hormones with which to influence inflammation; and, of course, the physician
can use these substances for treatment whenever
the body's own response is imperfect. But this is
possible only after we have learned just how these
hormones work and exactly where such treatment
is indicated or contraindicated.

No conscientious physician would like to take the

risk of learning all this by chance observations on patients. That is why experimental medicine had to step in and devise *similes of human diseases which could serve as experimental models,* so that the elementary lessons might be learned on animals.

Normally the inflammatory response is rather irregular and unpredictable; it does not lend itself to exact experimental research. You can produce inflammation in animals by simply dropping some irritating material under the eyelid, by rubbing it onto the skin, or by injecting it into internal tissues. But the results are quite unpredictable, because much of the material rubs off the eye or the skin and, if you inject it into deeper tissues, it distributes itself so irregularly that the response can never be predicted. From all we have said about inflammation, it is clear that what we really needed at this point in our research was an experimental model of it in animals, one which could readily be produced and possessing the following features: (1) it must not permit the causative irritant to escape, otherwise it would be impossible to establish the quantitative relationships between irritant and response; (2) it must have a predictable, regular shape and size, so that it can be accurately measured; (3) the two major components of inflammation, the cellular barricade and the inflammatory fluid, must not be intermixed (as are the solid and fluid parts of a wet sponge), so that each may be separately measured, because each has different functions; (4) the barricade must form a sac of even and predictable thickness, so that its functional value as a barrier may be measured— for instance, by injecting microbes or corrosive chemicals into its cavity and determining how much the pouch wall can stand before it perforates.

This is quite an order, and I had spent many years trying to devise such a test without success. I always felt that some kind of mold could do it, as for instance, a glass bead or a small ball of metal which, when inserted into connective tissue, would force it to take up a regular, spherical shape. But it would have to be a very bland and elastic foreign body and one which would eventually disappear, so as to leave a cavity for fluid accumulation. All the molds I had tried were hard and caused the surrounding skin to perforate wherever the rat pressed against them; besides, there still remained the problem of removing the mold after the barricade had formed. It seemed a more theoretic than practical idea to use this type of a procedure, until finally a lucky accident showed the way.

The Inflammatory Pouch Test

In patients suffering from consumption, it is often useful to inject air (or some other gas) into the chest cavity, so as to collapse a diseased lung and give it a rest to promote healing. Since, on the other hand, any kind of stress is particularly bad for tuberculous patients, I was interested in finding out exactly how stressful the air injection itself would be. To determine this, I injected air into the chest cavity of rats, with the intention of then measuring their adrenal response as an indicator of stress.

It happened that while I was doing this, a group of Brazilian physicians, who visited our Institute, were shown into my lab by one of my assistants. As I turned around to greet them, my needle slipped out of the chest cavity of the rat I was just injecting and all the air went under the skin; there it formed a perfectly regular, roughly egg-shaped, connective tissue sac. Why not *use air as a mold* with which to force connective tissue to form a sac of predictable size and shape? Air is very elastic and it need not be removed to permit fluid accumulation in the pouch. I then made such air sacs on purpose, and injected some irritant (usually croton oil) into the cavity, so as to transform the lining connective tissue into an inflammatory barricade. By giving more or less of the irritant, even the thickness of the surrounding barricade could be fairly accurately regulated at will.

This proved to be a very practical procedure. As soon as the lining was transformed into inflamed connective tissue, the cavity filled up with inflammatory fluid. After the rat was sacrificed, this fluid could be measured accurately by aspirating it into a graduated syringe, and the connective tissue barricade dissected and weighed separately. In fact, if the rat was shaved, the progress of inflammation could be followed every day by transilluminating the sac with an electric flashlight and measuring the height of the fluid column. Even function tests for the delimiting value of the barricade could be quite easily performed on this test object by injecting microbes or corrosive chemicals into the cavity of the sac and determining the highest concentration which could be tolerated without causing perforation.

To see how this kind of work is done, it would be

worthwhile to follow the manner in which certain
basic problems in the development and treatment
of inflammatory diseases could be analyzed with
this simple test. (*Figs. 21* and *22.*)

The Anti-inflammatory Hormones

Immediately after the introduction of ACTH and
cortisone into practical medicine, certain clinicians
were puzzled by the fact that these substances
influenced so many varied diseases. Dr. Phillip
Hench attempted to explain this by assuming that
the anti-inflammatory hormones acted like an
"asbestos suit," protecting various cells against
the "fire of disease" by somehow preventing the
disease-producing agents from getting into the
cells and tissues.

The validity of this assumption could easily be
checked by the inflammatory pouch test because it
permitted us to explore the problem under strictly
reproducible conditions, in what might be called *a*

Fig. 21   This is what the pouch looks like
on a rat.

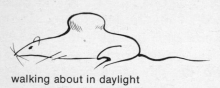

walking about in daylight

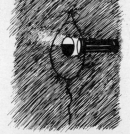

or held, head up, for
transillumination in the dark.

living test tube of connective tissue. For instance, by placing a chemical irritant, such as croton oil, into the subcutaneous connective tissue pouch, we could explore its effect upon the lining connective tissue as well as upon adjacent structures such as the skin covering the sac. In this way it was easily demonstrated that, in a normal rat, a given amount of croton oil transforms the lining tissue into an inflammatory barricade which protects the adjacent skin. In a COL-treated rat, on the other hand, the same amount of croton oil causes little or no inflammation; consequently, the irritant spreads into and destroys the adjacent skin. Far from acting as an asbestos suit, COL actually prevented the formation of a protective shield (that is, the inflammatory barricade) and thereby aggravated the situation in this test.

It was concluded that, in general, COL and similar anti-inflammatory hormones act nonspecifically because they inhibit the immediate inflammatory defense reaction to various agents. This may be advantageous when the irritant is mild and

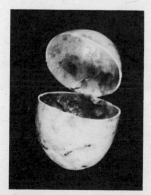

Fig. 22 Dissected inflammatory pouch. This is a pouch produced by injecting air and croton oil under the skin in the rat. This pouch has first been dissected, then—after removal of the fluid—cut open to show both inner and outer surfaces. Note the great regularity of the thickness of its wall. *(After H. Selye, courtesy of the "Journal of the American Medical Association.")*

unlikely to cause much destruction anyway, or it
may be detrimental when the irritant is severe and
likely to kill surrounding tissues if permitted to
spread into them.

The Proinflammatory Hormones

Similar tests with DOC or STH showed that these
substances actually increase inflammatory barricade and fluid formation; indeed if they are given
concurrently with anti-inflammatory hormones,
they neutralize the effects of the latter. In this
manner it was possible, within certain limits, to
titrate proinflammatory and anti-inflammatory
hormones against each other, using inflammatory
fluid and connective tissue formation as indicators
of activity.

Of course, whenever we clarify the mechanism
through which a biologic agent works, other questions arise. We now must ask, "Through what
chemical reactions do these hormones regulate
inflammation?" Much work along these lines is in
progress. Most probably, the hormones influence
certain enzyme reactions within the connective
tissue cell. Probably they can act upon disease in
many other ways as well. For instance, anti-inflammatory hormones have important effects upon
nervous activity, and they can suppress immune
reactions against microbes and other disease producers, as well as against grafts of foreign tissues,
such as heart or kidney transplants. Yet it is of
great practical value to know that one of the most
fundamental mechanisms through which these
hormones affect resistance to disease producers is
by inhibiting unnecessary defense reactions in

general. They promote peaceful co-existence with essentially harmless potential pathogens through their syntoxic actions.

Effect of General Stress on a Local Disease Condition

Various shock therapies and other nonspecific treatments have clearly shown that general stress can cure certain diseases; yet we also know that so often a latent disease tendency is transformed into a manifest malady by too much stress and strain. Could we not use the inflammatory pouch test as a simple model with which to analyze this apparent paradox?

I took two groups of rats in which an inflammatory pouch was produced under exactly identical conditions, except that in one group I put a weak irritant (dilute croton oil), in the other a strong irritant (more concentrated croton oil), into the air sac. Shortly afterwards both these groups of animals were exposed to a general stressor in the form of a frustrating experience. Without going into the technical details, let me say that, in such tests, the animals are forcefully immobilized, so that they cannot run around freely; this causes them to struggle and to become very angry. Cotton was put around their wrists and ankles where the shackles restrained them so that the animals could not even hurt themselves by pulling too strongly against the restraining bands. However, a rat wants to have his own way, just like a human being, and does not like to be prevented from doing what he wants to do. I thought that this kind of frustration and struggle would come about as close to the most common human stress situations as we can come in rats, and wondered how it would influence local tissue reactions to irritants.

The results were very illuminating and are illustrated in *Fig. 23*.

In the rats which received the weak irritant, there was little inflammation and the general stress actually cured the local disease by inhibiting this tissue response. The irritant was not strong

Fig. 23

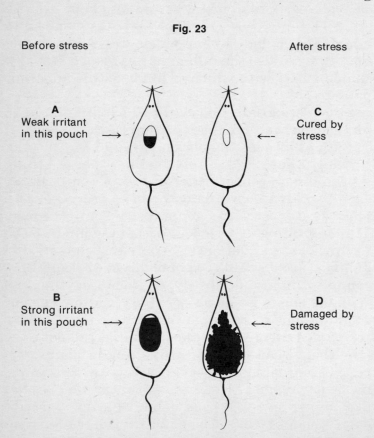

Before stress   After stress

A
Weak irritant
in this pouch →

C
Cured by
stress

B
Strong irritant
in this pouch →

D
Damaged by
stress

enough to destroy the covering skin in any case, so it did not matter whether the substance was allowed to spread or not. Inflammation was the whole disease here and, by inhibiting it, the rat was cured.

In the animals treated with the strong irritant, there was much more inflammatory barricade and fluid formation; still the adjacent tissues remained healthy, because the inflammatory barricade prevented the strong croton oil from spreading into the surroundings. Under the influence of general stress, however, the skin and all the adjacent tissues were infiltrated and destroyed by the spreading, concentrated croton oil solution. This was the crucial experiment showing that stress can either cure or aggravate a disease, depending upon whether the inflammatory response to a local irritant is necessary or superfluous.

I should add that there can be no doubt about the role of adrenal hormones in this type of general stress effect. We repeated the whole experiment on rats whose adrenals had previously been removed and found that, in them, general stress had no effect upon the course of inflammation, whether produced by weak or by strong irritants.

It is hardly necessary to underscore the importance of such observations as a guide to clinical treatment. Without this kind of information we would have been tempted to treat any inflammatory disease with anti-inflammatory hormones. The result would have been disastrous in certain maladies—for instance, in tuberculosis, or peptic ulcers, or acute appendicitis—where spreading must be prevented, whatever the cost. Yet, once we

understand the mechanism through which these
hormones act, even such patients can benefit from
them. For instance, in many cases, it is possible to
eliminate strong microbial irritants by suitable
antibiotic treatment; after that, destroying the
inflammatory barricade is no longer dangerous but
actually helps by removing the painful inflammatory tissue which has now become useless.

We have seen that inflammation is a feature of
the L.A.S., which develops in three stages, just as
does the G.A.S. (see pages 36-38 and 142). That is,
the microscopic structure and the function of inflammation vary, even while tissue is constantly
exposed to the same irritant. It seemed rather
important to determine at what point in its development inflammation is most sensitive to the
action of hormones.

Using again the inflammatory pouch technique,
I found that COL treatment is comparatively ineffective, if given on the day the irritant is introduced into the pouch. It is also quite difficult to
cause regression of an already fully-developed
inflammatory pouch with this hormone. But if COL
is given a few days after the irritant has been
applied, then inflammation can be suppressed very
easily. In other words, there is a definite critical
period during which inflamed tissue is especially
sensitive to this hormone. Almost exactly identical
results were obtained in animals exposed to some
general stressor; apparently, the COL secreted by
the rat's own adrenals during stress also acts best
during the critical period.

The hormones produced by endocrine glands are
discharged into the general circulation and conse-

quently every part of the body is supplied with
blood having the same hormone concentration.
Nervous impulses can be led selectively to one
region or another, but hormones are distributed
equally. At first sight, it would seem quite impossible that, in the same person, one region might have
too much and another too little of the same hormone. Classic endocrinology has recognized only
diseases caused by an excess or a deficiency of
hormones, but the question had never even been
raised whether, in the same patient, there might be
an excess in one place and a deficiency elsewhere.

The point seemed of fundamental importance,
and the just-mentioned experiments with the weak
and the strong irritants led me to suspect that this
question might well be worth a careful investigation. You will remember that COL treatment had a
curative effect in the rats bearing an inflammatory
pouch produced with a weak irritant, but that in
animals exposed to a strong irritant, it was
actually damaging. What would happen if, in the
same animal, we exposed one region to a weak and

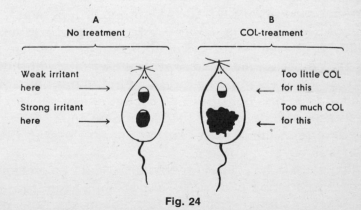

Fig. 24

another to a strong irritant? This was the sort of
problem that we could easily test with the inflammatory pouch technique. All we had to do was to
prepare two pouches in the same rat and put a
weak irritant into one, a strong irritant into the
other. The result of such an experiment is shown in
Fig. 24.

In both rats shown here, the weak irritant was
put in the pouch on the neck and the strong irritant
in the one on the back. The animal on the left was
not treated with any hormone; that on the right
was given subcutaneous injections of COL.
Obviously, after being taken up into the blood from
the subcutaneous tissue, the COL must have been
distributed equally to all parts of the body. Yet,
under the particular conditions of this experiment,
the amount of COL given was too little for the
pouch on the neck (it did not completely prevent
inflammation), and too much for the one on the
back (it caused tissue destruction worse than
inflammation).

The important lesson learned from this experiment is that there is no such thing as a definite
proper amount of COL for an animal or a person. A
certain quantity is appropriate only for a given
degree of local stress. To maintain the healthy,
steady state (homeostasis) of tissues, the amount of
stress hormone must be adjusted to the intensity of
the stress. It is definitely possible to have regional
excesses and deficiencies of hormones in the same
individual, as long as irritation (local stress) in the
various parts is uneven.

This again has considerable practical application
because, in man also, different regions are often—
in fact, usually—exposed to uneven degrees of

stress. We are now studying various techniques which permit us to concentrate COL activity in different parts of the body at will. In accessible parts this is easy: we merely apply the COL locally. We have not yet found any way to direct COL molecules selectively to various internal organs at will, but we can increase regional tissue sensitivity through the phenomenon of conditioning (page 123). For instance, certain blood vessel-constricting drugs sensitize limited regions of the body to the anti-inflammatory effect of COL.

Focal Infection Can Cause Generalized Disease

According to certain Egyptian tables—which date back to 650 B.C. and were found in the ruins of Nineveh—the great king, Annaper-Essa, suffered from a terrible disease, consisting of intense headaches and pains in the joints. No treatment known at the time was of any avail. Then, upon counsel of his physician, Arad Nassa, the royal patient had his bad teeth extracted and immediately all his troubles miraculously disappeared.

During the seventeenth century, the French surgeon Jean Louis Petit pointed out, in his famous *Treatise on Surgical Maladies*, that dental caries can produce all sorts of ailments throughout the body and that these can be treated by removing the infected teeth. As time went by, many physicians noted that infections in the mouth and throat can produce disease in distant organs, so that the discovery of this fact is certainly not new. Still, it was to the great merit of the American physician Frank Billings that, in his classic paper (1912),

"Chronic Focal Infections and Their Etiologic
Relations to Arthritis and Nephritis," he first formulated the problem with sufficient precision to
bring it to the attention of the medical profession
throughout the world.

Professor Russell L. Cecil, in his standard *Textbook of Medicine* (W. B. Saunders Co., 1943), defines
a focal infection as "a localized infection which presumably produces symptoms in other parts of the
body and in which there are usually no demonstrable bacteria in the blood stream." The latest edition
of W.A.D. Anderson's classic text, *Pathology*, men-
tions the possibility "that focal infections, especially those produced by Streptococcus viridans,
may be responsible for a variety of complaints such
as rheumatic fever, rheumatoid arthritis, sciatica,
myositis, neuralgia, etc. Benjamin Rush probably
gave stimulus to this concept by his report in 1801
of the cure of a patient with rheumatism of the hip
following extraction of a tooth. Foci of infection
most often considered responsible for such diseases
are apical infections of the teeth."

It is still something of a mystery just how focal
infection works, but undoubtedly much depends
upon the architecture of the inflammatory barricade around the infecting microbes. It is well
known, for instance, that children who often suffer
from very bad sore throats are predisposed to rheumatic fever. This cannot depend wholly upon the
microbes in the infected tonsils because, when
these same germs are introduced elsewhere in the
body, they rarely cause rheumatic fever. Perhaps
the architecture of the inflammatory barricade
around the germs is such as to permit only very

small numbers of them (or small amounts of their poisons) to enter into the blood stream at one time. This prevents massive invasion of the blood with demonstrable living bacteria and may modify the course of the illness by protracting the effects of the infection. There are many other theories, but we need not waste time on them because none has been definitely substantiated.

A few decades ago it was fashionable to ascribe almost any ailment of unknown origin to some focal infection. But, to quote Cecil's textbook again: "Many thoughtful physicians ... who originally accepted the theory of focal infection with enthusiasm, have watched with interest and some trepidation its rapid development in the various fields of medicine and are now wondering if the time has not arrived for the re-evaluation of the theory. Many students today question seriously its validity and some are quite willing to throw it completely overboard. This is particularly true in Europe, where the idea of focal infection has never met with enthusiastic acceptance. But even in America, many practitioners are becoming a little wearied of the theory which has been accepted as if it were an established fact."

You may wonder how there could be so much uncertainty about a condition which has allegedly been known since ancient Egyptian times. The trouble is that the development of focal infection is quite unpredictable. Sometimes a localized infection will be followed by rheumatic heart disease or arthritis and sometimes by nephritis or some other change in organs far removed from the site of infection. Sometimes surgical removal of the infected focus (for instance, the teeth or tonsils) leads to a cure and sometimes it does not. This being the case, it is difficult to prove a causal relationship between a localized infection and disease manifestations elsewhere in the body.

To prove definitely the existence and study the mechanism of the focal infection syndrome, we would first have to succeed in reproducing the condition regularly in experimental animals. This had never been done. It had been tried many times— ever since the discovery of bacteria—but the results had been just about as inconsistent and unpredictable in animals as is the effect of a sore throat upon the heart or of an infected tooth upon the joints, in human beings.

In the inflammatory pouch, though, we had a test which permitted us to regulate, more or less at will, the architecture of the barricade between the infected and the healthy tissues. By introducing different kinds of irritants, with or without microbes, we could force the wall of the sac to be built differently. Could one purposely construct a wall which would result in the consistent production of the focal syndrome in experimental animals?

This proved to be possible. Using certain combinations of irritants and microbes in rats, we finally managed to produce a syndrome characterized, among other things, by an inflammation of the heart valves (endocarditis), very similar to that which occurs in children suffering from rheumatic fever. Under certain circumstances, this was accompanied by inflammation of the kidney (nephritis) and excessive stimulation of the blood-forming organs. After we had learned how to produce this syndrome regularly, we could proceed to an experimental dissection of its mechanism, using essentially the same standard techniques that proved so useful in the analysis of the G.A.S. (removal of endocrine organs, injection of hormones, and so forth). It turned out, for instance, that the proinflammatory and anti-inflammatory hormones can modify the whole focal syndrome and that an excess of salt in the diet, after removal of one kidney, selectively aggravates the nephritis in the remaining kidney. This work is still unfinished and it would be premature to discuss it at great length. It is already evident, however, that here we are also dealing with some kind of disease of adaptation (which, in this case, is due to an improper adjustment of the body to invading germs); and now that we have constructed an experimental model of the disease in animals, it can be subjected to a systematic scientific analysis.

The Experimental Arthritis Tests

The inflammatory pouch proved to be very useful in the study of inflammation in general, but, of course, the character of inflammation largely depends upon the organ in which it develops. Chronic inflammation of the joints (arthritis) is one of the most common, crippling, wear-and-tear diseases of man. We still had no adequate procedure for reproducing this condition in animals, for the study of its mechanism and for the assay of hormones or drugs which may be used to treat it.

In searching for such a test, I noted that if we inject a drop of some irritant solution (Formalin, croton oil) under the skin of the sole of a rat's hind paw, there develops a *local experimental arthritis* (in technical language: *topical irritation arthritis*). First there is acute swelling at the site of injection, and then this gradually transforms itself into a chronic arthritis of the many small joints in the paw and, particularly, of the ankle joint. This arthritis, due to local stress, becomes a permanently crippling disease for the rat, because the joints stiffen with hard connective tissue, so that they can no longer be moved. On the other hand, if the rat develops an alarm reaction due to some stressor or if anti-inflammatory hormones (for instance, ACTH, cortisone, or COL) are given at the right time—during the critical period of development—the arthritis can be completely suppressed; and here again the proinflammatory hormones (STH, DOC) have an opposite, aggravating effect.

This test proved to be useful, among other things, in the routine screening of new hormone derivatives and other antiarthritic drugs, especially now that so many university laboratories and pharmaceutical companies are making such compounds. New drugs may be worthless or even dangerous and, of course, we must have an experimental assay procedure which permits us to select the best ones without having to try them out on people.

One disadvantage of this test is that an arthritis

produced by the local injection of irritants into a joint is not quite comparable to the kind of arthritis ("polyarthritis") that people develop. It was a great step forward, therefore, when Dr. Gaëtan Jasmin— while working for his Ph.D. degree at our Institute in 1955—discovered a more natural type of *multiple experimental arthritis*. Two of my earlier postgraduate students, Drs. A. Horava and A. Robert, had noticed that a peculiar inflammatory fluid was produced by certain experimental tumors when they were grown in the inflammatory pouch of the rat. Dr. Jasmin found that if one injects a single cubic centimeter of this tumor fluid into the blood of a rat, within a few days a pronounced inflammation appears in many of the joints, most frequently in the ankles, wrists, elbows, knee joints, and the many little joints between the vertebrae of the spinal column. It is impossible to say whether or not this experimental disease (which is probably due to the presence of certain so-called "PPLO" microbes in the tumor fluid) is closely related to the rheumatic or rheumatoid arthritis of man, but they certainly resemble each other in many respects *(Fig. 25)*. It was instructive, therefore, to learn that this induced generalized arthritic tendency of the rat also depends upon the function of the pituitary-adrenal defense mechanism. The principal findings were these:

1. In intact rats—which can respond to stress by anti-inflammatory hormone production—comparatively large amounts of tumor fluid must be used to elicit this arthritis.

2. In adrenalectomized rats maintained exclu-

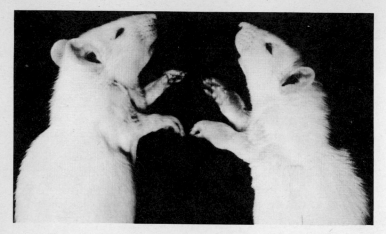

Fig. 25 Multiple experimental arthritis. On the left: untreated normal rat. On the right: rat which received a single injection of inflammatory fluid. Note the bilateral arthritis in the wrist joints. This animal also had similar lesions in the ankle and knee joints. *(After H. Selye and P. Bois, in The Stress of Life, 1956.)*

sively on the proinflammatory DOC, small amounts of fluid suffice to produce very pronounced and widespread arthritic changes.

3. In adrenalectomized rats treated only with the anti-inflammatory COL, even the largest doses of tumor fluid produce little or no arthritis.

4. In adrenalectomized rats treated with both COL and DOC, the anti-inflammatory effect of the former is neutralized by the latter hormone.

In conclusion, it seems that, in the intact rat, the injection of the tumor fluid produces enough stress to activate the pituitary-adrenal system, and the resulting increased secretion of anti-inflammatory hormones largely prevents the production of arthritis. In the absence of the adrenals, this protective response is, of course, impossible. Here the development of arthritis will largely depend upon the kind of hormone injected. DOC sensitizes, COL desensitizes for it. During subsequent years similar observations have been made with an immunologic type of polyarthritis. These findings confirm that certain potential pathogens will or will not induce arthritis, depending upon the body's hormonal defenses; whenever these self-protecting mechanisms are imperfect, we have it in our power to correct them by suitable hormone treatment.

Here again we have a typical tripartite disease production in that the malady depends upon: (1) the agents (microbes, immune bodies) which act as topical stressors for joints; (2) the amount of antiinflammatory hormone; and (3) the amount of proinflammatory hormone in the blood.

A few years later, my assistant, Dr. Pierre Bois, and I were able to show that some presumably infected inflammatory fluids (for instance, the liquid formed in the inflammatory pouch after local treatment with nonsterile solutions) can also acquire the property of producing multiple arthritis in ankles, wrists, elbows, knee joints, and the spinal column, when injected into the belly cavity of another rat. This brings up interesting points concerning the relationship between local inflammation in one part of the body and generalized inflammatory reactions in joints everywhere. The bearing of this observation upon the problem of focal infection is still unclear.

Figs. 25 and 26 illustrate what I have just said

and will help the reader to get a first-hand impression of the way these experimental models of disease actually present themselves to the investigator in the laboratory.

Rheumatic and Rheumatoid Diseases of Man

It takes no specialized medical training to realize that what we have said in the preceding passages about the role of hormones in inflammatory diseases is applicable to clinical problems. Rheumatic fever and rheumatoid arthritis, for example, are typical inflammatory maladies; their essence is inflammation in the joints, the heart valves, and other tissues. These diseases are not identical with the experimental conditions which we produced in rats—no spontaneous malady of man is identical with its artificial counterpart in animals—but they are certainly very closely related and presumably governed by the same general laws. The primary cause of rheumatic fever and of rheumatoid arthritis (the factor which would correspond to the croton oil, the Formalin, or the tumor fluid in our experiments) has still not been definitely identified; but their manifestations, like those of their experimental counterparts, depend largely upon the hormones produced by the patient.

This was perhaps most clearly demonstrated by Dr. Philip S. Hench and his associates at the Mayo Clinic in 1949, when ACTH and cortisone became available in sufficiently large amounts to be tested on patients. These investigators found that rheu-

A   B   C

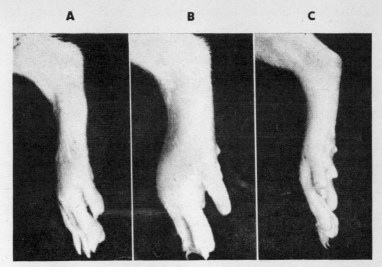

Fig. 26   Inhibition of local experimental arthritis by the alarm reaction in a rat. A. Paw of the untreated control. In the other two animals, Formalin was injected directly into the paw to produce local irritation. **B.** Full development of inflammation and swelling in an otherwise not treated animal. **C.** Almost complete inhibition of the arthritis by the stress effect of cold. Other stressors and anti-inflammatory hormones caused a similar inhibition. *(After H. Selye, courtesy of the "British Medical Journal.")*

matic and allied inflammations can be largely suppressed by anti-inflammatory hormones. Their observation opened the way for the clinical use of this type of treatment.

The extent to which such inflammatory diseases depend upon an insufficient mobilization of the body's alarm system *(Fig. 26)* is particularly well illustrated by the observations made by Drs. Wilhelm Brühl and Hans-Jürgen Jahn, at the Civic Hospital in Korbach, Germany. These physicians wanted to put the concept of stress therapy to practical use in patients suffering from very severe rheumatoid arthritis which did not respond to treatment with the usual anti-inflammatory drugs. They wondered whether the combined effect of naturally-produced anti-inflammatory hormones and the conditioning action of stress could not help here. In order to produce stress, they used a modified type of insulin shock which, at least temporarily, proved very effective in otherwise rather hopeless cases of this type. For instance, they describe the case of a 44-year-old woman, bedridden and crippled by an intense chronic rheumatoid arthritis in the joints of the hands, feet, and knees. After a series of insulin shocks, she was able to get up and walk about for the first time in three years. The German doctors ascribed this success to the production of an alarm reaction, with a discharge of ACTH and anti-inflammatory corticoids by the patient's own endocrine glands. Many similar observations have been published by other physicians who used different kinds of stressors.

All this makes it quite clear that the rheumatic maladies are really typical diseases of adaptation because, if the body's defenses are adequate, the disease is suppressed without any intervention by the physician. Here the primary pathogen (whatever it may be) is probably not very harmful in itself. When the inflammatory barricade against it is removed by hormones—be they secreted by the glands or administered by the physician—the causative agent (germ, poison) of the rheumatoid disease does not produce much tissue destruction.

These diseases are largely due to excessive adaptive reactions against comparatively innocuous injuries. They are caused by maladaptation.

Inflammatory Diseases of the Skin and the Eyes

We can discuss ailments of skin and eyes conjointly here because, generally speaking, they behave quite similarly in relation to stress and the adaptive hormones.

The great majority of all the skin and eye diseases are essentially inflammations, and many of them are caused by agents which would not be particularly harmful if the body did not react to them with unduly violent inflammatory responses. Here again we are apparently dealing with maladaptations, overreactions to cutaneous or ocular injuries. It had long been noted that during periods of intense general stress the predominantly inflammatory diseases of the skin and eyes tended to regress. Various nonspecific therapies have therefore been devised to combat such conditions and, more recently, even more striking improvements have been obtained by the use of antiinflammatory adaptive hormones (ACTH, cortisone, COL).

Of course, an excess of any hormone has harmful side-effects; the adaptive hormones are no exceptions. For instance, a patient heavily overdosed with cortisone tends to become very prone to infections and may develop high blood pressure, insom-

nia, gastrointestinal disturbances and so forth.
Indeed, often it is impossible to give enough cortisone to cure an inflammatory disease without also
automatically producing unpleasant side-effects of
hormone overdosage. But, in the cutaneous and
ocular diseases, cortisone or COL may be applied
locally, through ointments and eye drops, so that a
great concentration can be achieved in the diseased area without much getting into the blood. In
other words, here this kind of treatment can often
be applied without the usual dangers of overdosage.

Infectious Diseases

We have already seen that various germs, and particularly those of tuberculosis, can take a foothold
in the body more readily than is usual if inflammatory and immunologic defense reactions are
impeded by anti-inflammatory hormones. It is
important to keep this in mind when prescribing
ACTH, cortisone, or COL in the treatment of rheumatic, cutaneous, or ocular diseases because, so
often, a hitherto latent nodule of tuberculosis in
the lung begins to spread dangerously when, due to
these hormones, the inflammatory barricades
shrink throughout the body. It is, of course, a very
high price to pay for the improvement of a comparatively benign joint, skin, or eye condition if the
hormone opens the way for the spread of tuberculosis or some other lethal infection. Whenever there
is any danger of this, hormone treatment must be

stopped, or at least antibiotics must be given to fight the germs.

That the balance between proinflammatory and anti-inflammatory hormones is of paramount importance, even in tuberculosis, has clearly been shown by experiments performed in our Institute by Dr. Paul Lemonde. The rat is normally resistant to the human type of tuberculosis, but it can be made very sensitive to it by overdosage with cortisone. Dr. Lemonde found that this artificially-induced sensitivity to tuberculosis is in turn abolished if, simultaneously with the cortisone, large amounts of the proinflammatory STH are injected. In other words, the natural tuberculosis resistance of the rat can be abolished by an anti-inflammatory hormone and restored again by a proinflammatory one.

It would be difficult to furnish more eloquent proof of the important role played by adaptive hormones in determining disease susceptibility. It is an old and well-established fact that stress predisposes to tuberculosis. That is why patients suffering from this disease are advised to take long rest cures, in order to recover their resistance against tubercle bacilli. The analysis of the stress mechanism helped us to understand why this is so. Apparently, the anti-inflammatory hormones, which are produced in excess during stress, remove the protective barricades around the foci of tubercle bacilli and thereby permit them to spread.

Dr. B. Carstensen and his associates in Sweden have reported rather encouraging results with a certain type of STH in tuberculous patients. Unfortunately, up to that time, most of the STH-preparations were not suitable for routine clinical use. But now that better, human-type STH has become available, it will be interesting to see whether or not a tuberculosis resistance—such as that attained in animals—can also be induced in human patients. Of course, DOC has long been available, but unfortunately, for reasons which are not yet quite clear, it cannot substitute for STH in such animal experiments; nor has it been useful in treating the tuberculosis of man.

In this passage I have discussed tuberculosis at length because our own research work was mainly concerned with this infection. But essentially the same could be said about the role of stress and of adaptive hormones in other types of infection. All kinds of infections are met by the body with an inflammatory response which tends to delimit them. Therefore, the hormones regulating inflammation are evidently important in determining the course of various infections. Even the *saprophytes* (microbes which live in our lungs, gastrointestinal system, and on our skin without ever causing any disease) can become dangerous pathogens when our normal defenses against them are broken down by anti-inflammatory hormones. I have seen, for instance, that in rats treated with large amounts of ACTH, cortisone, or COL, such saprophytes can invade the blood and produce considerable tissue destruction, finally resulting in death. STH prevents all this.

These findings confirm the role of the hormones in determining just what microbe is pathogenic.

Almost no germ is unconditionally dangerous to man; its disease-producing ability depends upon the body's resistance.

Allergic and Hypersensitivity Diseases

Immediately after the discovery of the G.A.S., I spent a great deal of time trying to find out just how stressful various medical treatments are. Among other things, in 1937 I injected rats with a variety of drugs and assessed the resulting stress by the adrenal enlargement and by other signs of the G.A.S. In the course of this work one group of rats was injected with egg white, just to see how much stress this foreign protein would produce. Much to my surprise, egg white acted as a weak stressor, but produced a very specific and strange syndrome. Immediately following the injection the rats seemed to be quite all right, but soon afterwards they started to sneeze and sat up on their haunches, scratching their snouts with their forepaws. A few minutes later, their noses and lips became greatly swollen and red, giving the animals a very peculiar appearance. A friend of mine suffered from hay fever at that time, and he found his resemblance to my rats so striking as to be positively offensive. Well, in any case, this seemed to be a new experimental disease, due to some innate hypersensitivity of the rat to egg white.

To follow this up, I then injected other animals (guinea pigs, rabbits, dogs) with egg white, but they did not respond in this singular fashion.

Apparently, just as among people there are some who do, others who do not respond with hay fever to certain plant pollens, so among animals, the rat is sensitive to egg white, while most other species are not. This seemed to offer interesting possibilities for the study of what we call *allergic* and *anaphylactic hypersensitivity reactions*. Mind you, egg white in itself is not particularly damaging, even to the rat, because no special response to it is seen locally, wherever it is injected. In fact, when the substance is distributed to all parts of the body through the blood, it causes swelling and inflammation only in certain hypersensitive parts, such as the nose and the surrounding facial tissue. Usually the paws and the ears also become inflamed, but the rest of the body remains quite unaffected.

Even in 1937 when cortisone and COL were not yet available, it was quite easily proved that this inflammatory reaction also depended somehow upon adrenal hormones. We merely removed the adrenals of rats and then injected the egg white to see how the absence of corticoids would affect the reaction. The result was most spectacular. The rats which had no adrenals showed a much more intense inflammation; the swollen parts became bluish because of engorgement with venous blood, and within hours all these animals died.

This still did not prove that anti-inflammatory hormones made by the animals' own adrenals could combat such a hypersensitivity response. To prove it, I then produced marked alarm reactions in other rats, using a variety of stressor agents: invariably

the rats with the large, overactive adrenals tolerated egg white perfectly well, without showing any
hypersensitivity response. This type of anti-inflammatory effect is fundamentally the same as that of
insulin shock, liver disease, pregnancy or other
stressors in patients with rheumatoid arthritis; it
is due to the increased secretion of ACTH and COL-
like hormones by the endocrine glands.

Of course, now that we have highly potent, purified preparations of ACTH and of anti-inflammatory corticoids, it is much simpler to administer
these than to expose a patient to stress and make
his own endocrine glands produce the proper adaptive hormones. In fact, it is common knowledge
that, in a variety of diseases due to hypersensitivity, treatment with anti-inflammatory hormones
proves to be very effective. This is so, for instance,
in many cases of hay fever and asthma, as well as
in certain types of dermatitis and conjunctivitis,
which are due respectively to allergic irritation of
the skin and eyes.

Incidentally, this test—just like the experimental arthritis and the inflammatory pouch tests—
has now become a standard technique in screening
for effective anti-inflammatory drugs. It is used
particularly in testing remedies which may prove
beneficial in the treatment of acute hypersensitivity reactions. The test is illustrated by *Fig. 27*.

In this chapter I have spoken about the effect of
stress and adaptive hormones in inflammatory
diseases. Inflammation is the most nonspecific
local response to the stress of tissue injury, and it
is understandable that the stress hormones have

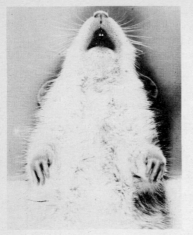 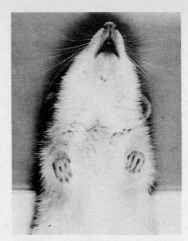

Fig. 27A   Fig. 27B

**Effect of ACTH upon hypersensitivity type of inflamma-
tion in the rat.** Both these animals have received the same
amount of egg white. **A.** Otherwise untreated rat, showing
pronounced swelling and congestion of the snout and
paws. **B.** Animal treated with ACTH. Note complete
absence of hypersensitivity type of inflammation. *(After H.
Selye, courtesy of the "Journal of the Canadian Medical
Association.")*

found their most spectacular applications in this
type of malady. But, of course, these hormones also
have many other effects, and our report would be
quite incomplete if it failed to consider the role of
stress in such conditions as mental and sexual derangements, digestive diseases, metabolic diseases,
cancer, malformations, and resistance in general.

chapter 12

Other Diseases

Nervous and mental diseases. Sexual derangements. Digestive diseases. Metabolic diseases. Cancer. Diseases of resistance in general. Malformations and aging.

Nervous and Mental Diseases

It is common knowledge that *maladaptation plays an important part in nervous and mental diseases.* As we have said, such expressions as, "This work gives me a headache" or "drives me crazy," grow out of experience. Many types of migraine headaches or mental breakdowns are actually caused by work to which we are ill-adapted. Heredity can doubtless predispose to certain types of mental disease, but there are imperceptible transitions between the healthy, the slightly disturbed, and the insane personality. In people with a defective hereditary structure, it is often the stress of adjustments to life under difficult circumstances that causes a change from healthy to disturbed, or from disturbed to insane. Conversely, we have also seen that a sudden stress (shock therapy) can help a person to snap out of an abnormal behavior pattern.

I am not competent to discuss this from the psychiatrist's point of view, but, as an endocrinologist and a student of stress, I have naturally been interested in exploring whether or not there are any demonstrable *relationships between abnormal mental reactions and the objectively measurable features of the G.A.S.* Again—as in so many other investigations described in this book—my attention was called to this possibility by the accident of a spoiled experiment.

In 1941 I was working on the effects of various adrenal and ovarian hormones upon the sex organs. For this purpose I injected rats with DOC or progesterone (an ovarian hormone chemically related to DOC). These injections were given under the skin of the animals in the usual manner and, after a few weeks of treatment, the sex organs were removed for microscopic study. Eventually, I handed this work over to a technician who had just then joined our laboratory, but much to my surprise the next day she reported, with great embarrassment, that all the animals were dead. Since I had given the same amount of the same hormones before without any trouble, I thought she must have made some mistake in preparing her solutions and merely told her to repeat the experiment more carefully. But next day all her rats died again. I could not imagine what might have gone wrong, so I asked the technician to inject yet another group of rats in my presence. It turned out that, being unacquainted with our techniques, she injected the hormones into the belly (the peritoneal cavity) of the rats. I did not think this would make much difference, but while we discussed the point, all the rats became excited and ran around in the cage as if they were intoxicated. After a time they fell asleep, just as if they had received a strong anesthetic, and eventually all of them died.

Now this was very odd, and I repeated the experiment several times, using smaller doses of hormones. Always there was an initial stage of excitement, followed by deep anesthesia; but after injection with smaller amounts the animals woke up within a couple of hours and were perfectly all right. We had produced a true *hormonal anesthesia*, with sleep induced by the natural products of endocrine glands. There remained no doubt that hormones can affect consciousness and that, at least under our experimental conditions, they act very much like an excess of alcohol, ether, and certain narcotics, which tend to cause excitement followed by depression.

Could the corticoids secreted under stress influence mental activity? Could the delirium of fever be related to adrenocortical activity? Could we use such hormones in man as sleeping pills, tranquilizers, or for the treatment of mental derangements, or perhaps even for the induction of surgical anesthesia? A multitude of problems was raised by this incidental observation and hundreds of medical publications have since dealt with experiments designed to answer them. Here are a few of the more outstanding facts which have come to light:

1. *Various species, including man, can be anesthetized with hormones.* My associates and I found that hormonal anesthesia can be produced not only in the rat, but in every animal species (fishes, birds and all mammals, including the monkey) which we have used for this work up to now. In fact, in 1954 a team of investigators at the Department of Obstetrics and Gynecology of Ohio State University in Columbus (Drs. W. Merryman, R.

Boiman, L. Barnes, and I. Rothchild) showed that,
in women, sleep can also be produced quite regularly by giving them progesterone. Shortly afterwards, in the *Journal of the American Medical
Association*, there appeared a paper in which a
group of Californian physicians (F. J. Murphy, N. P.
Guadagni, and F. DeBon) reported their findings
on people who were successfully anesthetized for
surgical operations with a close relative of DOC,
known as *hydroxydione*. The advantages of this
compound over other anesthetics have been carefully explored in laboratory animals by Drs. G. D.
Laubach, S. Y. Pan, and H. W. Rudel. Hydroxydione has subsequently been used in man throughout the world for the induction of anesthesia and it
has proved to have many advantages over other
anesthetics, especially in that it causes great muscular relaxation which often helps the surgeon's
task considerably. However, when the preparation
is injected into a vein it sometimes causes unpleasant local reactions. These can be avoided by giving
a related preparation of hormone derivatives
called Althesin which presently enjoys great popularity, especially in Europe. It shares with hydroxydione the property of inducing marked muscular
relaxation which prevents contractions and
reflexes that may interfere with surgical operations. Furthermore, the anesthesia it induces
appears to be very similar to natural sleep from
which the patients awake mentally alert and fresh,
without the unpleasant aftereffects of most other
anesthetics.

   2. *Adaptive hormones can combat convulsions*.
In rats in which I had produced epilepsy-like convulsions with certain stimulants (Metrazol, picro-

toxin), DOC and related hormones acted as tranquilizers. Dr. D. M. Woodbury and his associates at the University of Utah discovered that if such convulsions are produced with electric current, their intensity could be diminished by DOC and augmented by COL. This was the first indication of an actual antagonism between anti- and proinflammatory hormones as regards a nervous manifestation. Quite recently a derivative of DOC and of the previously-mentioned anesthetic hormones, named Pancuronium, has been synthesized and is currently in clinical use, especially as a muscle relaxant.

3. *Under certain conditions an excess of DOC can produce brain lesions such as are often seen in old people.* We have already discussed the blood vessel damage that is produced in rats by DOC poisoning (page 190). But when the arteries of the brain are involved, the animals can suffer a stroke or even repeated strokes, which eventually destroy large parts of the brain and cause widespread nervous derangements *(Fig. 28)*. Interestingly, such rats become extremely irritable and aggressive, a change quite characteristic of certain senile mental derangements among people whose brains often show the same kind of destruction.

These findings showed quite conclusively that there are very obvious relationships between mental derangements and the adaptive hormones. The importance of this became even more evident when ACTH and cortisone were introduced into clinical medicine.

4. *Adaptive hormones can cause mental changes in man.* Many patients who take ACTH or COL first develop a sense of extraordinary well-

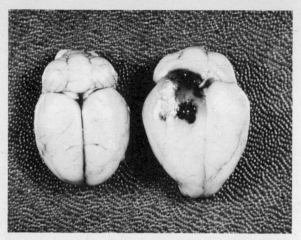

Fig. 28   Stroke produced by DOC overdosage in a rat.
On the left, normal brain of untreated rat. On the right,
swollen and congested brain of DOC-treated animal. Note
large bleeding into brain-substance (dark area). *(After H.
Selye, courtesy of the "Journal of Clinical Endocrinology.")*

being and buoyancy, with excitement and insomnia; this is sometimes followed by a depression
which may go so far as to create suicidal tendencies. In hereditarily predisposed people, profound
mental derangements may result, although fortunately, these are rare and always disappear when
the hormone treatment is interrupted.

At a conference organized by the CIBA Foundation in London, Professor Peter Forsham of San
Francisco discussed the effect of ACTH and cortisone upon "heightened perception" and the "dissociation of the ego and the id." He reported, among
other things, one observation which illustrates the
effect of adaptive hormones upon mentality so eloquently that I would like to quote it in full:

"The dissociation of the ego and the id has many forms. I had an American housewife with dermatomyositis [an inflammation of skin and muscles] who had been taught how to play the piano when she was little, and had continued for the entertainment of the children, but didn't get very far. When she started on large doses of ACTH she was suddenly able to play the most difficult works of Beethoven and Chopin—and the children of the neighbours would gather in the garden to hear her play. Here was a dissociation of the ego and the id that was doing good. But she also became a little psychotic, and so her dosage of ACTH had to be lowered, and with every 10 units of ACTH one sonata disappeared. It all ended up with the same old music poorly performed."

Many problems still remain unsolved in this field. Certain breakdown products of adrenaline can cause hallucinations. Could excessive adrenaline secretion during stress play a part in the production of mental changes, for instance, in patients who become delirious as a result of high fever or after burns?

5. *Perhaps adaptive hormones may even be used as tranquilizing agents in mental patients.* In chronic alcoholics, there sometimes develops a delirium characterized by terrifying hallucinations, great excitement, and trembling. This is known as *delirium tremens*. Preliminary observations of the French surgeon H. Laborit suggest that sometimes hydroxydione, the anesthetic DOC derivative, has a strikingly beneficial effect upon this condition. This type of treatment is far from giving reliable results, but it did raise the question of a possible causal relationship between adaptive hormones and certain delirious conditions in mentally deranged people.

The tranquilizing agents (chlorpromazine, reserpine), which are now so effectively employed in psychiatry, resemble in many of their actions the tranquilizing DOC derivatives. Could hormones be used in the treatment of confused and disturbed mental patients?

6. *DOC-like hormones can cause spells of periodic paralysis.* There is a rare hereditary disease which runs in families and tends to produce sudden spells of paralysis. It is called *periodic familial paralysis* and—apart from the fact that the predisposition to it is hereditary—very little is known about its cause. Interestingly, very similar spells of paralysis occur in patients in whom an adrenal tumor produces an excess of the DOC-like aldosterone (page 202). It is very probable that DOC-like mineralocorticoids have something to do with this condition. Many years ago a group of researchers at Columbia University in New York had discovered quite similar paralytic spells in dogs treated with DOC. Later Dr. C. E. Hall and I (making similar observations in monkeys) found that, in the DOC-treated animal, attacks can be precipitated and cured at will, merely by giving or withdrawing dietary sodium chloride. In monkeys the paralysis was often accompanied by intense or epilepsy-like attacks of convulsions. Obviously here again we are dealing with nervous derangements produced by DOC, and again these disturbances are aggravated by sodium chloride, just as the changes which the same hormone produces in the kidney and in the cardiovascular system. Is there a causal relationship here?

The many question marks in this chapter eloquently show how little we know and how much must still be learned. But they also indicate the ways in which we are using the stress concept as a guide to the study of the intriguing and mysterious borderline between mind and body. This has, in fact, been the subject of my book *"Stress without Distress,"* the essence of which will be summarized in Book V.

Sexual Derangements

That animals in which intense and prolonged stress is produced by any means suffer from sexual derangements was one of the first observations on the G.A.S. During stress the *sex glands* shrink and become less active in proportion to the enlargement and increased activity of the adrenals. Both male and female sex glands are stimulated by gonadotrophic hormones of the pituitary, just as the adrenals are activated by ACTH. It seemed probable, therefore, that during stress, when the pituitary has to produce so much ACTH to maintain life, it must cut down on the production of other hormones which are less urgently needed in times of emergencies. This change of emphasis was called the *shift in pituitary hormone production.* Our explanation seemed all the more likely since other functions which depend upon the pituitary are likewise diminished during stress. For instance, young animals cease to grow and lactating females produce no milk during intense stress. It will be recalled that growth and milk secretion are also governed by hormones of the pituitary.

It remains to be shown, however, whether these deficiencies are due to a diminished secretion or to a decreased efficiency of the pituitary hormones. Possibly when life itself is endangered, stress-induced metabolic changes could interfere with the hormone sensitivity of various organs whose function is not urgently required.

Clinical studies have confirmed the fact that people exposed to stress react very much like experimental animals in all these respects. In women *menstruation becomes irregular* or stops altogether, and during lactation *milk secretion may become insufficient* for the baby. In men both the *sexual urge and sperm cell formation are diminished.*

All this again reminds us of the finite nature of man's adaptability or adaptation energy. At times of imminent danger, in the face of extreme stress, the body must use all its reserves just to keep alive; while it does this the less pressing demands of reproduction are necessarily neglected.

In 1931 Dr. R. T. Frank described the *premenstrual syndrome,* a condition which tends to develop in women just before their monthly periods. It is characterized, among other things, by nervous tension and the desire to find relief in uncustomary, compulsive actions which are difficult to restrain. Many of Dr. Frank's patients also suffered from migraine headaches and swelling of the face, hands, and feet, with a definite increase in weight due to water retention. Other signs of the syndrome are: pain in the back and in the breasts, small hemorrhages in the skin, a feeling of stuffiness in the nose, asthma, and (very rarely) epilepsy-like seizures. All these symptoms disappear suddenly at the onset of the monthly cycle, but recur again as the next period approaches.

This long-overlooked syndrome is actually very common. A statistical study by Drs. W. Bickers and M. Woods revealed that, in one American factory employing 1,500 women, 36 per cent applied for treatment in the premenstrual phase; and Dr. S. L. Israel calculates that symptoms of this kind occur in 40 per cent of otherwise healthy women. The derangement deserves very serious attention also because it is frequently accompanied by a number of disturbing mental changes such as: periods of abnormal hunger, general emotional instability, and, occasionally, a morbid increase in the sexual drive. It is particularly noteworthy that, according to extensive statistical studies, 79 per cent (J. H. Morton and coworkers) to 84 per cent (W. R. Cooke) of all crimes of violence committed by women occur during, or in the week before, their periods.

Despite the frequency and severity of this condition, until recently very little had been done to alleviate it. "This is partly due to the attitude of the patients," say Drs. R. Greene and K. Dalton of London, England, because the syndrome is just accepted by them "as a necessary part of the business of being a woman, so still they pass through one week of discomfort in every month usually without complaining to their doctors but not necessarily without disturbing the tranquility of their homes."

Is there any relationship between premenstrual tension and stress? The great tendency to retain water, the predisposition for various allergic and

hypersensitivity reactions, the occasional occurrence of convulsive seizures, vascular disturbances, and rheumatic-like pains are, of course,
very reminiscent of the DOC intoxication syndrome. I might add that our DOC-overdosed monkeys also probably suffered from severe headaches
prior to the convulsive fits. At least I think so,
because they usually retired to a corner of the
cage, holding their heads between their hands; the
facial expression was one of intense pain, and their
attitudes quite unmistakably suggesting migraine. Autopsy of animals which died during these
spells revealed intense congestion and swelling of
the brain.

It is also of interest that, among all the drugs
with which I have so far tried to combat the DOC
syndrome in animals, ammonium chloride proved
to be most effective—presumably because this salt
washes out sodium and therefore acts like a salt-
free diet. It deprives DOC, the mineralocorticoid, of
sodium, the mineral substance through which this
hormone normally appears to act. In this manner it
helps to decongest and dehydrate the swollen tissues, including the brain. Now, interestingly, in
women with the premenstrual syndrome, ammonium chloride (7½—15 grains, about three times a
day during a fortnight preceding the period) is
often also very effective, especially if the patients
are at the same time using as little kitchen salt as
possible in their food. Furthermore, certain sex
hormones and antimineralocorticoids (such as spi-
ronolactone) and other diuretics which alter mineral metabolism and which we found to influence

the DOC syndrome in animals, affect the premenstrual syndrome of women essentially the same way. All these considerations led the Pakistani journal *Medicus* to state editorially that the "syndrome in our opinion should be designated as 'premenstrual stress,' because it represents a derailment of the general adaptation syndrome."

Be this as it may, there certainly are striking similarities between the manifestations of experimental DOC overdosage in animals, aldosteronism, eclampsia, and premenstrual tension in women. It would seem rewarding, therefore, to explore further the part played by adaptive hormones in this common and important derangement, so that we may perfect our means for treating it.

Digestive Diseases

The gastrointestinal tract is particularly sensitive to general stress. Loss of appetite is one of the first symptoms in the great "syndrome of just being sick," and this may be accompanied by vomiting, diarrhea, or constipation. Signs of *irritation and upset of the digestive organs* may occur in any type of emotional stress. This is well-known, not only to soldiers who experienced it during the tense expectation of battle, but even to the students who pace the floor before my door, waiting—with, I assure you, much less justified but almost equally great tenseness—for their turn in oral examinations.

It is also common knowledge that *gastric and duodenal ulcers* are most likely to occur in people who are somewhat maladjusted to their work or family life and suffer from constant tension and frustration. These chronic peptic (that is, digestive) ulcers are perhaps not quite the same as the acute, bleeding surface defects which developed in the lining of the stomach and duodenum during the alarm reaction in our rats. Still, even such acute ulcers have their equivalents in man. People who have been severely burned often develop bleeding duodenal ulcers within a day or two after the accident. This condition was known in medicine as *Curling's ulcer* long before the discovery of the G.A.S.; but it always remained a mystery just why and through what pathways a skin burn could so affect the intestinal lining. During World War II, veritable epidemics of "air-raid ulcers" occurred in people living in some of the heavily blitzed cities of Great Britain. Immediately after an intense bombardment, an unusual number of people would appear in hospital, with bleeding gastric or duodenal ulcers which developed virtually overnight. Many of the affected persons had not been physically hurt in any way during the attack but, of course, they suffered the great stress of extreme emotional excitement.

With this background, it was not quite unexpected that, when ACTH and cortisone were introduced into clinical practice, in patients receiving large amounts of these stress hormones—say, for an inflammatory disease—preexistent gastrointestinal ulcers often became worse, and sometimes actually perforated through the gut. Indeed, even any latent tendency to develop such ulcers was prone to turn into manifest disease.

This revived my interest in the *mechanism*

through which the lining of the stomach defends itself against self-digestion. Meat is digested in the stomach; why does the gastric juice not digest the lining itself? This problem has occupied many generations of physiologists, but no definite solution was found. The great Russian physiologist Ivan Petrovich Pavlov (already mentioned in connection with his classic work on conditioned reflexes) thought that perhaps some antienzyme is formed in the lining which inactivates the digestive enzymes of the stomach. Another view held that any healthy living tissue is immune to attack by gastric juice. This, it was thought, would also explain the fact that the crater (the floor) of a gastric ulcer—which is denuded of its allegedly antienzyme-containing lining—normally remains resistant to gastric digestion.

I wondered whether perhaps, here again, the inflammatory pouch test could help us to understand the situation. It may seem odd to think that an inflammatory pouch, produced on the back of a rat, could give information about gastric digestion—but judge for yourself.

I first took some rats and made air sacs on their backs—in the usual manner, but without introducing an irritant. Immediately after this, I injected 5 cc of fresh gastric juice. The adjacent tissue of the skin was digested within a few hours. This proved that normal living tissue can be attacked by gastric juice.

Then I made a similar air sac, but injected some croton oil into it, so as to transform the lining into an inflammatory barricade before introducing the gastric juice into the cavity. Now no digestion of adjacent tissue occurred. This proved that the inflammatory tissue itself is an adequate barricade to protect against gastric digestion. Obviously, an inflammatory barricade, such as always paves the crater of gastric ulcers, is in itself adequate protection against digestion, under normal conditions.

Next I repeated exactly the same experiment (introducing the gastric juice into an inflammatory pouch whose lining was transformed into an inflammatory barricade by pretreatment with croton oil), but then exposed the animals to the frustrating immobilization test *(Fig. 29)*. Now I witnessed the singular phenomenon of a perforating peptic ulcer on the back of the rat. During stress—presumably due to the secretion of anti-inflammatory hormones—the barricade became so weakened that the gastric juice digested it easily. Apparently in man chronic gastric ulcers, which normally are well under control, also perforate during stress, because an excess of anti-inflammatory stimuli breaks down the resistance of the barricade.

Finally, to prove this theory, I repeated the last-mentioned experiment on adrenalectomized rats. Here the condition was exactly the same as before (an irritated pouch possessing a well-developed inflammatory barricade was exposed to the general stress of frustrating immobilization), but these animals had no adrenals which might have responded by increased anti-inflammatory hormone secretion. Now the pouch remained unaffected by the digestive juices even during stress. This was definite proof of adrenal participation in this type of tissue breakdown.

That essentially the same mechanism is involved

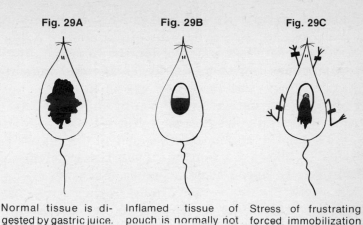

Fig. 29A	Fig. 29B	Fig. 29C

Normal tissue is digested by gastric juice.

Inflamed tissue of pouch is normally not digested by gastric juice.

Stress of frustrating forced immobilization causes perforating peptic ulcer on the pouch. Inflammatory fluid escapes.

in the production of peptic ulcers in man has been clearly shown by various physicians. Particularly instructive findings have been reported by Professor Harold G. Wolff, the well-known neurologist of Cornell University in New York. In a patient with a gastric fistula (an artificial opening through which the stomach can be directly seen), he observed that "during a period of prolonged emotional conflict involving hostility and resentment on the part of the patient," the lining of the stomach became engorged with blood and eventually began to bleed through minute erosions which formed on its surface.

The nerves of the stomach probably also play an important role in the formation of this kind of ulcer during stress; but the part played by adaptive hormones is likewise well established now. Dr. Seymour J. Gray, of the Peter Bent Brigham Hospital in Boston, furnished perhaps the most clear-cut evidence of this. He showed that patients under stress, or treated with anti-inflammatory hormones, excrete increased amounts of peptic digestive hormones in their urine. This would indicate that, through the intermediary of adaptive hormones, the resistance of the inflammatory barricade is not only weakened by stress, but, at the same time, the attacking influence of the digestive juices is increased because the stress hormones stimulate the production of peptic enzymes.

Of course, there are many other digestive diseases which can be influenced by stress and adaptive hormones. There would be no point in discussing them all here, but at least one more should be mentioned, and that is: *ulcerative colitis.* This—as the name implies—is an inflammatory disease of the colon (a part of the large intestine). It is characterized by bleeding intestinal ulcerations and, in fatal cases, the entire colon is almost invariably involved. The gut is denuded of its lining and death may then result from perforation or some other complication. It is often impossible to determine the cause of this disease, but physicians have always suspected that emotional tension plays an important role in its development. Significantly, this malady is often accompanied by signs of chronic rheumatism and, like the latter, it frequently responds very well to treatment with anti-inflammatory hormones.

Metabolic Diseases

Many of the so-called metabolic diseases are also largely diseases of adaptation. We have seen that

loss of weight is one of the most nonspecific consequences of chronic stress. It is due partly to loss of
appetite, but partly also to a kind of "self-combus-
tion" facilitated by a surplus of anti-inflammatory
hormones. In times of great stress, much caloric
energy is needed to face emergency demands and,
since food intake is usually diminished, it is very
important for the preservation of health that the
body should burn its own tissues to supply calories
for resistance. But, of course, if this goes on for a
long time, pathologic emaciation will result.

Conversely, excessive *obesity* may also be a manifestation of stress, especially in people with certain types of frustrating mental experiences. A
person who does not get enough satisfaction from
work or from his relations with other people may be
driven to find consolation in almost anything that
may provide comfort. This is just one aspect of the
general principle of *"deviation"* or diversion which
will be analyzed later (page 416). Some people are
driven to food just as others are driven to drink.
Many a person eats for lack of anything better to do,
or as an excuse for not doing anything better; besides, a stomach full of food also soothes by draining
the blood away from a disgruntled and maladapted
brain.

Of course, some people have such a strong hereditary predisposition to obesity that they become fat
even if they eat very little. Others become obese
because of some acquired organic disease in the
same brain region of adaptation (the hypothalamus) which also regulates pituitary activity. Still,
the large majority of fat people overeat because of
derailed adaptive reactions. Through this pattern

of response they hurt themselves in the same sense as a derailed hormonal adaptive reaction to tissue injury can predispose to inflammatory disease.

It is important to know that obesity can often be avoided by some self-analysis which may help the patient to stop overeating. Just how to do this will be explained later (page 405). Here I only want to point out that this is possible and certainly worthwhile, because obesity is not only deforming, but it also greatly increases the likelihood of contracting other diseases of adaptation, particularly hypertension and diabetes.

The predisposition to *diabetes* is also inherited, but it depends largely upon the way the body reacts to stress whether or not a latent diabetic tendency will develop into a manifest disease. The outstanding feature of diabetes is an increase in blood sugar, so that eventually much sugar spills over into the urine. Insulin is given to diabetics because this pancreatic hormone diminishes the blood sugar and improves its utilization as fuel for the tissues. This does not mean that diabetes is always due to an insufficiency of insulin formation. Often, it is caused by an excessive production of such adaptive hormones as ACTH, STH, or COL, all of which tend to raise the blood sugar. In fact, it has been possible to treat particularly insulin-resistant diabetics by removing their pituitary or adrenal glands. I have already mentioned the important work of Olivecrona and Luft, who had removed the pituitary in hypertensive diabetic patients and had obtained an amelioration of both the hypertension and the diabetes.

Hypoglycemia, an abnormally low blood sugar,

has also been considered to be a stress disease. It is usually associated with chronic fatigue. It has received perhaps somewhat excessive attention, especially in the USA. Many patients, and even physicians, ascribe the complaints of virtually anyone who chronically grumbles about having no energy to hypoglycemia. Since the GCs tend to augment sugar formation and raise the blood sugar level, these hormones have been recommended as a treatment for the "hypoglycemia chronic fatigue" syndrome.

Curiously, its proponents insist that crude adrenocortical extracts are more effective than the highly potent and purified GC preparations (cortisone, prednisone, prednisolone etc.) now on the market. Undoubtedly, the increased energy requirements created by any type of demand for adaptation can be expected to consume blood sugar, but this is unlikely to be the decisive factor in most cases of easy fatigability.

In connection with these disturbances in carbohydrate metabolism it is noteworthy that Dr. S. R. Bloom has recently summarized a good deal of evidence indicating that *glucagon*, an anti-insulin substance of the pancreas, is a "stress hormone." Stress increases energy requirements and creates a demand for an increased supply of energy-yielding glucose, which is satisfied by glucagon. In fact, a sudden rise in blood glucagon concentration has been demonstrated both in animals and in man under the influence of many stressors.

Hyperthyroidism is another disease which is often due to stress. Here, the thyroid gland becomes enlarged (goiter) and is driven to excessive activity by the thyroid-stimulating hormone of the pituitary (page 157). Sometimes this condition develops immediately after a particularly shocking mental experience; but in man the relationship between hyperthyroidism and stress is not always evident, because—probably due to differences in hereditary predisposition—only some people respond this way.

This whole problem was greatly clarified when Dr. J. Kracht of Borstel, Germany, discovered a breed of wild rabbits which regularly develop hyperthyroidism after being frightened, for instance by a barking dog. Here—presumably again due to some hereditary predisposition—the G.A.S. regularly derails, in the sense that the pituitary tends to produce an excessive amount of thyroid-stimulating hormone and correspondingly does not secrete enough ACTH. As a result of this, the thyroid enlarges and the eyes protrude, just as in certain hyperthyroid patients with Graves' disease or exophthalmic goiter. In fact, such rabbits may literally die from fear because of this abnormal endocrine response to stress.

There are also interesting relationships between stress and the *diseases of the liver*. It has been shown by Dr. Paul Lemonde at this Institute that during the alarm reaction the usual liver function tests reveal a marked hepatic insufficiency. This finding was of particular interest to stress research, because the corticoids are normally metabolized and destroyed in the liver. I first observed this in connection with the hormone anesthesia studies (page 249). At that time nothing definite was known about the way corticoids were destroyed in our tissues, but since the liver had always been regarded as the "central chemical laboratory of the body," it was reasonable to suspect that this organ might play an important role in corticoid metabolism. To prove this, I injected the same amount of DOC into intact rats and into animals from which I had first surgically removed three-quarters of the liver. It turned out that an amount of DOC which caused little or no anesthesia in the intact animal produced long and profound sleep after most of the liver had been eliminated. Volatile anesthetics (ether, for instance) do not produce more intense sleep in liver-deficient than in intact rats. It was assumed that DOC-like hormones are normally destroyed by the liver, so that they remain in the blood longer when hepatic function is artificially cut down.

These findings have been confirmed with a variety of techniques in other animals, but it is mainly thanks to the biochemical investigations of Professor L. T. Samuels of Salt Lake City that we learned to appreciate the important part played by the liver in destroying excesses of corticoids in healthy and diseased people. He has shown, for instance, that, in certain clinical liver diseases (such as cirrhosis, or morbid scar formation in the liver), the metabolism of corticoids is often deranged and excesses can be found in the blood and urine.

It is also obvious that, if during the alarm reaction, hepatic function is diminished, the disposal of corticoids must be impeded. This is one mechanism of conditioning through which the body can aug-

ment corticoid activity during stress. By diminishing the normal destruction of these hormones, a
given amount secreted by the adrenals can last
longer and do more good.

The importance of the liver in determining resistance to a great variety of toxic substances has
become particularly evident with the discovery of
the catatoxic steroids (see pages 84, 114, 408). As we
have explained, these substances induce a variety
of detoxifying enzymes capable of inactivating
many damaging substances which circulate in the
blood.

To illustrate the manifold relationships between
metabolic and inflammatory diseases, let me mention just one more derangement of metabolism,
gout, in which inflammation and maladaptation
appear to play important roles. This is yet another
example of a disease in which both hereditary predisposition and stress are involved. Gout is essentially a derangement of uric acid metabolism, with
the deposition of uric acid crystals in and around
the joints. It tends to run in families, and
extremely painful spells of it occur, frequently
after some stress, especially in the joints of the big
toe. The uric acid deposits act as local irritants and
the pain is due to excessive inflammation around
them.

Here again, treatment with anti-inflammatory
corticoids has proved to be of great value. It is not
yet quite clear why attacks of gout tend to occur
immediately after (not during) stress, but most
probably, a derailment of hormonal defense reactions is at least partly responsible for this condition.

Cancer

We still know very little about the possible relationship between stress and cancer. This is the way I would sum up what little we have managed to find out:

Many types of cancer develop at sites of chronic tissue injury. Prolonged exposure of the skin to sunrays or heat may lead to cancer formation at the place of irritation. In an inveterate pipe-smoker, cancer of the lip tends to develop at the place where he holds his pipe. The interesting statistical studies of Dr. F. Gagnon of Quebec City have shown that cancer of the entrance to the womb is virtually never observed among cloistered nuns, although it is quite common in married women, especially after repeated childbirth.

Experimentally, it has been possible to produce extremely malignant cancers by chronic irritation with croton oil in the inflammatory pouch.

These, and many other personal observations, have led Dr. J. Ernest Ayre of the Cancer Institute at Miami, Florida, to conclude, in his editorial in *Obstetrics and Gynecology* (June, 1955), that cancer production is an abnormal consequence of the local adaptation syndrome to tissue injury.

On the other hand, *general stress tends to suppress cancerous growth.* The progress of various types of clinical and experimental cancers is often greatly retarded during stress elicited by infections, intoxications, and various drugs which cause much nonspecific damage.

It has also been possible to *inhibit the growth of*

certain cancers by treatment with large doses of anti-inflammatory hormones. One of the salient actions of these substances is to diminish the response to local injury. Now, if cancer really represents a morbid response to tissue damage, it is understandable that the hormones which induce tissues to ignore injury should interfere with cancer production.

ACTH and COL have proved to be particularly effective in slowing down lymphatic cancers and the *leukemias*, certain of which are essentially cancers of the white blood cells. Interestingly, during the alarm reaction and after treatment with anti-inflammatory hormones, the growth of lymphatic tissues and of certain white blood cells (lymphocytes, eosinophils) proved to be most intensely inhibited (page 23).

There are many other observations which suggest *some dependence, at least of certain cancers, upon the adrenals.* The important observations of Professor Charles Huggins of Chicago have made it clear that removal of the adrenals can greatly delay the growth of some cancers, especially those of the male and female sex organs. This would suggest that there are adrenal factors which actually stimulate cancer formation.

It should be clearly understood, however, that all these are isolated observations which merely indicate some relationship between stress, the adaptive hormones, and cancer; these findings are sufficiently suggestive to justify further research from this new point of view, but not yet to formulate any coherent theory.

Diseases of Resistance in General

By *general resistance* I mean the ability to remain healthy—or at least alive—during intense stress caused nonspecifically by various agents. The most nonspecific breakdown of resistance is the condition which we call *shock*. A person who has been seriously burned, wounded, poisoned, or otherwise gravely damaged may develop a syndrome in which the blood pressure drops so much that the pulse can hardly be felt, the temperature falls way below normal, and the patient may even become unconscious. This often ends in death, without obvious selective injury to any one of the vital organs. This is what makes shock an eminently nonspecific stress condition. Accordingly, in such cases, autopsy reveals the characteristic triad of the alarm reaction: adrenocortical enlargement, thymicolymphatic atrophy, and bleeding erosions in the gastrointestinal tract. There can be no doubt about this being a disease of adaptation; it is due to a breakdown of the body's defenses in general rather than to the specific action of any one particular pathogen.

Treatment with corticoids has proven beneficial in certain cases; but it is not always effective, because a lack of corticoids is not the usual cause of the breakdown in shock. Presumably, during extreme stress, in most people, the pituitary-adrenal system performs optimally anyway; only occasionally (for instance, in very severe burns and infections) is it inactivated by exhaustive overstimulation, and it is especially in such cases that corticoid therapy has proven to be effective.

A special kind of what we now call a disease of adaptation was described by Thomas Addison in his famous treatise, *On the Constitutional and Local Effects of Diseases of the Suprarenal Capsule* (the adrenal), more than a century ago (in 1855). Addison worked at Guy's Hospital in London, just as did Richard Bright, who discovered Bright's disease a quarter of a century earlier (see page 185).

Addison's disease is due to a destruction of the adrenals, and one of its most outstanding consequences is an almost total breakdown of resistance. Patients with Addison's disease are not hypersensitive to any one thing in particular, but to virtually any change in and around them. Any infection, intoxication, or exposure to cold, nervous tension, or fatigue can put these people into a state of shock, in which they usually die unless suitable treatment with corticoids is given. Nowadays people whose adrenals are removed (say, for the treatment of cancer or extreme hypercorticoidism) become continuously dependent upon treatment with corticoids, because an artificial Addison's disease is produced in them by this operation. In Addison's disease, the thymus and the other lymphatic organs tend to become very large. Both in human patients and in animals, it is the lack of corticoids which prevents the shrinkage of lymphatic tissues during stress. We still do not know, however, whether the decline in resistance to stress has anything to do with this irresponsiveness of the lymphatic organs.

A somewhat related, but at this time still very mysterious condition is known as the *thymicolymphatic state*. It usually occurs in apparently healthy boys and girls. Such children may never have shown any indication of disease until, suddenly, after some slight stress (say, a plunge into cold water) they die instantly without any warning. Even autopsy reveals no obvious derangement, except that the adrenal cortex is small and the thymicolymphatic tissues are overdeveloped. It is reasonable to suspect that the low stress resistance of these children is due to some deficiency in the adrenal cortex, but this has never been proved.

It is now well-established that the thymus plays a crucial role in immunologic defense reactions such as the development of serologic resistance against microbes or the rejection of foreign grafts. It still remains a mystery, however, to what extent, if any, the thymus atrophy characteristic of the stress response decisively affects these phenomena.

Malformations and Aging

There is good evidence that exposure of pregnant women to unusually severe stressors may cause developmental anomalies and *malformations* in their fetuses, even if it does not lead to abortion. This phenomenon has been called the "syndrome of transmission." Similar changes have been produced experimentally in various animals.

It has also been claimed that, among the newborn infants of foreign women employed in Germany as "guest workers" during an economic

boom period, the malformation rate was unusually
high, and this has been ascribed to the stressor
effect of relocation into an unusual environment.
Similarly, a statistical study on a relatively small
sample of mongoloid children in Prague was interpreted as indicating that emotional stress during
pregnancy predisposes the embryo to this type of
idiocy.

In guinea pigs and mice exposed to heat during
certain stages of pregnancy, embryonic mortality
and malformations—particularly brain damage—
were often detectable. Various malformations of
the brain have also been reported in the offspring
of pregnant mice kept under extremely crowded
conditions.

Aging itself—and particularly premature
aging—is, in a sense, due to the constant, and eventually exhausting, stresses of life. But since I have
spoken of aging elsewhere (see pages 427-433), I
mention it here merely for the sake of completeness.

chapter 13

"When Scientists Disagree"

On scientific debate.   Debates about the stress concept.

On Scientific Debate

In the last three chapters I have tried to outline how we arrived at the concept of the "diseases of adaptation." To do this I had to correlate my own experiments on animals with clinical observations on the role of stress and of the adaptive hormones in the production and treatment of disease. The concepts of stress and of the adaptive hormones have had a definite influence upon the progress of contemporary medicine, and the observations reported here can easily be verified. But this is not a textbook of medicine and I have made no attempt to give a complete list of all the diseases influenced by stress and by adaptive hormones. Consequently, my selection of data may well be criticized. I have discussed only some of those maladies in which, to my mind, a derailment of adaptive reactions plays a particularly important role, and I have listed only the evidence which convinced me of this. It is hardly unexpected, therefore, that many physicians—and among them some highly competent ones—do not agree with certain aspects of my theory. My presentation of my concepts would lack the impartiality which must always guide medical research if I did not also present the views of those who disagree. Doing so necessarily implies a discussion of conflicting personal opinions—and the cold precision of provable fact ends where opinion begins.

Some of my friends have advised me not to mention dissident opinions in this book, because controversies among scientists would only confuse the general reader and could hardly hold much interest for him. I disagree. I think anyone sufficiently interested in medical research in general—or in stress in particular—to read this book would want to make up his own mind about the issues at stake. In any event, he will learn more about what is in doubt if the views of the opposition are not censored. I shall spare no effort to describe all major causes of contention in an understandable manner, because, to my mind, no one can really grasp the essence of research without trying to comprehend the reasons for disagreement among scientists.

Toward the end of his life, W. B. Cannon—the great American physiologist whose work has so markedly influenced my own—wrote a semibiographic book about his investigations. He knew from bitter personal experience what it means to be the target of constant, violent attacks by other scientists; this is probably why he wanted to tell the public something about the human element in research. In *The Way of an Investigator* (W. W. Norton & Company, 1945), he reminds us that, after all, science is the product of people, of scientists. Scientists, like all people, possess not only intellectual and technical skills, but also emotions; they

can be happy or angry, honored or humiliated.
Some scientists keep their emotions and motives to
themselves; others regard them as inherent parts
of investigative activity, which should not be suppressed if a research project is to be fully evaluated
for the benefit of future investigators.

Cannon devoted an entire chapter of his book to
debates about his work. He entitled it, "When Scientists Disagree." It is a remarkably instructive
and inspiring chapter and I could not resist the
temptation of using this same caption for the
thoughts I would like to put before you here. Not
only Cannon's work, but also his way of life, have
been a great inspiration to me, and I am certain—
were he here today—he would not mind my bor-
rowing his title for the use I want to make of it.

Cannon consoled himself for having been so
much attacked with the thought that original scientists have always been the victims of vicious
criticisms, and often by highly competent colleagues. He points out, for instance, what happened to one of his distinguished predecessors
among the professors of physiology at Harvard.
When Oliver Wendell Holmes, Sr., was still a very
young physician, he presented evidence that
childbed fever "is so far contagious as to be frequently carried from patient to patient by physicians and nurses." Meigs, a prominent and much
older Philadelphia obstetrician, contemptuously
commented on this foolish suggestion of "some
scribbler," and declared that he was not impressed
by the opinions of "very young gentlemen."
Instead of weighing the evidence judiciously,
Meigs righteously declared: "I prefer to attribute

cases of childbed fever to accident or Providence, of which I can form a conception, rather than to a contagion, of which I cannot form any clear idea." This must have sounded very cautious and proper at the time; but the fact is that young Holmes was right and Meigs was wrong. Ignaz Philipp Semmelweis, the Hungarian obstetrician who subsequently proved the contagious nature of this disease, saved the lives of countless mothers by prescribing antisepsis in the delivery room. Yet even this great benefactor of humanity was so violently attacked and ridiculed by his peers that he eventually became mentally deranged.

In discussing these problems, Cannon did not refer to himself, but the intimate feelings of the much criticized Father of Homeostasis come through to the reader when he mildly adds: "Any aspersions, any slurs cast upon the skill or ability or the personal uprightness of the man whose work is being corrected are sure to stir resentment."

Cannon was my first critic. I can still vividly remember his reaction when—just after having completed my initial experiments on stress—I talked to him about them. We discussed stress twice: first briefly, when I visited his laboratory in Boston, and again a few years later, in more leisurely fashion, in the Faculty Club of McGill University, just after he had delivered a remarkable lecture to our students. I felt quite frustrated at not being able to convince the Great Old Man of the important role played by the pituitary and the adrenal cortex in my stress syndrome. He gave me excellent reasons why he did not think these glands could help resistance and adaptation in gen-

eral and even why it would seem unlikely that a
general adaptation syndrome could exist. But
there was no trace of aggressiveness in his criticisms, no sting that could have blurred my vision to
the point of refusing to listen. His comments only
sharpened my eye for the limitations in the part
played by the pituitary-adrenal axis during stress.
They helped me, among other things, by inspiring
experiments which established that certain stress
manifestations could still be produced in the
absence of this gland system.

Of course, even the most objective scientist is not
infallible. One of the greatest physicists of all
times, Michael Faraday, said, "That I may be
largely wrong I am free to admit—who can be right
altogether in physical science, which is essentially
progressive and corrective?" This is, of course, even
more true in a less precise science, such as medicine. A detached analytic debate helps to point out
and correct errors; but criticism must always
remain objective. It should be offered in the
friendly tone which behooves colleagues in the
same field of learning, who merely want to promote
science by mutual constructive advice. Above all,
debate must, as far as our human limitations permit, not be directed by considerations of personal
prestige. The question is not, "*Who* is right?" but,
"*What* is right?" An old Hebrew proverb maintains
that "the envy of scholars will increase wisdom."
Even debate inspired by jealousy can stimulate
research; but it is less efficient and certainly less
pleasant than cooperation.

Great progress can be made only by ideas which
are very different from those generally accepted at

the time. Unfortunately, it is not only literally true that the more someone sticks out his neck above the masses, the more he is likely to attract the eyes of snipers. "The new truth," says Jacques Barzun, "invariably sounds crazy, and crazier in proportion to its greatness. It would be idiocy to keep recounting the stories of Copernicus, Galileo, and Pasteur, and forget that the next time the innovator will seem as hopelessly wrong and perverse as these men seemed." (*Teacher in America*, Doubleday Anchor Book, 1955.)

Very few fundamentally new ideas manage to by-pass the heresy stage. Among the really outstanding discoveries, only procedures which have immediate and important practical applications are relatively immune to violent criticisms at the start. This is illustrated by the discovery that penicillin (Fleming, Florey, and Chain), streptomycin (Waksman), and the sulfonamides (Domagk) have marked antibacterial actions, that antihistamines can suppress allergies (Halpern), or that ACTH and cortisone are useful in combating arthritis (Hench and Kendall). Although all these were truly great contributions to knowledge, they have stimulated only minor debates, mostly about limitations of the usefulness and about the damaging side-effects of these remedies.

On the other hand, a new concept in biology, such as Darwin's theory of evolution, is almost certain to provoke what Huxley called a "public war dance."

When Pasteur proclaimed that infectious diseases were due to germs, when Clemens P. Pirquet and Charles R. Richet discovered allergy, the literature was full of biting, hostile remarks, in which those who did not have the originality of creating—or even understanding—new concepts in medicine, tried to compensate by displaying their wit.

In his biography of Freud, Ernest Jones points out that the psychiatrist Walther Spielmeyer had, at first, denounced the use of psychoanalysis as "mental masturbation." Indeed, by 1910 the mere mention of Freud's theories was enough to start Professor Wilhelm Weygandt—then chairman of a medical congress in Hamburg—to bang his fist and shout: "This is not a topic for discussion at a scientific meeting; it is a matter for the police." (*The Life and Work of Sigmund Freud*, Basic Books, 1955.)

Even the greatest physicians may, especially as they grow older, become quite blind to new concepts. A much-quoted example of this was the unqualified rejection, by the great pathologist Rudolf Virchow, of young Robert Koch's theory that the little rods he saw under the microscope were the cause of tuberculosis.

Of course, the more uncontroversial discoveries, the finding of facts immediately applicable to practical medicine, can be made empirically, that is, through observation and experiment, more or less by chance, without using any theory. But this is rare; you cannot count on it. Such discoveries are like winning a fortune on a lottery ticket; no matter how great the practical gain, the accomplishment is immediately finished and offers no promise of future success at the same game. "The history of science demonstrates beyond a doubt that the really revolutionary and significant advances come

not from empiricism but from new theories."
(James B. Conant, *Modern Science and Modern
Man,* Doubleday Anchor Book, 1952.)

On the other hand, it is equally true that most
great theories originate from chance discoveries
made empirically by people who intuitively feel
which new fact lends itself particularly well to the
construction of a fruitful new concept.

Some scientists make important, immediately
applicable discoveries, using the technique of sheer
trial and error, somewhat as the old-fashioned
inventors used to work. This becomes increasingly
less profitable in modern medicine; even when in
the past the discoverer himself did not have to
formulate a theory to arrive at a result, he was
almost invariably guided by current concepts previously formulated by others.

So theories are indispensable. They stimulate
controversy, but this is all to the good because it
brings out the weak points in our concepts, showing where further research is needed. Even a theory that does not fit all the known facts is valuable,
as long as it fits them better than any other concept. To quote Conant: "We can put it down as
one of the principles learned from the history of
science that a theory is only overthrown by a better theory, never merely by contradictory facts."
(*On Understanding Science,* Mentor Book, New
American Library, 1953.)

It is not true that "exceptions strengthen the
rule," but they do not necessarily invalidate it
either. Sometimes facts which at first seem to be
quite incompatible with a theory gradually find
their natural place in it when more facts come to
light. In other cases the theory is sufficiently plas-

tic to be readily adjusted, so as to cover apparently paradoxical, incongruous new observations. As I ventured to say elsewhere, "the best theory is that which necessitates the minimum amount of assumptions to unite a maximum number of facts, since it is most likely to possess the power of assimilating new facts from the unknown without damage to its own structure." (*Second Annual Report on Stress*, Acta Inc., 1952.)

There is a great difference between a sterile theory and a wrong one. A sterile theory does not lend itself to experimental verification. Any number of these can easily be formulated to explain virtually anything, but they are perfectly useless; they lead only to futile verbiage. A wrong theory, on the other hand, can still be highly useful, for, if it is well-conceived, it may help to formulate experiments which will necessarily fill important gaps in our knowledge.

During the last century, the great French neurologist, Pierre Marie, discovered that, in certain kinds of giants (called *acromegalics*), the pituitary is completely replaced by cancer. He immediately formulated the theory that the pituitary produces some growth-inhibiting hormone, since destruction of this gland results in overgrowth. This theory was not only wrong, it was exactly the opposite of the truth. Actually, the pituitary produces STH which, as we have said, is a growth hormone. Now, the cancers Marie saw did replace the pituitary, but they did not destroy its activity; on the contrary, they consisted exclusively of abnormal pituitary cells which produced an excess of STH. Marie's interpretation could not have been farther from the truth. Yet it was his wrong, but highly

fertile, theory which first called attention to an
unsuspected, yet very real, relationship between
the little gland under the brain and the growth of
our tissues in general. The original faulty interpretation was later adjusted by Marie himself to fit
the known facts. To do so, he actually had to
reverse his first formulation; still, it should be
remembered that it was the initial wrong theory—
not the corrected modification—which acted as a
starting point for research on the endocrine activity of the pituitary. It was this line of research
which, when carried forward by subsequent investigators such as H. M. Evans, P. Smith, B. A. Houssay, J. B. Collip, C. H. Li, and A. E. Wilhelmi, eventually led to the isolation of highly-purified STH
from animal glands and the analysis of its chemical
structure.

Science cannot be fully appraised without understanding scientists. The way a person sees a thing
depends equally upon the person and the thing.
The motives and consequences of scientific debates
are of paramount importance to the creative investigator: and hence to his investigation. This is one
reason why I thought I should discuss these points
at length in this section. Besides, the same considerations also apply to debates about facts and theories touching everyday life; in this sense they concern everybody directly.

Debates about the Stress Concept*

Many of the objections to the concept of stress and
of the diseases of adaptation which have played a

*These debates are described in greater detail in my mono-
graph: *From Dream to Discovery*, McGraw-Hill, 1964, and Arno
Press, 1975.

major role between 1936 (when my first paper on
stress appeared) and 1956 (when the first edition of
this book was published) now seem completely
unfounded; since they no longer have any proponents the reader may feel that they could have
been eliminated in the present edition. Yet I kept
this section virtually unaltered, because I think
that it is most instructive, especially for young
scientists and those interested in the history of the
new ideas, to review them in retrospect and learn
from the simple errors in logic that can delay progress.

As far as I know, no one today would doubt that
there are such things as stress, a G.A.S., diseases of
adaptation and a difference between GCs and MCs;
nor would they continue to claim that MCs are not
secreted by the adrenal under any circumstances
but represent artificial products, etc. Yet, each of
these problems has been raised by competent
investigators.

Let us first take the principal arguments which
have stood in the way of acceptance of this concept
in the past; then we shall turn to the gaps which
still remain in the theory and hence represent
fruitful fields for further investigation.

What is new in this concept? At first, several
investigators actually denied the very existence of
the G.A.S.; others thought that these three letters
functioned merely as a new catchword for something that had been definitely proven long ago.
These two criticisms could not both be right. Since
the first no longer has any serious proponents nowadays, we shall consider only the second.

Almost every nation and every specialty of medi-

cine has mustered at least one biologic reaction
which, at one time or another, has been claimed to
be identical with the G.A.S.: the so-called *irritation syndrome*, described by the French bacteriologist Reilly; the *vegetative reorientation* of the
German internist Hoff; the defense through *conditioned reflexes*, so ably explored by the eminent
Russian physiologist Pavlov; the *defensive neurosis* theory of the Austrian psychiatrist Freud;
the hippocratic concept of *pónos*, which dominated
ancient Greek medical thought; and Cannon's
emergency reaction, are only a few representative
examples. We could add an almost endless list of
scattered observations, which have been made so
often and by so many people that they were never
attributed to any one author in particular. For instance, it had long been common knowledge that
animals infected with diphtheria usually have
large *adrenals*, that one or another drug can produce *gastric ulcers*, that in children the thymus can
undergo *accidental involution* under the influence
of this or that agent. Then there are all those *shock
therapies* and *"nonspecific therapies"* about which
we spoke in Book I. But the G.A.S., the stress syndrome, could not very well be identical with all
these individual observations, since they are certainly very different from each other.

Many of these earlier findings are of paramount
importance in themselves and, in retrospect, it is
easy to see that they are all somehow related to the
G.A.S. After what we have said about the ubiquity
of stress, it is clear that no human being could have
failed to note some of its individual manifestations.
The chief value of the G.A.S. concept is precisely

that it gives a *common basis which unifies all these, hitherto apparently unrelated, observations.*

Of course, you could say that the first cave man who saw lightning had already observed what later merely received the catchword *electricity.* The first woman who made her hair crackle by combing it vigorously even knew how to generate electricity at will. Yet these, as all other early observations on electric phenomena, remained puzzling, disconnected curiosities, because they could not be subjected to quantitative scientific study until Galvani began to define the basic concept which gave them unity.

Are experimental observations on animals applicable to man? Some reactions of animals just do not occur in man. For instance, it is impossible to study the effects of vitamin C deficiency in the rat. The tissues of this animal can make vitamin C themselves, but a human being is dependent upon the dietary ingestion of this foodstuff because his body cannot make it. Each species has its own peculiarities. Yet, the whole of *experimental medicine is based upon the fact that most of the fundamental biologic reactions are essentially the same in man and in other mammals.* This is true not only of bodily responses but also of the psychologic and behavioral lessons that we have tried to develop from our observations on cellular and molecular reactions in Book V. In this respect the G.A.S. is no exception.

First, take the *manifestations of stress.* The adrenal changes caused by various stressors are quite similar in man and in the usual laboratory

animals. The same is true of other manifestations
of stress, for instance, of the characteristic disappearance of blood eosinophils, the involution of
lymphatic tissues, the increased urinary elimination of corticoids, and the inhibition of inflammation. All these changes occur both in laboratory
animals and in man during acute stress.

Now take the *actions of adaptive hormones*. In all
species, including man, removal of the adrenals
greatly decreases resistance to stress, and treatment with corticoids can again restore it toward
normal. The anti-inflammatory adrenal hormones
(such as cortisone) inhibit inflammation, while the
proinflammatory corticoids (such as DOC) and the
adrenalines raise the blood pressure. All this has
proved to be true in man just as in laboratory
animals.

Finally, since the mechanism of the *diseases of
adaptation* was worked out in animal experiments,
it had been questioned whether it would be essentially the same in man. Is it possible actually to
prove, for instance, that an inappropriate secretion
of pituitary or adrenal hormones can become the
decisive factor in the development of diverse
diseases due to hitherto unidentified causes? Can
we combat any spontaneous disease of man with
such a concept as a guide? I believe all this has
been answered most eloquently by the work of
those clinicians who showed us how to treat so
many apparently unrelated maladies of cryptic origin with ACTH, corticoids, hypophysectomy,
adrenalectomy, or salt-poor diets.

*Is there really an increase in corticoid pro-
duction during stress?* After all I have said, you

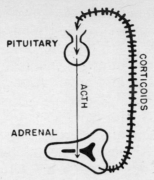

Fig. 30 ACTH stimulates the corticoid secretion of the adrenals; the corticoids inhibit the ACTH secretion of the pituitary.

may feel that there could hardly be any doubt about it. Well, the fact is that, even as late as 1954, some competent investigators still doubted the existence of a real increase in corticoid secretion during the alarm reaction.

This is why, if a patient receives large amounts of cortisone his adrenals involute, because the greater the concentration of corticoids in the blood, the less ACTH is produced by the pituitary. There evidently exists some sort of a *feedback mechanism* through which the corticoids automatically depress the secretion of that amount of ACTH which normally stimulates the adrenals to produce corticoids. This arrangement (illustrated in *Fig. 30)* is very important to maintain a steady corticoid concentration in the blood under basal conditions.

It had been claimed a few years ago that— because of this self-regulation—a real increase of corticoids in the blood could never develop during stress. This feedback mechanism would necessarily prevent a rise, just as the thermostat in an air conditioning system protects a room against overheating, even if the outside temperature rises.

Years ago, the well-known American physiologist Dwight J. Ingle discovered this self-regulating mechanism through which the adrenals normally protect themselves against overstimulation. Since that time, there has never been any doubt about the existence of such a feedback arrangement. But, as I found to my surprise in 1940, *during stress this moderator system is largely bypassed*. It turned out that the alarm signals (discharged from the various cells of our tissues during stress) can stimulate ACTH secretion, even when the concentration of corticoids in the blood reaches the highest attainable levels. This, incidentally, is most fortunate because much more than the normal blood concentration of corticoids is necessary to maintain life during stress. If the feedback mechanism were perfect we could never survive a seriously stressful experience. Besides, there are evident signs of corticoid excess during stress. There is, for instance, an inhibition of inflammation, a tendency for the spreading of infections, an involution of the lymphatic organs, and so forth.

To circumvent this difficulty, those who were still reluctant to accept my concept brought up another possibility. They said that, despite all this, the secretion of corticoids may not be actually increased; perhaps these hormones merely become more effective during stress. Of course, the activity of these hormones can be augmented by certain metabolic changes—the so-called *conditioning factors*—which sensitize our tissues to corticoids. This conditioning undoubtedly does occur in stress, but it cannot explain everything. Surely the adrenal enlargement and the chemically-demonstrable increase in the corticoid content of the blood are sufficient proof that, during stress, there is also a real increase in adrenocortical activity.

The "unitarian theory" of adrenocortical function. Although fractions possessing mineralo-corticoid activity had been prepared from cattle adrenals some forty years ago (F. Hartman, E. C. Kendall, T. Reichstein), most of the experts believed, even as late as 1952, that the adrenal does not actually secrete such compounds. It was thought, in line with the "unitarian theory" of adrenocortical function, that only the glucocorti-coid type of life-maintaining hormone is actually poured into the blood. The other corticoids which had been extracted from adrenals were assumed to be mere precursors of hormones, stored in the glands but not released into the circulation.

This theory greatly handicapped progress by branding as futile any search for new corticoids in the blood. Yet, unfortunately, it enjoyed great popularity because it was supported by two seemingly weighty arguments: (1) with the techniques available at that time only glucocorticoid activity was demonstrable in the blood; (2) after adrenalectomy the signs of adrenal insufficiency were thought to be perfectly corrected by COL (a glucocorticoid); the body did not seem to need anything else.

Had these conclusions been correct, they would have invalidated my theory that diseases can be due to excessive mineralocorticoid activity. *In the light of the unitarian theory, DOC and other miner-*

alocorticoids were considered to be wholly-artificial compounds, and consequently my experiments with these substances were claimed to have no bearing upon clinical problems. For instance, the renal and vascular lesions which I had produced in animals with DOC were attributed to some allergy against this "unnatural compound," or to some infection which I might have introduced accidentally together with the DOC.

Later, my coworkers and I reproduced the same renal and cardiovascular changes by treating animals with pituitary extracts (rich in STH), with a distant relative of DOC (called MAD), or even with stressors (for instance, cold). Significantly, all these agents also caused histologic signs of adrenal stimulation. The opponents of my views immediately took this to mean that the effect of DOC is not specific and has nothing to do with its mineralocorticoid properties. Evidently many things can act like DOC, but there was one important difference: only DOC produced disease even when the adrenals were surgically removed. This compound—unlike the other agents (pituitary extract, MAD, cold)—evidently does not act through the adrenals.

We concluded that, *under the influence of various treatments, some DOC-like mineralocorticoids can be produced by the adrenals* of the intact rat; the adrenalectomized animals are saved from disease simply because in them, the source of these damaging hormones is removed. No alternative explanation was offered by anyone, but many physicians still did not feel they could go along with my interpretation because it was contrary to the "unitarian theory."

The unitarian theory eventually lost its basis. First, using perfected techniques, *aldosterone*, a typical mineralocorticoid, was detected both in the tissue of the adrenals and in the blood which leaves these glands (S. A. Simpson, J. F. Tait, T. Reichstein). Second, it became evident, as time went by, that adrenalectomized patients were not as well maintained on cortisone alone as when they were also given small amounts of DOC or aldosterone. Third, MCs related to DOC (e.g., 18-OH-DOC) were detected in body fluids. Fourth, a natural disease (Conn's syndrome) was discovered in patients whose adrenals secreted an excess of aldosterone.

Now, of course, nobody could doubt any longer that *mineralocorticoids are natural hormones* of the adrenals, but it took much work on the part of a great many scientists to get that far. These investigators persisted in their search despite the discouraging effect of the unitarian theory. Why did they try so assiduously to isolate this aldosterone rather than any one of the many other suspected, but still undiscovered, hormones? The effort would hardly have seemed worthwhile if the goal had been merely to prepare yet another DOC-like compound. On the other hand, any effort to learn more about mineralocorticoids was certainly justified to prove whether these hormones really do play a decisive role in the production of the most commonly fatal wear-and-tear diseases of mankind, such as the cardiovascular and renal diseases.

How much DOC is too much? Another reason for doubts about the clinical implications of my work was that I had to use very large amounts of

DOC to produce disease manifestations. It was held that such enormous quantities could never be secreted by the adrenals, in health or disease.

Well, first of all, *it was disease we produced with DOC so that the dosages used were naturally incompatible with health.* Moreover, nobody knew how much the adrenals could produce during disease. In view of this, who could tell how much was too much? If I wanted to see whether an excess of this hormone would produce disease, I had to give an excess. The appropriate amount, I thought, was that which would give us an experimental reproduction of some known human malady.

In any case, this objection also lost its basis as new facts came to light. It turned out, for example, that the same *disease manifestations can be induced with much less DOC than I had originally given,* provided the compound is administered not by injection of solutions but by the implantation of solid hormone pellets. From these the hormone is taken up very constantly into the blood and this probably corresponds much more closely to the way the adrenals would continuously secrete it. Injections suddenly flood the body with DOC, but between treatments the hormone content of the blood is not kept very high.

Apart from this, *the natural mineralocorticoid, aldosterone, proved to be much more potent than DOC,* so that the adrenals would have to produce comparatively little of it to cause a severe overdosage. Finally, it was found a few years ago that many patients with demonstrably-increased aldosterone production often suffer from kidney damage (nephrosis, nephrosclerosis), just as the theory predicted (see page 201).

In view of all this, there can hardly be any question today about the ability of the adrenals to secrete large amounts of mineralocorticoids. Furthermore, adrenal hyperfunction in disease can induce the same kind of cardiovascular and kidney damage in man that DOC produces in animals. Finally, removal of the adrenals has had a curative value in patients suffering from such diseases, prior to the development of various useful drugs which counteract the resulting damage.

Can there really be an imbalance between anti- and proinflammatory corticoids? In 1949 the extraordinary anti-inflammatory effectiveness of ACTH and cortisone was first demonstrated in patients with rheumatoid arthritis. In view of the animal experiments which had demonstrated the proinflammatory effect of DOC, this new observation supported the idea that an imbalance between two types of corticoids plays a part in the production of inflammatory diseases. When inflammation is excessive, as, for instance, in rheumatoid arthritis, the situation is corrected by treatment with ACs. Conversely, an adverse effect could be expected from such treatment in diseases characterized by a relative inability to put up adequate inflammatory barricades or immunologic defense against invaders, as, for instance, in tuberculosis.

To many of us this seemed to be a rather natural—in fact, the only possible—explanation of the facts known at that time. Yet some physicians still

felt that the idea of a balance between proinflammatory and anti-inflammatory hormones was pure
speculation, designed to reconcile the newly-discovered anti-inflammatory effects of ACTH and
cortisone with the earlier observations on the
proinflammatory actions of DOC.

There can be no doubt now that the two types of
hormones can mutually antagonize each other's
actions on inflammation. Many observations have
shown this, but it will be enough to mention two: (1)
the aggravation of various experimental infections
with anti-inflammatory hormones (which remove
inflammatory barricades and inhibit immunologic
defense), and their amelioration with proinflammatory ones (which strengthen inflammatory barricades and stimulate immunologic defense); (2) the
protection against anaphylactoid inflammation,
topical irritation arthritis, inflammation in the
inflammatory pouch, etc., with ACTH and cortisone, and the abolition of this protection by simultaneous treatment with STH or DOC.

Is there such a thing as a disease of adaptation? Here the answer depends on how you define
a "disease of adaptation." *No disease is exclusively
caused by maladaptation*, but derangements of our
adaptive mechanisms do play a decisive role in the
development of many diseases.

You might just as well question whether there is
such a thing as an "infectious disease." We are
constantly exposed to all kinds of germs which
could make us sick, but often do not. Why not?
Because the entry of the germs into our system is

not in itself the disease. All depends on how much the germs can damage us and how much we can damage them. We cannot injure some of the microbes at all, but if they have no way of doing us any harm either, there is no disease. These germs live peacefully in our intestines, lungs, or throats without causing any trouble.

Other microbes could damage us, but before they get the chance, our tissues quarantine them within impenetrable inflammatory barricades, or actually kill them with chemicals known as *immune bodies*. Some people remain in perfect health although they carry germs of typhoid or diphtheria. Such persons can, nevertheless, infect others, who may then die of one of these diseases because their defenses are weaker. Almost every adult human being has, at one time or another, been infected with tuberculosis, but the germs usually cause no inconvenience because they are walled off by fibrous inflammatory membranes somewhere in the lungs.

Significantly, an overwhelming stress (caused by prolonged starvation, worry, fatigue, or cold) can break down the body's protective mechanisms. This is true both of adaptation which depends on chemical immunity and of that due to inflammatory barricades. It is for this reason that so many maladies tend to become rampant during wars and famines.

If a microbe is in or around us all the time and yet causes no disease until we are exposed to stress, what is the "cause" of our illness, the microbe or the stress? I think both are—and equally so. In most instances *disease is due neither to the germ as such, nor to our adaptive reactions as such, but to the inadequacy of our reactions against the germ.*

I have used infectious diseases as an example here, but the same could be said about many other diseases. If a company goes bankrupt and the owner develops a gastric ulcer, what is the cause of the disease, the bankruptcy or the owner's inability to adapt himself to his losses? When a joint becomes crippled by constant inflammation and scarring, is it not correct to blame our own bodily reactions (inflammatory responses) for the deformity? You may say that, had there been no defensive inflammation, the causative germ or allergen might have had other and possibly more serious effects. Quite so; but we are not talking about those. The germ or allergen which stimulated inflammation might or might not have caused another disease had there not been any tissue reaction against it; but the illness which did in fact develop was an inflammatory disease. Moreover, when inflammation is suppressed with ACTH or corticoids, often—for instance, in allergies and in rheumatoid arthritis—no other disease develops in its stead.

It still remains to be shown to what extent maladaptation participates in each individual disease, since it seems to play a role in all of them, but a decisive part only in some. Another task for future research will be to show how far man can improve upon Nature's own adaptive reactions.

Let me point out here parenthetically that Pasteur was sharply criticized by many of his enemies for failing to recognize the importance of the *terrain* (the soil in which disease develops). They said he was too one-sidedly preoccupied with the apparent cause of disease: the microbe itself. There were, in fact, many debates about this between Pasteur and his great contemporary, Claude Bernard; the former insisted on the importance of the disease producer, the latter on that of the body's own equilibrium. Yet Pasteur's work on immunity induced with serums and vaccines shows that he recognized the importance of the soil. In any event, it is rather significant that Pasteur attached so much importance to this point that on his deathbed he said to Professor A. Rénon who looked after him: *"Bernard avait raison. Le germe n'est rien, c'est le terrain qui est tout."* ("Bernard was right. The microbe is nothing, the soil is everything.")

But today, work along these lines has progressed far enough for us to say that, like all the reactions of the human body, those concerned with adaptation are not always perfect, and at least some of the resulting diseases of adaptation can be corrected. They can be combated, for instance, by the administration of hormones, the removal of endocrine glands, or by treatment with drugs which suppress endocrine or nervous activity.

These were the principal problems which had to be settled before accepting the stress concept. Now let us turn to the *weak points in the theory which still exist today.* Such gaps in our knowledge are particularly important; they focus attention upon the limitations of our concept and thereby point to fruitful fields for further research.

What are the alarm signals and how do they act? What is the "first mediator" of stress? In Book II I have already presented the observations which led me to suspect that some *alarm signals are discharged by various cells, as a side-effect of both activity and damage.* We have seen that each type of cell has its own specific reaction forms: the muscle contracts, the eye sees, the connective tissue holds our parts together and responds to injury with inflammation. The sum of these characteristic responses could not be computed directly because they have no common denominator. Yet the visible degree of stress in a man is proportionate to the sum of everything that is going on in him at the time. How could the body calculate the sum of, say, that much contraction plus that much vision plus that much inflammation? All biologic reactions— no matter how different they are from one another—must produce some nonspecific by-product which adds up and thus serves as an indicator of all the activity that goes on throughout the body. There must be a first mediator of the stress response (see page 106).

This, you will note, is pure speculation. Nobody has ever seen or otherwise demonstrated this by-product by direct methods of observation. Nevertheless, it seems to me that the existence of this indicator is just as definitely established by logic as if we had seen it. No one has ever seen electricity either, but the reality of it is demonstrated beyond doubt by its manifestations. The same is true of the alarm signals. We cannot see them directly, but we can readily prove their existence, and even mea-

sure their amount, indirectly, by their effects. The
discharge of ACTH, the enlargement of the adrenals, the involution of the lymphatic organs, the
corticoid hormone content of the blood, the feeling
of fatigue, and many other signs of stress can all be
produced by activity or injury in any part of the
body. There must be some way of sending messengers from any cell to the organs which are so uni-
formly affected by all stressors.

To my mind, our ignorance about the nature of
these alarm signals is one of the most serious handicaps in the study of stress; but how can we find out
more about them? Well, to begin with, we might
examine what *pathways* they could use. There are
two, and only two, all-embracing coordinating systems which connect all parts of the body with one
another: the nervous system and the blood vessel
system. The alarm signals could be carried everywhere *through nerves*, but it is virtually certain
that this is not the only route they could take,
because organs can send out alarm signals even
when their nerves are cut. It is probable that often,
if not always, the signals travel *in the blood*. We
know that certain compounds, such as proteins,
occur in every cell; parts of protein molecules may
split off and then act as blood-borne transmitters of
the stress message. Any other product of cell activity might fulfill the same function, but it is equally
possible that *the alarm signal is not a substance, but
rather the lack of one*. During activity, cells consume a variety of chemicals, and the withdrawal of
such compounds from the blood could also act as an
alarm signal.

Intensive research along these lines is now under way in many laboratories throughout the world. Several investigators have published observations allegedly proving that one or another substance (proteolytic enzymes, polypeptides, histamine, acetylcholine, or adrenaline derivatives) is the first mediator of the stress response. In my opinion, none of these assumptions has as yet been adequately supported by facts.

It is even possible that *no one substance or deficiency has the monopoly of acting as an alarm signal.* A number of messengers may carry the same message. The actual facts which led us to postulate the existence of the alarm signals would be in agreement with this view also. The various cells could send out different messengers, as long as their messages would somehow be tallied by the organs of adaptation (as, for instance, by the pituitary). To explain, let us assume that the acidity of the blood is what counts. We have no reason to think that this is actually the case, but if it were so, any acid compound discharged by cells (or even the consumption by cells of alkalis) would forward the same message; yet the total amount of it could be computed as "acidity."

All these possibilities must be envisaged in designing experiments to identify the nature of the signals which gear the body for defense.

In the complex picture of a disease, what is due to what? If we look at disease from the viewpoint of the stress concept, a number of additional questions arise which cannot yet be definitely answered. Let us take rheumatoid arthritis as an example. We must ask:

1. What is the causative agent of this disease: a germ, an allergen, or nervous tension?

2. Why does a particular agent (say, a germ) to which everybody is exposed produce rheumatoid arthritis in one person and not in another?

3. We have seen that the most striking feature of rheumatoid arthritis is an excess of apparently useless inflammation. Is this due to excessive local irritation of the joint by the direct action of the causative agent? Is it due to an excessive production of proinflammatory or a deficiency of anti-inflammatory corticoids? Is it the consequence of those conditioning factors which sensitize the tissues to the former and desensitize them to the latter hormones? Or do several of these factors play a part here? The disease consists mainly of inflammation, a tissue response which is easily influenced by a variety of circumstances, so that the problems presented by every case are naturally complex.

4. Why has it not been possible to show any striking derangement in the corticoid content of the blood and the urine in rheumatoid arthritis? Why is inflammation so readily inhibited in this disease by anti-inflammatory hormones and yet not significantly aggravated by proinflammatory corticoids? Why is it that, in nephrosis, an increase in aldosterone production is associated with water retention (dropsy) and a certain type of kidney damage, with no increase in blood pressure, whereas in the so-called "primary aldosteronism,"

it is often associated with another kind of kidney damage (nephrosclerosis), high blood pressure, and no dropsy?

Of course, in theory it is always possible to get around such apparently incongruous facts. Possibly they could be due to differences in the speed of development or the intensity of the hormonal derangement, or to variable conditioning by other hormones, heredity, or diet. It is very probable that explanations should be sought somewhere along these lines, but it is well always to keep in mind that these are still unanswered questions.

The important thing is that now these questions can be asked clearly; once this is possible, sooner or later they will be answered. True, it may take a long time, but this need not discourage us. The concept of the microbial transmission of disease was outlined more than a hundred years ago; yet, even in this field, we are still faced with very similar problems today. Despite all the progress made in bacteriology, all we know of some diseases is that they are infectious. Of other maladies we know the causative germ, but have no remedy against it; or we fail to understand why the same germ causes disease in some people but not in others. Yet, as soon as Pasteur formulated the basic problems of infection, this field began to emerge from centuries of darkness.

The science of stress is much younger and correspondingly less well worked out than that of bacteriology, but we have already learned a good deal. For instance, we have recognized the role of the endocrine glands and hormones in the causation and treatment of the most varied diseases. With the greatly improved means for scientific research in our century, we have every reason to expect rapid progress along these lines now.

What is adaptation energy? Here we are touching upon what is probably *the* most fundamental gap in our knowledge about stress. I say "fundamental" because adaptability, or if we want to give it this name, "adaptation energy," is a basic feature of life itself. The length of the human life-span appears to be primarily determined by the amount of available adaptation energy. A better understanding of it promises to show us how to improve recovery from any kind of exhaustion and perhaps even to prolong life. Yet all we really know about this mysterious quantity is that constant exposure to any stressor will use it up. That much is certain; we can verify it by experiment. We can observe that anything to which adaptation is possible eventually results in exhaustion, that is, the loss of the power to resist. Just what is lost we do not know, but it could hardly be the caloric energy—which is usually considered to be the fuel of life—because exhaustion occurs even if ample food supplies are available.

To my mind, these are the most important gaps in our knowledge about stress—which means that these are also the most promising fields for further study.

BOOK IV

Sketch for a Unified Theory

Summary

The study of stress has shown how important it is to *distinguish clearly between specific and nonspecific vital responses.* Can they both be embraced by some unified theory?

Specific responses are simple in kind; they affect one or a few elements only. Nonspecific responses affect numerous elements without selectivity. In life, differences in kind (as different tones on a piano) cannot occur at the level of the elements (any one key); *the impression of a qualitative change is created by blending the responses of the unchanging fundamental units.*

But what are the elements of life? *The cell* is only a structural, not a functional unit: yet it can perform different functions at the same time. *The atoms* which make up our body are not true units of life either. They do not possess any characteristics of life; it is only their interconnections in living bodies that somehow endow them with vitality. When fitted into the pattern of living matter, individual chemical units cannot react to stimulation selectively. Anything which affects one of them also influences a number of other closely-connected chemical units.

The *reacton* is defined as "the smallest particle of life"

which can still respond selectively to stimulation. In other words, biologic matter cannot be specifically affected in lots smaller than a reacton. In this sense, the reacton concept is not a theory, but a description of observed facts. The limits of the reacton are comparatively vague, but a quantum has no sharp borders either, yet it is an elemental unit of energy.

The significance of the reacton concept is that it opens to experimental analysis that range of units between the cell and the chemical element; at the same time, it bridges the gap between specific and nonspecific vital responses.

All manifestations of life in health and disease are viewed as simple combinations and permutations of individual yes-or-no responses in these ultimate units of life, the reactons.

The impression of virtually any color, shape, or movement can be created on an illuminated panel by turning off and on different combinations of colored light bulbs, though each is capable only of one kind of response. As far as we can see, the human body represents an essentially similar, though enormously more complex, three-dimensional panel, in which all the manifestations of life can be evoked by activating various combinations and permutations of primary reactive units, the reactons.

I am particularly indebted to a number of scientists (among them: L. V. Bertalanffy, C. H. Best, G. Biörck, C. Cavallero, W. E. Ehrich, Albert Einstein, U. S. v. Euler, C. Fortier, I. Galdston, L. Hogben, B. A. Houssay, Pedro Lain Entralgo, C. D. Leake, A. Lipschütz, G. Marañon, J. Needham, J. Ortega y Gasset, R. Pasqualini, A. Pi-Suñer, L. Prado, A. Szent-Györgyi, E. Tonutti, P. Weiss, and J. H. Woodgers), who were good enough to peruse the original version of Book IV, "Sketch for a Unified Theory," in the manuscript of the first edition before it appeared (in more technical language) in the *Third Annual Report on Stress.* Many of these investigators made valuable suggestions which have greatly influenced my presentation of this topic in the present volume.*

*This section is intended only for those who are keenly interested in the nature of normal and morbid life. Like Book II, it is somewhat heavy, but those who would rather skip the details can do so by reading the preceding outline which will provide the necessary continuity.

chapter 14

The Search for Unification

The value of unification.   Stress and the relativity of disease.

The Value of Unification

Whenever a large number of facts accumulates concerning any branch of knowledge, the human mind feels the need for some unifying concept with which to correlate them. Such integration is not only artistically satisfying, by bringing harmony into what appeared to be discord; it is also practically useful. It helps one to see a large field from a single point of view. When surveyed from a great elevation, some details in the landscape become hazy, or even invisible; yet it is only from there that we can see the field as a whole, in order to ascertain where more detailed exploration of the ground would be most helpful for its further development.

Efforts to arrive at a unified concept of disease have been made by physicians ever since the beginning of medical history. Of course, any attempt at a perfect unification would *a priori* be doomed to failure. The various diseases differ, both in the mechanism of their development and in their detectable manifestations: they could never be reduced completely to any one common denominator. Nevertheless, whenever any new, ubiquitous structural or functional characteristic has been detected in all parts of the body, or in all diseases, efforts have been made to single out this attribute (the cellular structure of living things, enzyme functions, metabolism, and so forth) as a lookout post from which to obtain a coordinated view of biology and medicine as a whole.

If we do not go any further than this—if we do not look upon these unifying constructions of the mind as anything more fundamental than an elevated position from which we can get a synoptic view of disease—such efforts are, to my mind, quite permissible and often of great practical value in guiding research.

We have seen that stress plays an important part in many diseases. Its general (G.A.S.) and localized (L.A.S.) forms encompass the very essence of what we call disease. It is rather tempting, therefore, to explore the possibility of using the concept of stress as a basis for some degree of unification.

Stress and the Relativity of Disease

We have illustrated, with many examples, that the most varied manifestations of disease depend upon a tripartite mechanism consisting of: (1) the direct action of the external agent—the apparent pathogen; (2) factors which inhibit this action; and (3) factors which facilitate this action. All potential disease producers cause some degree of stress. Through this they can modify the body's response by altering the internal forces of resistance and of submission. This appears to be the basic pattern of defense when the body itself fights disease through stress. To improve upon Nature's self-healing efforts of this type is also the object of the physician, who uses stress therapy in the form of shock, tranquilizing agents, adaptive hormones, and so forth.

In essence, stress therapy (whether used by the body itself or by the physician) is a *tactical treatment*, such as was hitherto practiced almost exclusively in surgery. In surgery it was always customary to use it whenever the pathogen could not be eliminated. For instance, when an inoperable cancer occludes the gut, the surgeon makes an artificial opening to by-pass the obstruction. This is no cure, but it helps the patient to live in relative harmony with his disease. Here we accomplish by purely mechanical means what stress therapy achieves through biochemical processes.

Stress therapy is *not offensive;* it is not specifically directed against any one disease producer (as are specific serums, antibiotics, and other chemotherapeutic or catatoxic compounds).

Stress therapy is *not symptomatic, nor strictly substitutional;* it does not act by merely eliminating any one specific symptom (as does aspirin in a headache), or by patching up a defect (as when a loss of skin is repaired with a graft, or a lack of vitamin with a curative amount of it).

Stress therapy is instead *tactically defensive* in that it adjusts active defense (for instance, barricading off a pathogen with inflammation) and passive submission (as permitting local death of limited cell groups, or the spread of inoffensive pathogens in a manner favorable to the organism as a whole).

Some agents are virtually *unconditional disease-producers* in that their influence upon the tissues of the body is so great that they cause disease, almost irrespective of any conditioning or sensitizing circumstances. (For instance, all "direct pathogens": ionizing rays, great extremes of temperature, intense mechanical injuries or certain microorganisms to which everybody is susceptible.)

Still, most of the agents which can make us sick are, to a greater or lesser extent, *conditionally-acting pathogens:* that is, they cause maladies only under special circumstances of sensitization. Their disease-producing ability may depend upon hereditary factors, the portal through which they enter into the body, the previous weakening of resistance by malnutrition or cold, and so forth. Here, it is impossible to decide which, among the many factors necessary for the production of disease, is actually the cause and which the conditioning factor: a complete *pathogenic situation* must be realized before the malady can become manifest. For instance, whether a microbe which could produce disease actually does so or not depends largely upon the forces of resistance and submission which will face it after it penetrates the body. It may have free entry into the blood and cause death by blood poisoning, or it may be completely quarantined within a thick barricade of inflammatory tissue which renders it innocuous. In a case like this, it is meaningless to discuss whether the microorganism itself or the body's response is the final cause of the outcome. Here the development of illness depends upon a whole constellation of events. This is what I have called a *"pluricausal disease."*

This interpretation was still not wholly satisfactory as a unifying concept of disease, mainly because it failed to encompass the *noninflammatory maladies.* With the characterization of the L.A.S. it became evident, however, that local stress produces not only inflammation but also degeneration and death, or stimulation, enlargement, and multiplication of cells at the site of its action. All these changes can be regulated by proinflammatory and anti-inflammatory hormones whose actions (as well as the corresponding effects of nervous stimuli) might therefore be viewed more generally as favoring or inhibiting reaction to injury in general. Finally, it should be noted that catatoxic compounds do not act upon tissue reactions at all, but simply destroy offensive pathogens. Therefore, the concept must certainly not be restricted to the purely inflammatory diseases.

The question remained, however, *whether the manifold specific effects of agents could also be integrated into this concept.* These appear to be qualitatively different, both from each other and from the nonspecific (stress) effects: they did not seem to lend themselves to any unified interpretation. But then we saw that there were imperceptible transitions between the most and the least specific actions, so that the difference is actually not one of kind but merely one of degree. *If we could somehow also express specific actions in terms of stress, all disease manifestations would be reduced to a common denominator.* They could result, for instance, from differences in the intensity, sequence of action, anatomic distribution, and the relative proportions of the three basic components of disease: the stressor, the forces of resistance, and the forces of submission.

Apart from the relative proportions between the three basic factors of disease, the manifestations of individual maladies would then only depend upon *when, where, and how much* this tripartite situation depends: upon (1) *time* (the duration and possibly repetitive nature of stress), (2) *space* (the location of the stress situation), and (3) *intensity* (the degree of the whole tripartite phenomenon). To my mind, the link between the manifold specific and nonspecific reactions is that they are all composed of the same kinds of elementary responses to demands made upon our tissues.

During the past thirty years, I have attempted to formulate the conceptual foundation for this view through the *reacton theory.*

Although biologic reactions tend to give the impression of oneness, they actually represent mosaics of simple activation and inhibition by demands (stress) in a great variety of preexistent, elementary, subcellular biologic units: the *reactons.** Each of these is capable of only one kind of

---

*The word *biophore* (Weismann) has already been used to describe a hypothetic "smallest body of matter capable of life." Allegedly such particles may be successively aggregated into larger groups called: (1) *determinants*, still beyond the limits of microscopic vision and equivalent to genes, and (2) *ids*, identified with the visible chromatin granules in cell nuclei. The biophore is more or less equivalent to the *bioblast* (Altmann), the *pangene* (Hugo De Vries), the *plasome* (Wiesner), and the *biogen* (Verworn). The idea of *reactons* is also related to that of *drug receptors* and, much more distantly, to the concept of the *monads* (Giordano Bruno and later, Gottfried Leibniz).

response, but, by blending these elementary reactions in different combinations, qualitatively distinct aggregates result.

To illustrate this with an example, let us remember that one can create a virtually unlimited variety of melodies on the keyboard of a piano by merely activating or inhibiting its chords—varying time, site, and intensity of simple touch on preexistent keys—each capable of only one kind of response. We hope to show that reactons, not cells, are the elementary "keys" of living matter, and that all the manifestations of normal and pathologic life depend only on when, where, and how much (or how many of) these biologic elements are stressed.

This concept is closely related to that of the German Gestalt school of psychology. *Gestalt* means literally "form" or "shape," and is used in this sense for a configuration of separate structures or systems (physical, biologic, or psychologic), so integrated into a pattern as to constitute a functional unit. One may therefore conceive of physiologic, biologic, or psychologic events as occurring, not through the mere summation of distinct elements, but through the functioning of the *Gestalt* (shape) as a single unit. The shape of each disease strikes us as one thing, as a single unit, although it is made up of innumerable simple reacton responses.

In thinking about the fundamental nature of any phenomenon, man invariably tends to analyze it from two essentially distinct viewpoints: its *primary cause* and its *primary constituent elements*.

For instance, if an intelligent member of a primitive tribe was first confronted with an automobile in motion, he would ask, "Who made it?" (that is to say, what is its cause?) and "What is it made of?" (that is, what are its constituent elements?).

This innate quest for the primary is also quite evident during the period of mental awakening in every child. It manifests itself by what might be called the "serial why," which leads to the following type of conversational pattern: "Why is it dark at night?" "Because the sun sets." "Why does the sun set?" "Because the earth turns away from it," and so forth until the hard-pressed adult succeeds in changing the topic.

Our craving to climb up along such question ladders does not diminish with maturity, but our hope of reaching the top rung fades away with age, for we come to realize that it is just as inherent in human nature to be blind to the primary as it is to look for it. Yet, as soon as man understands that, for him, the ladder of comprehension has no end, he can find comfort in the realization that consequently there is no limit to his possible progress; no matter how advanced his wisdom, he remains capable of yet another step forward.

We have little to say about primary causes in biology, yet experimental work has led us to a point where we feel that a better understanding of the primary elements of disease could be of great assistance in sketching a more unified picture of medicine.

What are those concepts of medicine whose distinctness is in question? Let us take five pairs of twin concepts as examples, first, because they are rather basic in biology and medicine, and second, because they seem to defy any effort to reduce them to one common denominator:

(1) health and disease, (2) disease itself and its signs or symptoms, (3) specific and nonspecific phenomena, (4) qualitative and quantitative differences, (5) units and complexes.

Health and disease. Textbooks usually define health as the absence of disease, and vice versa. These "definitions" rest upon the assumption that the two conditions are opposites of each other. Is this really so? Are they not rather different only in degree and in the position of vital phenomena proceeding within time-space?

Bleeding, inflammation, loss of weight, or fever could be mentioned as typical manifestations of disease, in that they supposedly represent deviations from the condition of health which we call the norm. But menstruation is accompanied by bleeding and inflammation in the womb, and the failure of its occurrence is what we would call a disease in a young adult woman. If she bled excessively during her period or menstruated from any place other than the womb (as happens in a malady called *endometriosis*), that would also be a disease, as would be the beginning of the monthly periods at an abnormal time (for instance, in precocious puberty).

A low body weight or a high temperature can likewise be considered as morbid only in relation to some norm of health; but even health and biologic normalcy are not synonymous. A man born with an undeveloped toe, or with a disfiguring scar across his face, is neither normal nor unhealthy. A defect is not a disease.

It may be argued that the examples given (bleeding, inflammation, loss of weight, a rise in tempera-

ture) are merely manifestations of disease, and not
disease itself. Perhaps we should try to clarify the
difference between the two.

Disease itself and its signs or symptoms.
The dictionaries tell us that *disease* is "a definite
morbid process having a characteristic train of
symptoms. It may affect the whole body or any of
its parts; its etiology, pathology, and prognosis may
be known or unknown."* On the other hand, a
symptom is "any functional evidence of disease,"
and a *sign* is "any objective evidence of disease."
(*Dorland's Illustrated Medical Dictionary.*)

These definitions, though quite generally
accepted, are hardly satisfactory to the analytic
mind. Is the high blood pressure of ordinary
("essential") hypertension a disease or a sign? If it
is a disease, it is also its own sign, and if it is a sign,
what is it a sign of? The same doubts arise in
connection with nephritis or pneumonia. These
conditions could be called diseases, but their consequences (for instance, protein excretion and hypertension with nephritis, fever and loss of breath
with pneumonia) might be regarded as their signs.
Yet, if the same renal and pulmonary changes happen to develop in the course of, say, scarlet fever,
they are no longer considered diseases in themselves, but signs of the latter malady.

---

*Significantly, *Blakiston's New Gould Medical Dictionary*—a
standard modern reference volume in medical schools—defines
disease as "the failure of the adaptive mechanisms of an organism to counteract adequately the stimuli or stresses to which it
is subject, resulting in a disturbance in function or structure of
any part, organ, or system of the body."

Actually we have a generally subconscious but very practical reason which largely justifies this usage. When we speak of *disease* we actually mean that, in the light of available knowledge, there is no hope of ascending any higher in the causality chain of the condition before us. When we speak of a *sign*, we mean that there is hope that we could climb, at least one rung higher, toward the understanding of the primary cause.

In view of this, the difference between disease and its symptoms or signs does not appear to be very fundamental. We are tempted to ask whether some unifying interpretation of these derangements could not help us to arrive at a more basic understanding of morbid processes in general. Of course, when it comes to signs and symptoms, the first preoccupation of the physician is the degree of their specificity: their reliability as indicators of any one disease.

Specific and nonspecific phenomena. The original meaning of the term *specific* is "that which characterizes or constitutes a species." For instance, we speak of specific (characteristic) differences between the dog and the wolf, although both belong to the genus *Canis*.

The concept of specificity is of particular importance in stress research, since we have defined biologic stress as a nonspecific demand made upon the body. In this sense, stress is a condition elicited preponderantly by nonspecific agents, that is, those which act on many organs without selectivity. By contrast, a specific agent acts only on one or few parts and therefore provokes selective (specifi-

cally-formed) effects. Agents causing very selective, that is, specific changes in strictly circumscribed parts are comparatively rare; most stimuli
cause rather diffuse (nonspecifically-formed)
responses in many parts of the body. Therefore the
somewhat loose expression *specific agent* generally
implies both specificity in the causation and in the
form (or composition) of the change it evokes.

Any one part can stand only a limited amount of
wear and tear, but if many parts are nonspecifically affected, the total demand for adaptation
adds up. That is why agents affecting many parts
without specificity in the form of their action are
the most effective stressors. I have mentioned the
thyrotrophic hormone as an example of a specific
agent because few, if any, other substances share
its ability to stimulate the thyroid gland selectively. Conversely, many of the changes elicited by
severe infections, ionizing rays, or intense worry—
for instance, fatigue, gastrointestinal upsets, loss
of weight—are rather nonspecific, because they
can be duplicated by many agents. And still *it
would be impossible to give any example of an absolutely specific or absolutely nonspecific agent.*

Here again we get the impression that the two
partners of the conceptual pair, specific and nonspecific, are only apparently different in quality,
but actually distinct merely in degree, that is, in
some quantitative aspect of their composition.

Qualitative and quantitative differences.
This brings us to the very crucial problem of distinguishing between qualitative and quantitative differences in general. One would think, for instance,

that mild and severe blood pressure rises differ only in degree (quantity) whereas a nervous stimulant and depressive drug would differ in quality. But this distinction appears to be self-evident only because of the terms used. Speaking about excitation and depression implies that we view these conditions from an intermediate level, which we recognize to be the norm. If we begin from absolute lack of activity, we can construct an ascending scale, which rises from zero through the increasingly less pronounced degrees of depression all the way to excitation.

It is perhaps not wholly unjustified, therefore, *to ask whether quantitative and qualitative differences are not likewise merely a matter of degree* and of the distribution pattern of vital phenomena in time and space. One could imagine, for instance, that the impression of virtually any qualitative difference could be created by mere combinations and permutations of induced activity in a limited number of biologic elements, each capable only of a single kind of response.

Think of those gigantic, illuminated advertising panels in Times Square: the impression of virtually any color, shape, and movement can be created on them by mere combinations and permutations of induced "activity" in a limited number of light bulbs each capable of only a single kind of response. Does the human body represent an essentially similar, though enormously more complex, three-dimensional panel, in which all the manifestations of life can be evoked by activating various combinations and permutations of primary reactive units, the reactons?

This brings us to the last and perhaps the most important twin concept which we shall have to analyze before attempting to arrive at some unified interpretation of biologic phenomena: the problem of the fundamental unit of life.

Units and complexes. The difficulty of distinguishing sharply between units and complexes is, of course, by no means peculiar to biology and medicine. We encounter it also in chemistry, physics, algebra, and geometry. We speak of a unit of matter, or of energy; a number can be taken as a unit, and so can any element of structure or form. To take a classic example, the atom has long been considered to be the unit of matter. Yet, in view of recent progress, particularly in physics and mathematics, this apparently indivisible building block has been shattered and, from its fragments, has emerged the most general theory of unification which the human mind has yet been able to create. Still, the atom is a unit though not, however, the ultimate or fundamental unit of matter.

In biology a species is a unit among living forms, and so is an individual within this species, an organ within this individual, a tissue within this organ, or a cell within this tissue. Traditionally, the cell has been considered to be the primary or fundamental unit of life, and yet it is still a highly complex aggregate.

I do not know—nor does it really matter— whether or not the basic arguments in support of my views have already been expressed by philosophers. Probably they have. Priority of discovery, in the sense in which it exists in the natural sciences, hardly has a true counterpart in the science of thought itself. Every pattern of argument compatible with the structure of the human brain has probably been formulated at some time, in some language or form, by some author, especially as regards such basic principles as those with which we shall have to deal. But there is a great difference between a thing that has been seen (or even described) and one that is known to those whom it concerns. The basic procedures of reasoning are equally applicable to all sciences; yet, in order to use them for the creation of new knowledge and understanding in any one domain, they must first be translated into a language which is understood and accepted by the workers in that particular field. To us biologists and physicians, *generalizations are acceptable only if they are demonstrably substantiated by many measurable individual data.* We instinctively shy away from philosophic arguments, because the mind works much more rapidly than the hand, and as soon as we risk the formulation of some generalizations about our science, we realize that verification in the laboratory cannot keep pace with the imagination.

Ours should be an *experimental philosophy*, since it is only the teachings of objective observation that we can really assimilate. As its natural counterpart, such an experimental philosophy would create a *theoretic medicine*, which, I believe, could become just as enlightening and practically useful to physicians as theoretic physics has been to our colleagues in the sciences which deal with the inanimate world.*

---

*Since the first edition of this book appeared, a *Journal of Theoretical Biology* has come into existence.

To lay the foundations for this will necessarily be a time-taking endeavor, likely to require the concerted efforts of several generations. The following pages can be regarded only as a very tentative attempt to draw a preliminary sketch, based on the limited number of facts which I have been able to verify in the laboratory.

chapter 15

Unification through the Stress Concept

Stress and adaptation. Stress and growth. Stress and specificity. The structural unit of life: the cell. The functional unit of life: the reacton. Analysis and synthesis of cellular disease. Possibilities and limitations of the reacton hypothesis. The continued importance of in vivo research.

Stress and Adaptation

Our earlier work on the G.A.S. and particularly the more recent observations on the L.A.S. have brought out clearly the essential difference between what I called *specific resistance* (resistance to an agent induced by pretreatment with the same agent) and *crossed resistance* (resistance to an agent produced by pretreatment with another agent).

The *stage of resistance* (see page 37) received its name because, here, resistance to the particular agent which produced this stage of the (general or local) adaptation syndrome is at its peak; yet, at the same time, resistance to most other agents tends to fall below normal. It seems that the adjustment of our tissues to perform one function detracts from their adaptability to new circumstances. These observations convinced me that we must distinguish between two fundamentally different types of adaptation:

1. *Developmental adaptation* (in technical language: homotrophic adaptation), that is, a simple, progressive, adaptive reaction, accomplished by mere enlargement and multiplication of preexisting cell elements, without qualitative change. This response occurs whenever a tissue is required only to increase its activity as regards a function to which it is already adapted at the onset, as, for instance, when a muscle is forced to perform more than the usual amount of mechanical work.

2: *Redevelopmental adaptation* (in technical language: heterotrophic adaptation), in which a tissue, organized for one type of action, is forced to readjust itself completely to an entirely different kind of activity. This happens, for instance, when bacteria or the debris of dying cells come in contact with a muscle cell and the latter must transform itself so as to engulf and destroy these materials (in technical language: metaplasia for phagocytosis). It is interesting that, whenever such redevelopmental adaptation is called for, cells specifically shaped to perform certain functions first lose their acquired characteristic attributes. They must first dedifferentiate, become simple in structure and similar to very young cells, before they can acquire new characteristics to adapt them for other functions. Local stress is very powerful in promoting this dedifferentiation and rejuvenation of cells; it thereby paves the way for a reorganization of their individuality. This should be kept in mind when we discuss, from a more philosophic point of view, the stress factor in the origin of individuality (page 433) and the role of stress as an equalizer of activities in general (page 414).

Here I have used as examples structural rearrangements for adaptation to demands made by local stress. But it is evident that the same considerations also apply to functional responses (since these likewise must have some material—structural, chemical—basis), as well as to adaptive reactions of the body as a whole (which are essentially composed of many coordinated local responses).

All these diverse adaptive reactions are, in the final analysis, due to the demands caused by exposing different combinations of tissue elements to stress. There emerges the impression of some fundamental unifying law. But this is still only an impression. As the picture stands at this point, perhaps its most disturbing feature is the difficulty of correlating the "morbid" phenomena of transformative or redevelopmental adaptation (for instance, of a regular muscle cell into an irregular structure which engulfs foreign particles) with the "physiologic" type of simple tissue development (growth and maturation). The evolution of our tissues from infancy to adulthood appears to be directed primarily by the laws of heredity, but it is also manifestly dependent upon the demands that we must face, that is, stress.

Stress and Growth

It is remarkable that many so-called adaptive hormones, or stress hormones, are also important regulators of *general growth*. ACTH and COL are potent growth inhibitors, and STH is so effective in the opposite sense that it has actually been called the *growth hormone*. It is not unexpected, therefore, that stress itself can affect the growth of the body as a whole. If children are exposed to too much stress, their bodily growth is stunted and this inhibition is, at least in part, due to impaired STH activity and an excess secretion of ACTH and COL.

But is there any link between stress (or adaptive hormones) and the selective *local growth* of certain parts, which leads to qualitative changes by molding the shape of the body? Of course, inflammation, one of the most striking features of local stress, is accompanied by selective tissue growth at the site of injury. Some of this is purely developmental (increase in the size and number of cells), but some is redevelopmental (transformation of connective tissue cells into other types which can engulf bacteria).

In growing rats I found it possible to inhibit selectively the growth of even one ear, one paw, or part of the snout by local treatment with COL. These are true postnatal malformations. The applicability of this principle to the treatment of abnormal overgrowth of organs in children is now under investigation.

Local growth of certain tissues may be selectively influenced by stress (or by adaptive hormones) even at a distance from the site of injury. We have seen that, through the anti-inflammatory hormones, local stress applied anywhere in the body can cause involution of distant lymphatic structures or of inflamed tissues, while the proinflammatory hormones have opposite effects.

Often the local effects of stress and hormones—either upon inflammation or upon growth—are manifest only under certain conditions. For instance, local malnutrition due to constriction of blood vessels sensitizes to the growth-inhibitory and anti-inflammatory effect of hormones, and dilatation of the vascular system has an inverse effect. It has become a major branch of stress research to explore mechanisms through which these conditioning factors alter regional tissue responsiveness, and thereby permit selective reactions to hormones which are distributed equally to all parts of the body through the blood.

It is also possible that during local stress certain cells may develop a special affinity (attraction) for growth-regulating adaptive hormones. Now that radioactively-tagged hormones are available it will become possible to establish this point with certainty. All these factors could endow certain tissue regions with a selective sensitivity for one or the other type of adaptive hormone and, in this manner, permit stress to mold the structure of the body.

Perhaps the most important local stimulant of growth is the demand for activity. A muscle cell forced to perform much mechanical work or a glandular cell stimulated to excessive secretory activity will become enlarged. *Could the stress of local hyperactivity itself act as a conditioning factor for growth-regulating adaptive hormones?* We have already shown that the growth hormone causes more growth in a hard-working than in a resting muscle. But selective activity in a limited muscle group is a rather specific type of reaction and, by

calling this *stress*, we may appear to obscure the
limits between specific and nonspecific actions—a
distinction which is the very basis of our stress
theory.

Stress and Specificity

We have seen how specific local stimulation of certain parts (the eye through light, the ear through
sound, a muscle through its motor nerve) can produce general stress by sending out alarm signals
from the stimulated tissues.

We have also seen that selective local stimulation of any part can produce demonstrable manifestations of local stress. For instance, excessive
stimulation of a muscle can produce local inflammation. Indeed, the Swedish investigator R. Bar-
any has shown that intense muscular work can
even modify the ability of the overworked tissue to
undergo inflammation, following the local application of various irritants. There can be no doubt
that the specific stimulation of organs is inseparably interwoven with nonspecific, local, and general
manifestations of stress.

Another important point is the *relationship
between specificity and quality of response*. Nonspecific agents have been defined as stimuli "which
affect many targets and are devoid of the ability to
act selectively upon any one." By definition the
reverse is true of specific agents. Similarly, a nonspecific change is one which can be elicited by
many agents, while a specific change can only be
produced by one, or at the most by a very limited
number. The two types of agents appear to be quite

unrelated and different in quality. Indeed, we have come to consider them as opposites.

Yet even this apparently fundamental difference between the specific and the nonspecific is perhaps more apparent than real. It has been proposed, for a great many reactive elements in living organisms *(receptors* or *targets),* that they can respond to irritation in only one manner. This type of reaction is conditioned by their own structure, not by the stimulus which activates them, although they may be more sensitive to some agents than to others. Whether stimulated by heat, mechanical injury, or electricity, a muscle fiber reacts with contraction, an optic nerve fiber with the sensation of light, a glandular cell with secretion, and so forth. Could it be that the apparent multiplicity of specific reactions is merely due to combinations and permutations of such single reaction types of which the various biologic elements of the body are capable? If so, all the manifestations of life—from the regional to the general, from the entirely nonspecific to the most highly specific—could be brought down to a common denominator. They would merely represent various groupings of simple, qualitatively unidirectional responses in the diverse biologic units (organs, cells, cell parts) of the body.

Viewed in this light, the fundamental uniformity of any vital response—growth and adaptation, reaction to regional (local) or to general stressors— begins to emerge in a more definite form. One great problem which remains is to formulate the precise nature of the interrelations between the specific and the nonspecific responses. I believe that the clarification of this has been particularly handi-

capped by the general acceptance of the theory
which assumes that the cell is the ultimate unit of
living matter. *Even a single cell can respond in
qualitatively different (specific or nonspecific)
ways.* It would be difficult to understand this without accepting that the ultrastructural smaller
units within the cell are still relatively independent of each other in their reactivity.

The Structural Unit of Life: The Cell

In 1667, looking through his primitive microscope,
Robert Hooke saw minute compartments in living
plant tissues. These appeared to be empty spaces
separated by walls; he therefore called them *cells*.
What we now understand to be a cell is actually
filled with apparently living matter: a nucleus and
some cytoplasm (cell body).

More than a century and a half after Hooke's
discovery, the German biologists Matthias J.
Schleiden and Theodor Schwann noted that all living matter, including both plants and animals, was
made up virtually of cells alone. This led them to
propose (in 1839) the first great, truly unifying scientific concept in biology: the *cell theory*. In brief,
they assumed that the cell is the fundamental unit
of all that is alive—just as, for some time, the atom
was considered to be the fundamental, indivisible
building block of matter. The stimulating and fer-
tilizing effect of this concept was as great for biology and medicine as that of the atomic theory was
for chemistry and physics. Most of our fundamental biologic concepts are based on the cell theory.
To mention but one outstanding example, the

Father of Morbid Anatomy, Rudolf Virchow, could not have formulated his famous *cellular pathology* without it, since this doctrine holds that every disease is essentially a disease of cells. It is the essence of science to explore causal and spatial relations between units. No wonder that the recognition of a visible unit of life helped the progress of biologic science!

And still, subsequent research revealed many *facts incompatible with the cell theory* of life. Certain slime molds, for instance, grow to considerable size and, although they contain many nuclei, they show no signs of a subdivision into cells. Conversely, the red blood cells of man contain no nucleus. The configuration of viruses is even more remote from the cellular structure. Still, they do appear to be alive. And why should we consider intercellular substances as inanimate?

Despite these and many other facts which are patently incompatible with the cell theory, the latter was so useful that it became too deeply ingrained in the minds of biologists to be displaced by any other concept. Findings which did not fit into it were merely discarded as unimportant exceptions to the rule. After all, the atomic theory, which postulated the inconvertibility of elements into each other, also had its exceptions.

But now we know that the atom *is* divisible and does not represent the fundamental unit of matter. This explains why it is possible to effect qualitative changes in elements—although each of them consists only of one kind of atom—by rearrangement of their true fundamental units. Yet for a long time work along these lines was actually handicapped by the otherwise fruitful atomic theory of matter. Could these same considerations also apply to the cellular theory of life?

There can be no doubt that certain targets or receptors of biologic stimuli are of subcellular dimensions. *It is inconceivable that the cell should be the fundamental unit of living organisms because, in a single cell, various portions can perform diverse vital functions independently and simultaneously.* For instance, a single cell can concurrently move about, secrete, engulf a foreign particle, digest food, and perceive external stimuli. An agent can undoubtedly influence one part of the cell (for instance, an organelle, visible only under the electron microscope) or one biochemical unit (for instance, an enzyme) selectively.

The Functional Unit of Life: The Reacton

The cell is undoubtedly a building block, a structural unit, of life. It has a visible membrane which separates it from its surroundings and emphasizes the distinctness of this element in space. But it is not the elementary unit of biologic function.

The living undoubtedly consists of matter, but life is only one of its characteristics. The great strength of the cell theory is that one can see the limits of these "building blocks" and demonstrate that virtually all living matter is made up of them. *But this only shows that the cell is a structural unit. It is not necessarily the fundamental primary unit of life.* The organs are units in the body; the tissues are units in the organs; the cells are units in the tissues. Why must we stop our dissection of living matter at this particular level? The possibility of demonstrating clear borders by optic or even electron microscopy is hardly an adequate reason. A quantum has no such sharp borders either, yet it is an elemental unit of energy.

Where then should we draw the line? Living, just as inanimate, matter consists of chemical elements, but these cannot be regarded as being alive. They are specific units of matter, but not necessarily of living matter. Only certain combinations of the elements engender the characteristics of life. A specific element of any organization is the smallest part still specially fashioned to fit a certain composite structure. (For a mechanical analogy illustrating this principle, see *Fig. 31*.) Since this is undoubtedly true, *why not recognize, as the fundamental specific elements of life, those smallest organizations which still exhibit selective reactivity to biologic stimuli and manifest the generally-accepted criteria of life?*

In analogy with the larger biologic units (such as the *nephrons* of the kidney, the *neurons* of the nervous system), I have called these *reactons*. The reacton is defined as *the smallest biologic target which can still respond selectively to stimulation*. They might be compared to interdependent synergistic teams of receptors. The limits of these units are not visible under the microscope; in fact they may not have any sharp, structural limits. But, irrespective of their position, they can function in unison, since certain agents act selectively on one type of reacton in many cells or intercellular sub-

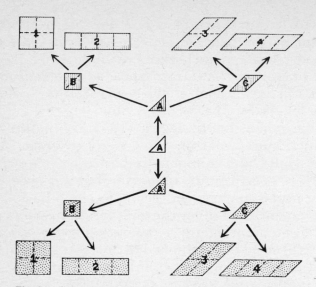

**Fig. 31 Illustration of the view that a specific element is
the smallest part still specially fashioned to fit a certain
composite structure.**

The central white triangle A is a common element of A
hatched and A stippled. The latter two differ from the
parent structure only in shading, not in form. A whole
series of structures can be created with either type of
shading, by joining the elements of A and its increasingly
more complex aggregates in different ways. Therefore, in
either series shown here, A is a specific element of B, as
well as of C.

On the other hand, B is a specific element of 1 and 2,
but not of 3 and 4, since the latter two could not be
constructed from it.

Let us emphasize particularly that A is not a *specific*
element of any among the structures 1, 2, 3, or 4, but only
of their precursors B and C, since it is only up to this level
that the shape of the small triangle (dotted) is still dis-
tinctly implied by the outlines of the whole. In the same
sense, the specific element of a species is the individual
animal (not the cell), that of a tissue is the cell (not the
reacton), and the smallest but still specific element of
living matter is the reacton (not the atom).

stances throughout the body. Here the functional organization into reacton units is more important than the structural subdivision into cells.

Are reactons "alive"? In the absence of evidence to the contrary, we must at least consider the possibility that they are, because they exhibit the features regarded as characteristic of life, just as the complete cell does. Among other things, reactons can grow and reproduce their own kind. They also have a great tendency to maintain their characteristic individuality, despite changes in the milieu; that is, they are highly adaptable. For instance, much-used parts of a cell can enlarge and become more numerous within the cell.

Let me point out clearly that none of my observations would justify the conclusion that these elementary targets are necessarily bodily structures, that is, matter. It is equally possible that the reacton is only a focus of interaction, a functional plan or pattern which governs the organization of matter. A plan possesses, to an exquisite degree, such accepted characteristics of life as the ability to grow, to reproduce its own kind, and to adapt itself to changing requirements.

Let us see now whether this hypothesis of the reactons could help us to understand phenomena which the cell theory does not explain. The hypothesis of the reactons postulates that:

1. *The fundamental specific elements of life are of subcellular dimensions.* They may not have visible limits; they may merely be focal points of interactions between the constituents in living matter (somewhat like the bonds which hold atoms together in inanimate matter). These reactons are

defined as the smallest targets capable of selective biologic reactivity.

2. *Each reacton can give only one kind of response.* The nature of this response depends upon the inherent structure of the reacton itself. Hence, at the level of these ultimate units, reaction patterns cannot yet be separated into the specific and the nonspecific. In other words, the concepts of quality and specificity of response have no meaning at this elementary level.

3. *Specificity of action (causation of effect) depends upon the degree of selective affinity* which an agent exhibits for certain reacton types.

4. *Specificity of response (kind of effect) depends upon the degree of freedom with which certain reactons can be activated* independently of others.

5. *Intensity of response depends upon the number of reactons activated.* It is still to be determined whether the degree of activation has any importance at this fundamental level, or whether reactons are subject only to the "triggering" type of yes-or-no response, which necessarily leads to the complete discharge of the accumulated action-potential. In the latter event, intensity of response would depend exclusively upon the number of reactons of any one kind that are fired.

6. *Developmental adaptation depends upon simple growth and multiplication of certain preexistent reactons.*

7. *Redevelopmental "transadaptation" depends upon growth and multiplication of certain previously-undeveloped reactons, at the expense of inactivity-atrophy in others, which were previously* *developed.* It is this type of response which we have been accustomed to regard as a "qualitative" change. The schematic drawings in *Figs. 32–37* illustrate these thoughts by a simple mechanical analogy.

At first sight it may be difficult to understand *how mere quantitative responses in a limited number of reactons might give the virtually unlimited number of qualitatively distinct reaction patterns of which living matter is capable.* Yet this is not without precedent in biology.

For instance, according to the famous Young-Helmholtz theory of color vision, there are only three fundamental color sensations: red, green, and violet. By suitable combinations of these, all other colors can be formed. To explain this, it was assumed that three kinds of nerve elements exist in the retina of the eye, each of which is specifically responsive to the stimulus of waves of a certain frequency corresponding to a particular color. If the nerve elements which correspond to red and green were simultaneously set in action, the resulting sensation would be orange or yellow; if mainly the green and violet, the sensation would be blue or indigo, etc. Actually, no such nerve fibers or elements are known, but the theory is equally valid if the stimuli affect three photochemical substance units. The innumerable melodies which can be derived from the simple keyboard of a piano (although each key can produce only one tone) have already been mentioned as another suitable analogy.

In modern terminology, the individual reacton comes close to what we call a pharmacologic recep-

Schematic drawings illustrating the reacton hypothesis as applied to the interpretation of specific and nonspecific actions.

In all the drawings that follow, the individual reactons are schematically represented by round bodies, and the connections between them (interactions) by straight lines. This is similar to the customary representation of atoms and bonds in chemical formulas. Although, actually, reactons are arranged three-dimensionally in living matter, they are shown here in a single plane. Only reactons representative of special conditions are numbered.

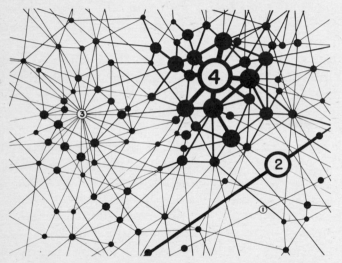

Fig. 32   A field containing numerous reactons (dots) in various stages of development. Reactons are associated with each other by interactions of varying importance (straight lines). We might visualize them as the focal knots in a complex network of more or less obligatory or rigid interactions. Evidently pressure exerted upon any focus will displace others as well, and the extent to which local tension can spread will depend upon the number and strength of the connections between the directly affected focus and the rest of the system.

(1) Undeveloped reacton, directly connected with only two others.

(2) Highly developed reacton, directly connected with only two others.

(3) Undeveloped reacton, directly connected with many others.

(4) Highly developed reacton connected with many others.

This illustrates that stimulation at a point such as 1 will have a selective specific effect (change to type 2): it will develop only the directly-affected reacton and its two immediate connections. On the other hand, stimulation at a point such as 3 will have a very generalized nonspecific effect, even though the agent again acted at one point only (change to type 4).

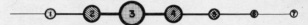

Fig. 33 Sample of seven resting reactons not exposed to any agent. One (No. 3) is most developed and the prominence of the others diminishes as we approach the periphery of the former's activity range. This is intended to be a graphic expression of a situation in which (due to hereditary factors or previous activity), even at rest, one type of reacton is most developed, while the others have evolved only in proportion to the importance of their interactions with the former. (For instance, in a developed muscle, the reactons directly and more or less indirectly related to contractility.)

SPECIFIC AGENT I

Fig. 34 Specific effect with developmental adaptation. Specific Agent I has acted upon the system represented in the previous drawing, stimulating it to perform the particular function for which it is specialized. This leads to simple *work hypertrophy*, with a proportionate development of all the pertinent reactons and of their interactions. (For instance, in the just-mentioned example of the muscle, the repeated specific stimulation through its motor nerve.)

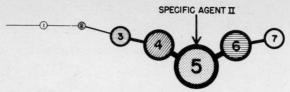

Fig. 35 Specific effect with readaptation. Here Specific Agent II has called upon the system to perform a function qualitatively different from that for which it had been specialized. Now the chief demand is upon a previously not fully-developed reacton (No. 5). This leads to a shift, a *transadaptation,* with varying degrees of inactivity-atrophy in previously-developed reactons (near the left end of the chain) and a corresponding qualitative change in structure and function. (For instance, selective exposure of a single muscle group to microbes, with a resulting transformation of the muscle cells into so-called "cleaning cells" or *phagocytes* especially adjusted to engulf foreign particles.)

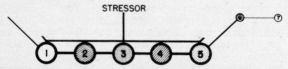

Fig. 36 Stress due to a nonspecific action. Here the nature of the stressor is such that it makes demands on five reactons and their interactions. The corresponding dedifferentiation, or equalization, is illustrated by an enlargement of the previously-underdeveloped reactons at the expense of involution of the previously most-developed reactons. (For instance, exposure of a large tissue area to heat which directly affects all its cells.)

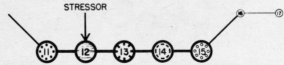

Fig. 37 Stress due to a nonspecific reaction. This also affects five reactons (and their bonds) in this field, although the stressor acts selectively on one (No. 12) alone. The reason for the generalization of the stress effect is the complete interdependence of the units (Nos. 11–15) in this particular field. Therefore, the response of one (No. 12) immediately produces marked repercussions in all others within the system. (For instance, overstimulation of a sensory nerve whose direct effect is highly specific, but the resulting pain produces a widespread stress response.)

tor (receiver). In Ehrlich's theory of immunity, the receptor is one of the side chains of the cell which combines with foreign substances. Sherrington used the term for individual sensory nerve endings in the skin or the sense organs. In modern pharmacology, they represent the smallest chemical units within a cell or molecule that are capable of receiving a biologic stimulus. As such, the reacton and receptor theories are closely related, though not completely identical, because a reacton (unlike a receptor) does not necessarily imply a definitely-formed chemical entity, but may merely be a functional focus of reactivity.

It is not too difficult to imagine that the many reaction patterns of which any cell is capable could thus be synthesized by simple yes-or-no responses of its constituent reactons. In all these instances, the quality of the true fundamental element (as the electron, neutron, pure color or pure tone) is invariable. *Differences in kind cannot be induced at the level of the elements; the impression of a qualitative change is created by blending the responses of unchanging fundamental units.*

Analysis and Synthesis of Cellular Disease

The reacton concept suggests experiments to test the feasibility of an analysis and synthesis of cellular disease. For example, it should be possible to analyze and identify, by their characteristic actions upon the cell, common stimulating elements *(actons)* in various complex disease producers (microbes, drugs, rays), because these will affect one type of reacton preferentially. To explain what I mean, we may take an example from chemistry. The acidity (or the oxidizing power) of various molecules affects cognate receptive groups of various materials in essentially the same manner and, to a large extent, irrespectively of other characteristics of the acid (or the oxidizing) molecule.

Conversely, it should be possible to synthesize cellular disease by the application, in suitable order and intensity, of several agents containing the requisite combination of elementary disease producers (actons), even if none of these agents were in itself endowed with the whole desired pathogenic combination. In chemistry this would correspond to the synthesis of NaCl from NaOH and HC1. The inflammatory pouch (page 216) furnishes a convenient model on which the simplest biologic reactions of this kind can be examined. We have shown already that, by conjointly introducing several simple irritants—each of which produces different kinds of simple tissue responses—rather complex vital reaction forms can be synthesized. Furthermore, just as in chemistry we can identify elements of matter by the reactions they undergo in contact with various substances in the test tube, so also we can detect elementary units of living matter (reactons) by the simplest cellular reaction forms which can be provoked in the cells of the "living test tube": the inflammatory pouch.

Possibilities and Limitations of the Reacton Hypothesis

The greatest weakness of the reacton concept is— as previously mentioned—that the *units which it postulates have no sharp limits.* But this is true of most biologic units. It would be equally difficult to delimit between two sharp pencil-lines what we mean by "the trunk" or "the neck." Of course, this fluidity of transition between various constituents of the body is even greater when it comes to functional units. For example, the respiratory system undoubtedly includes the lung, yet this organ also has many other metabolic functions which have nothing to do with respiration; the ribs are necessary for breathing, but they also belong to the skeletal system, and the marrow in them is part of the blood-forming system.

Functional units can only be defined and demarcated by their activities, not by their substance. The same glucose molecule can become part of the respiratory, nervous, or locomotor system, depending upon the function for which it will happen to furnish energy.

A glance at *Fig. 32* (page 344) shows clearly that each reacton is connected, at least indirectly, with many others. It represents a focal point of activity, whose functional radius overlaps with that of other reactons. This situation could be compared with a complex telephone system, in which there are focal points (the exchanges) and connecting wires. You could point out a building in New York or in Montreal as a focal point of exchange, but the wires between these two cities would belong no more to one than to the other. It would be impossible to analyze the system without recognizing these focal points as units, and yet these would be meaningless without the connecting wires, which in turn make the sharp delimitation of the focal points impossible in a functional sense. It is the great weakness of the cell theory that it recognizes only the "exchanges" and not the "wires" of life.

The study of stress has shown us how important it is to distinguish between specific and nonspecific biologic actions. We could not differentiate between simple, specific, and complex, nonspecific responses of living matter without formulating some idea of the primary elements of activity, the only ones which can be truly simple and specific. That is why we have compared our problem with the task of the chemists, who first had to find the elements of matter before they could distinguish between simple compounds (consisting of one type of atom only) and complexes (consisting of many kinds of atoms). We found that the cell is still much too complex to act as a true functional element of life. On the other hand, the atoms and molecules which make up the human body do not yet possess, in themselves, any characteristic organization for life; it is precisely their interconnections in living bodies that endow them with the features of vitality.

> In studying life, you keep diving from higher levels to lower ones until somewhere along the way life fades out, leaving you empty-handed. Molecules and electrons have no life.
>
> Albert Szent-Györgyi,
> *Internat. Sci. Techn. June 1966.*

The sum of all the elements and molecules in a man does not constitute the man unless they are interconnected and arranged in a certain manner. When so fitted into the pattern of living matter, individual atoms cannot react to stimulation selectively. Anything which affects one of them will also influence a number of closely-connected chemical units. In other words, biologic matter cannot be specifically (selectively) affected in lots smaller than a reacton. In this sense, the reacton concept is not a theory, but a description of observed facts. Only the limits of the reacton are comparatively vague. But this degree of vagueness is an inherent characteristic of any biologic unit; and *the significance of the reacton concept is that it opens to experimental analysis that range of units between the cell and the chemical element.*

The Continued Importance of In Vivo Research

These considerations led me in 1967 to write a special book entitled *In Vivo: The Case for Supramolecular Biology.* There I have summarized our observations showing that, despite the enormous gains made by rapid progress in molecular biology, observations on the living patient or experimental animal, that is, studies on the supramolecular level, will always remain essential for progress in the life sciences.

Most of the normal and morbid manifestations of life depend upon the coordinated excitation of given sets among the simplest elementary constituents of living matter. Our work on pluricausal diseases showed that these depend not upon any one causative agent, even if they manifest themselves in the form of highly specific lesions, but upon the *time, site, and intensity* in which a finite number of elementary pathogenic stimuli can be applied.

In theory even a single molecule may contain several biologically-active parts, e.g., one for the production of stress, another for the induction of cartilage formation or tumor development. But it would hardly be possible to break up individual molecules into their suspected elementary pathogenic functional groups when the latter might not even be separate parts but merely distinct physical or chemical properties, such as the electric charges of atoms, or distances between atoms in a single molecule.

Hence, it may be better to speak of "elementary qualities" rather than particles or subatomic loci that combine to produce different physiologic and pathologic phenomena. To use an illustrative analogy, grains differing in size, weight, magnetic force, color, or temperature can be identified in a mixture by appropriate means (sieves, centrifuges, magnets, color filters, or thermometers). Once isolated, they may even be manipulated as blocks for the planned synthesis of qualitatively distinct structures, although each grain is homogenous and devoid of any characteristic regional differences or loci that could be compared to the functional groups of a molecule participating in chemical reactions. Thus, we are led to postulate that even individual atoms contain several types of actons if they demonstrably possess different combinations of qualitatively distinct potencies—for example, one for the quality of the response, the other for its localization in one or the other region of the body.

It would go beyond the scope of this book to present the actual experimental evidence which led us to formulate these views; besides, this has been done in the above-mentioned volume *In Vivo*. As I have said there:

> Time will tell to what extent this hypothesis can be substantiated by further experimentation. Now, all we can say is that meanwhile it served well as a guide to facts which we could not have found otherwise. But we are not bound to remain loyal to the concept of actons and reactons; we shall desert it without the slightest scruples as soon as we find an interpretation more compatible with the facts.
>
> In any case, here, we are at the subatomic level of biology. We are beginning to explore with simple techniques entities even more minute than the subjects of today's molecular biology that could be studied only through the most sophisticated modern approach of quantum mechanics.[*] It is ironical that I should have to end up here in my defense of the old-fashioned coarse methods recommended for the exploration of broad correlations and the gross phenomena of life!

[*]Szent-Györgyi, A.: *Introduction to a Submolecular Biology.* New York: Academic Press, 1960.

chapter 16

Apologia for Teleologic Thought in Biology and Medicine

What do we mean by "understanding"
something? Purposeful causation.
Recapitulation and conclusions.

What Do We Mean by "Understanding" Something?

It is evident that our whole unifying concept is based upon teleologic thought: the principle of purposeful causality. Many of the most outstanding investigators of our time, however, believe that one can, and should, merely register scientific observations, refraining from all considerations of purpose. I cannot accept such arguments. To my mind, the sensations of causality with purpose are inherent in the structure of the human brain. Understanding itself is but the feeling of having securely attached a thing to our treasury of known facts, by solid bonds of obligatory cause-and-effect consequences. In fact, understanding is always relative, and the more perceptions knowledge predictably

unites, the truer it is. The fullest possible understanding of a thing is the most constant manner of
connecting the largest number of perceptions
relating to its essence and causation. Of course,
nobody has any quarrel with causality; only purposeful causality (teleology) is under attack. Causality becomes objectionable if interpreted not
merely as the achievement of a result, but as the
fulfillment of a wish.

Knowledge includes purely descriptive information (the answer to, "What is it like?"), but we can
"understand" only the cause of a thing (the answer
to, "What brings it about?"). In other words, we can
know a thing by its characteristics (a house), or by
the instinct of self-evidence ($6 \times 6 = 36$), but we can
understand it only operationally (cf. operational
definitions, page 61) in terms of its cause. In conversational English, the two terms are somewhat
loosely used. For instance, we say that we "understand" a foreign word, but what we actually mean
is that we know its meaning. This is really mere
recognition by characteristics, and essentially different from true causal understanding.

This can be illustrated by *Fig. 38.*

Purposeful Causation

But teleologic (from Greek *telos* = end plus *logia* =
science) thought implies more than mere causality.
It suggests purposeful causation (i.e., intention) to
achieve an end or aim. It is really because of this
aspect that so many biologists refuse to accept it.
As applied to our topic, the problem is rather
clearly put in Professor P. Schwartz's remarkable
essay on inflammation. He says:

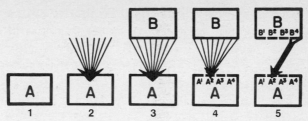

Fig. 38 Usual sequence of problems met as we attempt to approximate the understanding of primary causes and primary elements in experimental medicine.

1. We discover a biologic target (say, the adrenal). This gives us knowledge, but not understanding.

2. We notice that the target can vary; it is capable of being changed by agents of as-yet-unidentified nature and origin (adrenal enlargement). This gives us more knowledge, but still no real understanding. We ask ourselves, "What is the cause of this change?"

3. We find that the cause is B (some action of the pituitary). This gives us the impression that we understand the cause of the change.

4. But we may find, upon closer investigation, that the apparent change of the whole is really due to an alteration of only one among its elements, A^2 (the adrenal cortex). Actually, B acts on A^2.

5. Then we learn that not the whole of B, but only B^4 is the cause of the change (in our example, not the whole pituitary, but only one of its hormones, ACTH). This gives us the sensation of an increasingly better understanding. It is not a coincidence that, as understanding deepens, the sequence of causality becomes increasingly more obligatory. B does not always act on A, but only if it can reach A^2. The response is still more predictable if B^4 itself can be applied in abundance, since other elements of B are ineffective and may be inhibitory. The same argument applies to still more primary causes in the chain of events, when we begin to ask, "What acts on B?"

"One should think that the exalted Law of Nature—to vary a famous saying of Anatole France—recognizes no difference between microbes and man. One cannot consider inflammation as a specific 'cleansing' measure, that is one for the conservation of tissues, any more than one can envisage malignant neoplasia [cancer] as having the 'purpose' or 'duty' to destroy organs: both processes are—just as all manifestations of Nature—*in themselves* aimless and purposeless phenomena." Their "aim and purpose" (or, better, their consequence) is merely to bring about a result, not to fulfill a wish.

I can certainly not avoid dealing with this problem here. All my factual observations were made possible by experiments planned on the assumption that stress responses are purposeful, homeostatic reactions. We must realize that in both the examples just mentioned (inflammation in response to microbes and cancer) there are actually two *teleologic centers;* their interests are opposed but, within each of them, purposeful activity "for its own good" is clearly recognizable. On the one hand is the interest of the patient, on the other that of the microbe or of the cancer. Indeed, the very essence of cancerous growth is the setting up of a center whose own interests are largely opposed to those of its host.

Of course, one center of homeostasis can exist within another and then their interests can no longer be identical in every respect. To take an example, a citizen shares many interests with all his countrymen but, in ascending order, he shares even more with all those who live in the same city, the same district, or the same house. Not only microbes and cancer, but even our own normal tissues constantly compete with each other for nourishment and space. Consequently, every cell, even every reacton within the body represents a teleologic center, whose purposeful reactions must be analyzed in relation to all other centers. Indeed, the terms *teleology* and *purpose* can be meaningful only in relation to an identifiable center. "It is advantageous" means nothing unless we say for whom or for what.

The formation of what we might call *teleologic centers* within the universe appears to be one of the great laws of Nature. The stability of the most diverse structures seems to increase up to a certain optimum size or degree of complexity. The acquisition of this stability strikes us as an aim, since everything tends towards it. All structures tend to become unstable after they have reached their optimum complexity; then they "die" by falling apart, so that their elements may initiate another similar cycle. In its product, it is rare to find exactly the same elements arranged in the same manner as in the parent structure, because precisely the same conditions are not likely to prevail twice in succession. This leads to a constant, slow evolution towards increasingly more stable structures. This is merely a fact, but from the viewpoint of structure, a purposeful fact.

We see this in the case of small drops of mercury which, upon contact, tend to aggregate into a larger and more stable drop. This goes on until a certain optimum dimension is reached, then the drop becomes unstable because of its size and falls apart. We see this when a crystal develops, or an icicle, or an ameba, or a human being. They all grow and then fall apart—though in different ways. There can be simple shattering or disintegration (crystal, icicle), which makes all parts immediately available for totally different constructions.

There can be direct and complete division into smaller structures, similar to the parent body (ameba). Here, the falling apart of the old is, in itself, the birth of the new; there is no "corpse" from which to construct something totally different. Finally, an aggregate can fall apart by a combination of the two mechanisms (man), where a large section of the body (the "corpse") disintegrates yielding up its units for wholly different constructions, while other parts (the germ cells) are preserved by previously reproducing similar offspring, which are only relatively new.

Everything that has any degree of stability acts as a teleologic center in this sense, for this persistent activity does not need the continued direction of an intelligent external influence with a purpose. Even a man-made object, once finished—an automobile, for instance—can give the impression of being guided by teleology; of continually looking out for its own interests; it will meet hostile influences with "intelligently planned defense reactions." When driven along the highway it will cool its own motor to prevent damage by heat. On bumpy roads it will protect its body against shock with the aid of the springs and—if it has self-sealing tires—it can even be capable of true *wound-healing* after being punctured.

Of course, someone has to make the automobile and someone has to make the maker of the automobile; and this leads us to the point where our teleologically-constructed brain can no longer follow, for we cannot understand anything except in terms of creation, which fulfils the "purpose of its cause." Understanding is nervous activity and, in the maze of nerve fibers which make up our brain, every impulse comes from somewhere: its cause.

We sense a Creator mainly because we and our surroundings seem complex, and during our short life-spans we see no really complex structure built up by chance without the purposeful influence of a maker. But could not the organizing effect of a centralizing teleology be our view of the maker? Could it not—in the span of ages—eventually build up awe-inspiring complexities, such as a planet, a tree, or even a human being?

Having been built and being capable of building are the most inherent characteristics of our every part. We therefore see everything through an atmosphere of building which tinges all our perceptions, just as a red crystal ball—were it alive and capable of perception—would probably see everything as red, in and outside itself. Teleologic thought does not necessarily have to lean upon an individual, purposeful Creator, nor should it do so, even on religious grounds, since faith does not need the support of understanding. What we must clearly realize in biology is that teleologic analysis is applicable to every unit of creation.

Science cannot and should not attempt to embrace the purpose of the original Creator; but it can and constantly must examine teleologic motives in the objects of creation. Only by doing this can science progress from the mere accumulation of unintelligible facts to what we call *understanding*.

Here, the same arguments apply as have been brought out by many philosophers against Francis Bacon's attempt to base the "Scientific Method" of achieving understanding, upon the validity of proof by induction. As has been pointed out repeatedly (and with particular clarity by Karl Popper) no number of individual observations could logically entail an unrestricted general statement and, hence, one cannot form general laws on the basis of observed facts, no matter how numerous. If "A" is attended by "B" thousands of times without exception it still does not follow logically that this will always be the case in the future. Attempts to justify induction beg the question by taking its validity for granted to start with. However, the human brain is so constructed that it can think only by assessing the probability of future events on a statistical basis. Induction is not a logically valid principle, but all human knowledge is based on experience. Even the degree of assurance with which we can call something true is based on a number of earlier observations that are compatible with it and inversely proportional to findings (if any) which are incompatible with it. We must agree with Bertrand Russell that "induction is an independent logical principle, incapable of being inferred either from experience or from other logical principles and that without this principle science is impossible."* I do not know whether under these conditions we can call it a "logical" rather than an "illogical" principle. (Karl Popper calls it a myth, but if so it is certainly a useful one.)

Colin Pittendrigh designated the species-main-

---

*Russell, B.: *History of Western Philosophy*, Allen & Unwin, Ltd., London, 1967, p. 647.

taining value of natural selection "teleonomy," hoping that this new word would distinguish it from teleology as clearly as astronomy is from astrology. As Konrad Lorenz says, all complex structures of organic beings are influenced by the species-maintaining pressure of selection. When the biologist hits upon a structure of unknown value, he will ask, for example, "Why has the cat pointed and curved claws?" and the answer will be "To catch mice." Actually, the reply is only a simplified statement of the fact that natural selection has, through teleonomy, encouraged the development of this structural change.

As Lorenz goes on to say, in biology, unlike in physics and chemistry, we must recognize the principle of "species-maintaining purposeful teleonomy." Since much of selection is based on maintaining useful characteristics, the result appears as though it were the work of a wise "plannifying being," adapting things purposefully to this end. Human wisdom itself is the result of similar selective processes which affected the development of genes.

Recapitulation and Conclusions

We have seen that, although stress itself cannot be perceived, we can appraise it by the objectively measurable structural and chemical changes which it produces in the body. These manifest themselves as the G.A.S. (when stress affects the whole body) and as the L.A.S. (when only a limited region is affected). Evidently the whole body, as well as its individual organs and tissues, can respond specifically to special stimuli and nonspecifically to stressors.

These findings have naturally led us to compare the behavior of individual cells under stress and during adaptation to various specific stimuli. It became evident that even *a single cell can respond with many more or less specific, qualitatively different biologic reaction forms*.

All these studies have sharply highlighted the difference between developmental *adaptation* (simple quantitative progression along evolutionally established lines) and *readaptation* (which involves some regression or disintegration to secure building blocks for subsequent qualitative reconstruction). Since even a single cell has proved capable of readaptation (through a rearrangement of its biologic elements), it could not itself be the fundamental unit of living matter.

Thus we arrived at the hypothesis of the *reactons*, which postulates that *subcellular units can still exhibit the generally-accepted characteristics of life*. Of course, it is difficult to define life, because there does not appear to be any sharp line of demarcation between it and the inanimate. Life is perhaps best defined by the degree to which it has developed certain characteristics, particularly those of recreating its own kind (growth, reproduction) out of less highly-organized materials, and of maintaining its structure tenaciously, despite any environmental changes that would tend to destroy it (adaptation). These characteristics are recognizable, even in the most elementary subcellular biologic targets, the reactons.

Simple chemical compounds never exhibit these qualities to any great degree. That is why we do not regard them as living. The now most generally accepted theory postulates that the cell is the smallest unit that can still be considered to be alive. Yet many facts are incompatible with this view. Neither microbes, nor viruses, nor even the intercellular substances of man exhibit the characteristic features of cells, yet they appear to be alive in the classic sense of this word. Then too, a single cell can respond in qualitatively different ways to stimuli (perception, locomotion, secretion), and even its constituent parts exhibit the powers of growing (selective growth of ultramicroscopic organelles in an individual cell), of reproducing their own kind (regeneration of cell parts) and of maintaining their structure, despite external forces which tend to destroy it (new formation of lost secretion granules, healing). Real elementary units may be large or small, numerous or few (they may show quantitative differences) but, by definition, they cannot be composed of diverse elements (they cannot show qualitatively different parts).

There is no evidence that new reactons could be formed in any mold other than that of preformed reactons of the same kind. The Latin adage, *Omnis cellula e cellula ejusdem generis* (every cell comes from a cell of the same kind) did not really hold true for the cell: under stress a certain type of cell can transform itself into another one (in technical language this is known as *metaplasia*). It is more consistent with the facts known today to say: *Omne reacton e reactone ejusdem generis* (every reacton comes from a reacton of the same kind).

In the light of this hypothesis we have attempted to formulate some fundamental concepts in biology this way:

> *Growth* = multiplication or enlargement of reactons.
>
> *Specificity* = selective responsiveness of certain kinds of reactons.
>
> *Developmental adaptation* = response to a demand by further activation and growth of previously-developed reactons.
>
> *Readaptation (or transadaptation)* = response to a demand by activation and growth of dormant reactons, with relative regression of those which were previously most prominent.

As we see it now, the most fundamental task will be to find strictly objective means with which to test the validity of our principal proposition, namely that: *all vital phenomena depend merely upon quantitative variations in the activation of preexistent elementary targets.*

BOOK V

Implications and Applications

Summary

The most important *applications of the stress concept as regards purely somatic medicine* are derived from the discovery that the body can meet various aggressions with the same adaptive defensive mechanism. A dissection of this reaction teaches us how to combat disease by strengthening the body's own defenses against stress.

This also has important *psychosomatic implications.* Bodily changes during stress act upon mentality and vice versa. Only by dissecting our troubles can we clearly distinguish the part played by the stressor from that of our own adaptive measures of defense and surrender. We shall see how this helps us to handle ourselves during the stress of everyday life, and in particular, how to tune down when we are wrought up, how to overcome insomnia, and how to get out of certain grooves of stereotyped behavior.

Stress research also has far-reaching *philosophic implications.* We shall see that stress plays a role in such diverse manifestations of life as aging, the development of individuality, the need for self-expression, and the formulation of man's ultimate aims. Stress is usually the outcome of a struggle for the self-preservation (the homeostasis) of parts within a whole. This is true of cells within an individual, of individuals within society, and of

species within the whole animate world. After surveying
the emotions which govern interpersonal relations (the
thirst for approval, the terror of censure, the feeling of
love, hate, gratitude, and revenge), we come to the conclusion that the incitement, by our actions, of love, goodwill and gratitude in others is most likely to assure our
safety within society. Why not seek this consciously as a
long-range aim in life? No other philosophy has the
exquisite property of necessarily transforming all our
natural but reckless egoistic impulses into altruism
without curtailing any of their self-protecting value.

But human beings cannot think only of future safety;
we want more immediate rewards; we have a need for
self-expression; we want to enjoy the pleasures our sen-
ses can bring; we want the satisfaction and equanimity
which come from reverently contemplating the great
wonders of Creation. In the light of research on stress,
my advice would be:

> Fight for your highest attainable aim
> But never put up resistance in vain.

There is no ready-made success formula which will
suit everybody. We are all different. But, since humans
are essentially rational beings, the better we know what
makes us tick, the more likely we will be to make a
success of life. Our ultimate aim is to express ourselves
as fully as possible, according to our own lights.

chapter 17

The Stressors of Daily Life

Occupation.   *Climate and Environment.*

In formulating our definition of stress as the non-specific response of the body to any demand, we have repeatedly had to correct certain misconceptions which arose because people tend to think of the very general biologic phenomenon of stress, which occurs in all living beings, only in terms of human problems, and only in terms of its unpleasant, disease-producing effects. As a result, stress was identified with mental arousal, frustration at one's work or in private life, the necessity of facing responsibilities beyond one's capacities, physical exhaustion, and fatigue—and not with its agreeable, even curative actions. The stress mechanism, like the consumption of energy, and, indeed, nature in general, is quite indifferent to human concepts of good or bad.

However, the author and the readers for whom this book is meant are human beings and concerned with human needs and wants. Therefore, in this chapter, stress as it affects humans is naturally our main concern, and rightly so. We will leave to the zoologists, botanists and microbiologists the question of other species while, in the following pages, we shall concentrate on our own problems, especially those we are likely to encounter most frequently in daily life.

It may be said without hesitation that for man the most important stressors are emotional, especially those causing distress. Naturally, purely physical demands upon the tissues of our body, such as wound healing, restoration of lost blood, fighting of infections or poisonings, can also become of paramount importance. Yet these are far less commonly met in normal life than the emotional stimuli with which we are almost constantly faced; besides, even somatic reactions affect us largely because of the nervous responses (fear, pain, frustration) which they evoke. This is probably because among all living beings, man has the most complex brain and is the most dependent upon it. Thus, it is especially true that, in our life events, the stressor effects depend not so much upon what we do or what happens to us but on the way we take it.

It is virtually impossible to distinguish between stressors and conditioning factors in human life. It is mostly very arbitrary whether we think of an inherited weakness or any other physical defect (that is, internal conditioning) or food ingredients, atmospheric pollutants, contacts with other people (external conditioning) as the stressor or the conditioning factor. As a rule a problem arises because we are conditioned or predisposed to react in a certain way when meeting the stressors of daily life; but we could also say that normal life events may turn otherwise inconsequential conditioning factors into potent stressors.

According to our definition any demand upon the body, including those merely necessary to maintain life, act as stressors, but we will limit our discussion here to the generally health-threatening stressors we are most likely to encounter in daily life, especially those which we might be able to handle better if we knew more about them.

Occupation

We cannot select our parents and so influence our stress responses by the acquisition of the best possible internal hereditary traits. Therefore, probably one of the most practical considerations in this respect is the selection of our occupation, by choosing to do what we really think suits us best, including both the amount and direction of adaptation required to accomplish a maximum of eustress with a minimum of distress.

Here are a few facts, almost randomly gathered from the medical literature concerning stress in various occupations. Since eustress represents no threat to well-being or health, most of the medical and sociologic studies along these lines were concerned with distress, although for simplicity's sake this is commonly referred to merely as stress. In the exceptional cases where eustress is meant this is specifically mentioned.

Accountants. Serum cholesterol levels (a good indication of stress) among accountants consistently rose during heavy work periods, such as the preparation of income tax returns. This type of stress predisposes to heart accidents.

Invoicing clerks. Subjective feelings of fatigue and the urinary excretion of adrenalines were found to be increased whenever remuneration was changed from fixed salaries to piece wages, presumably because of the extra motivation to accomplish as much as possible in the shortest time. The stress of hurried concentrated work also tends to cause fatigue, backache, and pain in the arms and shoulders.

Industrial occupations. Job satisfaction was inversely related to the frequency of heart accidents. Furthermore, a good deal of evidence has been compiled to show the "curative effects of work satisfaction" on mental distress. Job pressure undoubtedly aggravates distress both in lower-level employees and in top management. New awareness of these problems has produced much literature on distress in industry caused by over-promotion, underpromotion, or managerial indifference to the personal problems of employees. According to such studies, severe distress in industrial work may even lead to sexual impotence and decreased fertility.

Executives. Many scientific studies were performed to establish the stressor effects of executive responsibilities in middle and top management relative to that of subordinate employees in various occupations. Undoubtedly, executive responsibilities, if taken very seriously, produce severe distress with somatic and psychic manifestations often conducive to actual disease. However, here, as in all considerations of stress manifestations, conditioning factors must be taken into account, for whatever a person's position in the hierarchy of command, the stressor effect of his decision-making depends mainly upon the way he reacts to it. This explains the many contradictory statements about whether being the boss or being bossed about is more distressful or eustressful. Some people are born leaders, others followers. The main problem each person must face squarely is to determine what he actually prefers to do and behave accordingly. Some of my most intelligent employees impressed me greatly by repeatedly refusing promotions because they had the insight to realize that a higher level of responsibility would have brought with it too much frustration and job dissatisfaction. However the executive responsible for his employees must usually make these decisions himself because most of his employees will not be able to resist such temptations of promotion on their own initiative.

It is common practice to keep promoting personnel from jobs in which they performed competently to higher positions until they have reached a level at which they are incompetent (the Peter principle). To prevent this, the best technique I have been able to develop has been to ask an employee temporarily to substitute for one in a higher position (to avoid disappointment by concealing my wish to promote him); I have then offered the higher post only after he has already shown his competence for it.

Shift work. It has been possible to show that the normal circadian rhythm of blood corticoids usually remains unaltered in night workers and blind persons; presumably, at least, this diurnal change is not considerably affected by light.

However, working long hours predisposes different occupational groups to heart accidents, with the exception of farmers and farm laborers; for unknown reasons, they appear to tolerate long working hours unusually well.

In one statistical study, it has been emphasized that peptic ulcers are particularly common among shift workers, probably because night work is especially fatiguing and conducive to mental distress. Even in this case adaptation tends to occur after a while, especially when the shift work does not provoke social problems. Rotating shift work probably produces the most severe disturbances in corticoid and adrenaline production.

Most investigators agree that shift work becomes less stressful in proportion to habituation and that being "excluded from society" is perhaps the most frequent complaint among shift workers.

Telephone and telegraph operators. The need for these workers to be constantly alert has resulted in a variety of stress signs detailed in several statistical studies. This leads to a comparatively high rate of absenteeism. As judged by replies to questionnaires, the most common complaints (rigid job supervision, noise, drug and drinking habits) were not so much due to the work itself but to the way the workers responded to their tasks. No clear-cut difference in the incidence of stress complaints could be established between telegraphists, clerks, mechanics, and high management.

Physicians. A statistical study on more than 2,500 physicians suggested that the incidence of heart accidents is higher among general practitioners and anesthesiologists than among dermatologists and pathologists, allegedly because the former two groups live on a higher stress level.

In many U.S. hospitals where medical interns have particularly strenuous work shifts, both their performance and their health are endangered because of excess stress. Radiotelemetric observations on physiologic functions among physicians and medical students performing stressful tasks almost invariably indicated rapid pulse rate, roughly paralleling urinary excretion of adrenaline and its metabolites. This was particularly evident in surgical personnel encountering operative difficulties.

A statistical study on British physicians revealed a special predisposition to drug addiction, suicide and mental disease.

Dentists. Several investigators have found that increased corticoid and adrenaline production as well as typical psychic manifestations of distress are readily detectable both in patients and in dentists, especially during complex and painful interventions. In such cases, the use of tranquilizers is often justified.

Nurses. Conscientious nursing of difficult patients is also highly distressful, particularly for the nurses of intensive care units.

Lawyers. Among lawyers, heart accidents have been claimed to be most frequent when their

work was associated with considerable stress. On
the other hand, answers to a questionnaire sent to
almost 2,000 attorneys in the Cleveland area correlated much better with the quality of the law school
they attended than with the stress-ranking
(defined by various tests) of their legal specialties.
These findings again support the often-repeated
principle that it is not so much the stressor agent
as your preparedness to meet it that counts.

Public speaking. As committee meetings,
round tables, congresses and political campaigns
proliferate, the stress of public speaking assumes
special importance. For some people, addressing an
audience represents a source of considerable distress with all of its physical manifestations, including increased adrenaline and corticoid production,
a rise in blood fats, accelerated pulse rate, raised
blood pressure, all of which may predispose for
cardiovascular accidents. These changes, if severe,
also interfere with the quality of public speaking;
hence it is of practical importance to learn how to
avoid them. This can best be accomplished by practice and by listening to good speakers. However,
several studies have shown that antiadrenaline
drugs may also help to overcome many of the distressing manifestations of public speaking without
interfering with the quality of the presentation.

Police work. It is hardly surprising that
highly responsible and dangerous police assign-
ments can be the cause of considerable distress. A
statistical study on 100 policemen of the Cincinnati
force was performed by one of the great experts in

this field, Dr. W. H. Kroes, along with his coworkers. Somewhat unexpectedly they found that the most significant stressors for policemen are those circumstances which threatened their sense of professionalism, such as being reprimanded by superiors. These were more frequently mentioned in questionnaires than directly life-threatening situations. Presumably, policemen accept the prejudice, fear, suspicion, and hostility directed at them by a large segment of society as part of their job, in addition to its inherent physical dangers.

Diving. The stressor effect of underwater demolition work has been well established. Among the typical biochemical indicators of stress, a rise in blood cholesterol and corticoids is often seen among divers. The effects of anxiety, increased barometric pressure and other stressors inherent in this occupation are further augmented by heat loss in the case of scuba divers practicing in cold water.

Armed forces. The relationship between life in submarines and the G.A.S. has been extensively explored. Even training in tanks for submarine work produces such typical stress manifestations as an increase in corticoid production. This is still more evident on prolonged submarine trips.

Medical studies of U.S. soldiers under combat conditions have been made in recent years. Increased secretion of adrenalines and corticoids occurred among infantry men, bomber pilots, and helicopter crews alike. To a large extent they occur also under simulated combat conditions. Peptic ulcers and other gastrointestinal derangements, and cardiovascular diseases are also frequent consequences of stress during warfare.

The most serious effects of combat stress are the so-called "war neuroses." Their development depends largely upon hereditary predisposition, preparatory indoctrination to boost morale and interpersonal relations within the fighting group, and motivation.

Considerable distress may also become evident among military personnel during peacetime, especially in those not used to life under disciplined, strictly-supervised conditions. Change in command appears to be a particularly stressful experience, both in peace and in war.

Aerospace work. Stress is perhaps one of the most important problems we meet in aerospace medicine. In selecting crews for planes and spaceships, it is naturally of the utmost importance to develop meaningful tests with which it could be determined—as accurately and objectively as possible—to what extent a candidate is likely to withstand the stresses of all the physical and mental demands made by this kind of work. Most of these tests are based on exposure to simulated flight conditions and subsequent measurement (by special instruments or questionnaires) not only of performance in properly-selected perceptual-motor tests, but also of physical and mental responses, as well as the analysis of circulation, pulse rate, electrocardiograms, etc. Several special "stressalyzers" have been devised for the concurrent determination of several among these variables.

Extensive studies in England during the Second World War showed that, after repeated missions over enemy territory, the initially great anxiety of the pilots gradually subsided, but consistent with the triphasic nature of the G.A.S., eventually their adaptation broke down and they developed a variety of neurotic manifestations. Even the most courageous and well-balanced fighters could perform optimally for only a limited number of sorties until their "adaptation energy" was exhausted. To a lesser extent, the phenomenon of "pilot fatigue" is also noted in civil aviation, especially under heavy work load. Of course, here again innate hereditary predisposition plays an important role, but the strain of battle brings out latent tendencies that would not be manifest under similar circumstances in civilian aviation.

Undoubtedly not only anxiety, but various other sensory stimuli participate in this phenomenon. In one interesting experiment it was noted that deaf persons with vestibular defects (depriving them of their sense of equilibrium) who accompanied experienced pilots on acrobatic flights failed to show the usual increase in corticoid and adrenaline production, presumably because of their impaired sense of hearing and balance.

Air traffic controllers. Despite their sedentary occupation, usually performed in air-conditioned, pleasant rooms and comfortable chairs, air traffic controllers (ATCs) experience considerable stress, especially during busy periods, presumably because they have to concentrate continuously on their task and are personally responsible for the lives of many people. The longer they are in their profession, the more they develop subjective feelings of disease, and also such objective indicators as rapid pulse rate, sweating, increased excretion of adrenalines and corticoids, etc. These manifestations may persist even on days of rest, and are especially intense during night shifts and at peak hours of airplane traffic.

Among ATCs, peptic ulcers, hypertension, and probably also heart accidents are particularly common. In one study, 32.5% of the ATCs suffered from peptic ulcers, and in another group the incidence was even higher.

Driving. The effects of this stressor have been measured extensively. From a practical point of view it is helpful to appraise its effects as if it were a single entity, but of course its stressor potential is due to a combination of factors: concentration (especially when driving at high speed in heavy traffic), anxiety, the physical discomfort of maintaining the same body position, and boredom during prolonged trips. In addition, there is the concern of reaching one's destination on time, and— depending upon the construction of the vehicle— vibration, noise, etc.

In general, it may be said that driving and other stressors elicit essentially the same physical and bodily manifestations, namely: a drop in blood eosinophil cells with increased corticoid and adrenaline production, physiologic signs of nervous tension or exhaustion, raised blood pressure, rapid heart beat, sweating, and gastrointestinal disturbances. All these changes are most pronounced under dan-

gerous conditions (e.g., auto races or very prolonged truck driving, especially if the cargo is flam-
mable, explosive or particularly valuable).

Climate and Environment

Air and water pollution. In view of its
increasing importance, much research is now in
progress on this subject. Chemical agents,
microbes, and noise are potent stressors. As yet,
however, few data are available on the measurable,
truly nonspecific stressor effects as such. Most of
the relevant publications deal with the psychologic
effects of life in polluted, overcrowded, urbanized
areas and in concentration camps or prisons.

Social and cultural stressors. These are difficult to separate from related agents such as
genetic factors, climate, diet, prevalent diseases,
overcrowding, isolation, and innumerable others
with which they often overlap.

For example, the fact that arteriosclerotic heart
accidents are uncommon in Japan in contrast to
the North American white population has led to
some speculation about the roles of social and cultural elements in the pathogenesis of this typical
disease of adaptation. However, the striking differences in nutrition and genetic predisposition must
also be considered.

Special attention has been given to what is
termed "culture stress" or "cross-cultural stress"
in relation to the G.A.S. These investigations dealt
mainly with the stressors encountered by
migrants, "guest workers," and others, often

regarded as undesirable intruders by the host population. Such newcomers may suffer from the lack
of friendly social contact in addition to being
obliged to follow customs, diets, and a general philosophy of life which is foreign to them.

Most of the investigators in this field have based
their assessment of the stressor conditions merely
on written answers given to standard printed
questionnaires and the frequency of typical "diseases of adaptation" such as hypertension, gastric
ulcers, and mental illness. Very few and inconclu-
sive data have come to light with respect to the secretion of stress hormones such as corticoids and
adrenalines, or of plasma fat constituents which are
said to be very sensitive indicators of interpersonal
stress.

A special index of culture stress was based on
comparison of traditions and social habits in 37
totally dissimilar societies and races. It was concluded that protest suicide, defiant homicide, drun-
ken brawling, and witchcraft attribution are suitable tentative indicators of this type of stress.

In any event, there appears to be agreement on
the fact that severe social and cultural stress predisposes to a number of maladies, not only to typical psychosomatic diseases but even to infections,
by decreasing general resistance. Comparative
studies in high and low stress areas of Detroit
revealed that social and economic factors predispose to hypertension, especially among blacks.

Social stress also occurs among animals. In
chickens, the establishment of a "pecking order" is
a source of social stress because it indicates dominance and power. The confrontation of two male

tree shrews immediately results in fighting associated with loss of body weight and other biochemical indicators of stress, which bring on kidney disease. This allegedly shows "the great significance
which social stress may have in the origin of renal
disease—possibly in man as well as in animals."
When a male tree shrew is defeated by a trained
fighter and separated from him by a wire mesh to
be protected from further attack, the conquered
animal's adrenals still enlarge and the blood corticoids tend to remain above normal. The defeated
shrew dies after about 20 days of such "psychosocial stress."

In colonized squirrel monkeys, the dominant animals had the highest corticoid but curiously the
lowest adrenaline levels, whereas the reverse
occurred in their subordinates. It was concluded
that high adrenocortical activity is perhaps necessary for the maintenance of dominance, at least in
this species.

It would be hazardous to draw far-reaching conclusions from such animal experiments concerning
comparable situations in man, but it is of interest
that observations made under strictly comparable
conditions in the laboratory do offer ample confir-
mation of the fact that social stress can elicit objective, measurable changes in stress hormone production.

Crowding. Typical manifestations of the
G.A.S. in animals as well as in man under crowded
conditions include adrenal enlargement and hyperactivity, thymicolymphatic and sex organ involution, decreased fertility, a special tendency towards

the formation of peptic ulcers, and sensitivity to infection. In this sense, crowding may even be useful for the species in maintaining a normal population density. In mice and rats, crowding at a very early age may cause lasting changes in the offspring of surviving females, perhaps as a result of deficient lactation.

The direct effect of crowding is usually complicated by the increasing importance of social rank within the community. For example, among wild mice, low-ranking subjects have the largest adrenals, possibly because they are subjected to more physical and psychologic stress than are their "social superiors."

In chickens, overcrowding definitely diminishes egg production concurrently with adrenal hypertrophy, and the population growth of wild rabbits is significantly inhibited in overcrowded colonies. Similar findings have been reported for a large number of other animals, as well as man.

A population study on human behavior suggested that, under crowded conditons, men become more competitive, somewhat more severe, and like each other less, whereas women tend to be more cooperative and lenient and like each other more. On the other hand, a study on young Swedish soldiers confined to a small shelter for more than two days revealed no significant adverse effects upon social compatibility or pistol shooting skill.

An especially interesting study has been done among hunter-gatherers in Botswana and South-West Africa. There, the Kung Bushmen live under crowded conditions by choice. The population density in the total area is one person per ten square miles, yet they form camps in which they occupy only about 188 square feet per person. Typically, their huts are so near that people sitting at different hearths can hand items back and forth without getting up. Yet their blood pressures are low, even at an advanced age, and their serum cholesterol levels are among the lowest in the world.

Allegedly, residential crowding in itself does not produce psychologic or physical symptoms of stress. In fact, under certain conditions interpersonal contact is supportive, as long as the people know they have the space to get away from each other whenever they want to. Of course, the interpretation of such studies is extremely difficult since the tribesmen do not suffer from air pollution, competitive strife, noise and the many other stresses associated with urban life in western societies.

Sensory deprivation and boredom. In maximal sensory deprivation experiments, the subject lies quietly in a very comfortably-cushioned bed, every effort being made to protect him against sound, temperature variations, air pollutants, physical or mental work, and all other stimuli that may make demands upon his adaptive mechanism. Yet he is far from being protected against stress. Actually, under such conditions, the subjects experience "an intense desire for extrinsic sensory stimuli and bodily motion, increased suggestibility, impairment of organized thinking, oppression and depression, in extreme cases, hallucinations, delusions and confusion." As we have so often said, living beings are constructed for work and if they

have no outlet for their pent-up energy, they must
make extreme efforts at adaptation to this unphy-
siologic state of inactivity which has been named
"deprivation stress" and has been incorporated
into the G.A.S. concept (Galdston, 1954).

Normal function of the brain depends on constant arousal generated in the reticular formation
by continuous sensory input. Hallucinations, which
may cause accidents, have been noted in pilots,
astronauts, and long-distance truck drivers, presumably because the monotony of their work acts
as a form of sensory deprivation.

Although virtually complete sensory deprivation
over a prolonged period is rare in daily life, a
decrease in sensory input below the normal level is
a common cause of boredom. It will undoubtedly
represent a major pathogen not only in astronauts
on long voyages, but in all those whose work
becomes increasingly monotonous as mass-produc-
tion techniques develop.

Furthermore, separation of infants from their
mothers and all other types of relocation which
leave few possibilities for interpersonal contact are
very common forms of sensory deprivation; they
may become major factors in psychosomatic disease.

Isolation and loneliness. In prisoners, during solitary confinement, isolation may produce a
change in subjective feelings but does not in itself
cause considerable mental or psychomotor deterio-
ration. Other studies have shown a definite difference between the stressor effect of perceptual isolation and that of social isolation. In comparing

the performance of people working alone or in small groups, it was noticed that task motivation, emotional composure, and social compatibility are the main determinants.

It is a common impression that isolation increases alcoholism. Objective observations in rats showed that isolation raises voluntary consumption of alcohol when drinking water is equally available as an alternative choice.

The statement that man is essentially a social animal has become a platitude, but man is certainly not the only social animal. Observations on confined puppies revealed that the presence of another puppy decreases the level of emotional distress and helps to maintain homeostasis. Most of the pertinent studies have been performed on mice, certain strains of which tend to become extremely aggressive in isolation and at the same time show a drop in blood eosinophils and characteristic changes in the brain content of adrenaline-like compounds. We can thus hypothesize that those changes may have an influence on the development of aggressiveness. Also the formation of gastric ulcers in fasting mice is facilitated by isolation. The aggressiveness of previously-isolated mice diminishes after adrenalectomy, but can be restored by corticoids.

In isolated people, the normal circadian rhythms of corticoid and adrenaline production are disturbed, but they become normalized soon after synchronization with the usual social stimuli.

Captivity. Sudden death may be caused by the so-called "shock disease" which develops in some captive wild animals even after exposure to such minor stressors as transfer to new quarters, or repairs in an adjacent cage. In these animals the lymphoid tissues are enlarged, the adrenals and heart small, and they are predisposed to hypoglycemia. The syndrome has been compared to the exhaustion phase of the G.A.S., but supportive evidence is not very conclusive.

Captive wild Norway rats have comparatively large adrenals and atrophic thymus glands with other typical manifestations of the G.A.S. in comparison with domesticated controls. These changes have been ascribed to the more sheltered existence of the laboratory rat. Studies on numerous other animal species showed that captivity decreases fertility and causes changes corresponding to those of the stress reaction.

In POWs repatriated after captivity in China or North Korea, the "prisoner of war syndrome" was described as being mainly characterized by apathy and withdrawal as defensive adjustments. However, comparatively little work has been done on these soldiers with respect to measurable indexes of the stress response.

Ever since the end of the First World War, a very large number of publications dealt with the problems of concentration camp inmates and with the "concentration camp survivor syndrome," which may develop long after liberation.

Principal emphasis has been placed upon the psychologic problems related to coping behavior, but, of course, it is difficult to distinguish the relative roles played by loss of freedom, poor nutrition, bad treatment, fear, and generally deficient hygiene.

In these studies, much attention was given not only to the psychologic defense reactions, which enabled the prisoners to endure the hardships, but also to the actions of their oppressors who had come to terms with their own entirely inhuman behavior by shifting the responsibility to those who gave the orders.

Internees in diverse concentration and labor camps developed remarkably similar symptoms: an initial reactive depression was followed by varying degrees of adaptation. New cases of psychoneurosis rarely occurred until after liberation.

Many of the survivors developed depression with irrational guilt feelings about having been able to survive while so many of their fellow inmates died. Several investigators mention that the damage was particularly severe in those imprisoned at an early age who suffered not only psychic injury, but often also physical trauma, malnutrition, or illness. A fairly constant and typical syndrome resulted from conflicts at an unconscious level between the wish to get well after liberation and the need to suffer for the purposes of revenge and expiation of the "guilt of survival." These observations show that it is incorrect to ascribe the late symptoms to a "constitutional inadequacy" and to reject compensation claims because the disturbance developed only after liberation.

In both male and female concentration camp survivors, the sexual urge and fertility were often diminished owing to deficiencies in sperm formation and amenorrhea. Psychosomatic skin disorders were also especially frequent.

Due to the unending process of mourning and the

emotionally depleted state of the inmates, life in a concentration camp sometimes even affected the second generation. Parents were often so handicapped that they regarded their children's normal robust activity as an interference with the morally prescribed mourning process or as an extra burden on their already taxed resources. Consequently, the children became anxious and aggressive.

Relocation and travel. The great shifts in population following wars or economic upheavals in certain countries centered attention on this stressor. Most of the corresponding scientific work is concerned with voluntary or enforced transfers of entire populations, often into an environment totally different from their own in climate, culture, and ethnic characteristics. The problems of nomads, migrant workers, and explorers of Arctic or tropical regions as well as the effects of long distance travel for business or pleasure have been analyzed. Other experiments have focussed on the difficulties of becoming accustomed to prolonged life in hospitals, homes for the aged, or schools far removed from home. For the aged, the stress of being transferred into "old folks' homes" is exacerbated by the feeling of being useless burdens on their families and of having no further purpose in life. However, most of these studies have been limited to psychosocial observations with only occasional references to somatic manifestations of the G.A.S.

In people transferred to unaccustomed polar or tropical regions, both psychic and biochemical indicators of stress are commonly noticeable. But most of the pertinent studies have been performed on small groups in which it was virtually impossible to separate the effects of relocation itself from those of numerous incidental factors, such as desynchronization, caused by sudden changes in time zones, variations in temperature, atmospheric pressure, and psychosocial factors which induce people to change their environment.

The classic indicators of relocation stress subject to quantitative measurements have received particular attention in experimental animals. In rats, a slight environmental change, caused by transfer from one room to another, suffices to alter blood corticoids and various additional objective biochemical signs of stress. They have also been detected in wild animals transferred to laboratories or zoologic gardens in totally different climates. In these latter cases, of course, captivity also acted as a potent stressor.

Urbanization. Scientific studies on the effect of urbanization are concerned mainly with problems of town planning and the avoidance of noise, pollution, and psychosocial complications resulting from life in a modern city.

Again, it is difficult to distinguish the stressor effect of urbanization as such from that of its individual components.

Apparently in a Zulu population, the stress of urbanization increased the incidence of hypertension, predisposing people to heart accidents. In Bedouins and other nomadic Arabs, ulcerative colitis has been noted after settlement in Kuwait City, presumably as a consequence of urbanization. The high incidence of neurosis in certain housing estates has likewise been similarly interpreted.

American blacks of both sexes have higher blood pressures and mortality rates from heart disease and strokes than do whites living under comparable conditions. Pertinent studies in different areas of Detroit suggested that "blood pressure levels were significantly correlated with different patterns of life stress for the essentially working class persons in the high stress area and for the middle class persons in the low stress area."

In the U.S. Department of the Interior's Year Book for 1968, Secretary Stewart Udall wrote that the "Gross National Product is our Holy Grail . . . but we have no environmental index, no sense of statistics to measure whether the country is more liveable from year to year." This Mr. Udall called the "tranquillity index," which should be carefully studied by finding out what people really value in their lives. It comes down to an index showing the balance between eustress and distress caused by different techniques of urbanization.

Catastrophes. The psychologic consequences of catastrophes and disasters of various kinds— particularly those brought about by bombings, earthquakes, floods, combat, tornadoes, or extreme emotional traumas after accidents—have certain elements in common which may be ascribed to their stressor effect. These have been described as apprehensive avoidance, stunned immobility, apathy, depression, docile dependency, and aggressive irritability. Scientific studies contain many interesting descriptions of behavior during catastrophes as well as suggestions on protective measures against irrational behavior at such critical times, yet comparatively little is known about the purely medical, especially biochemical, aspects that can be unquestionably attributed to stress.

Meteorologic factors. Numerous studies have dealt with stressor effects of solar eruptions, magnetism, and various types of cosmic rays, and special attention has been given to certain hot, dry winds of Israel called "sharav." These are similar to the African "khamsin" or "sharkiye" and the European "sirocco" and "Föhn." Weather-sensitive people can react to these winds with an "irritation syndrome" with a wide range of psychologic and somatic disturbances including migraine headache, cardiac infarcts, changes in mood, predisposition to automobile accidents, loss of sodium, increased corticoid excretion and other changes characteristic of the typical stress response.

Neuropsychologic stressors. As stated before, in man with his highly-developed brain, neuropsychologic stressors are of special importance. Most of the experimental work on the stressor effect of these factors was concerned with reactions to such experiences as problem solving, academic examinations, anticipation of surgery, social problems, and real or simulated panic situations. In the majority of these investigations only psychologic indicators of stress were employed and with these it is always difficult, if not impossible, to ascertain that they really reflect nonspecific biologic stress as presently defined.

Still—as expected—these studies made it clear that anxiety does cause distress and interferes with performance in various tests. For example, students who were praised (irrespective of their actual success) after a first examination, usually did better during a second test than those who were sharply criticized. But here again, conditioning factors play a decisive role, as shown by various questionnaires which predict coping behavior to a considerable extent. Some people are stimulated by sharp criticism to even greater efforts, while others are discouraged. In other words, here again, we meet the basic principle that what matters is not really what happens to you but the way you take it.

There is ample evidence of increased ACTH, GC, and, under certain circumstances, even aldosterone secretion as a consequence of fear and anxiety, for example, in students during oral examinations and in preoperative patients. And, of course, a raised adrenaline production during fear, demonstrated by Cannon as early as 1911, has become a matter of common knowledge. This is associated with so many biochemical and functional alterations characteristic of stress—including the typical drop in blood eosinophils and the production of stress ulcers observed in the population of London during air raids in World War II—that a detailed description is hardly necessary.

It would go far beyond the scope of this book to enumerate all the stressors and conditioning agents that may result in stress or diseases of adaptation. Many hundreds of scientific publications are now available on the stressor or conditioning effect of a variety of agents. Here are just a few: diet, temperature variations, burns, sound, ionizing rays, light, vibration, air blasts, compression, gravity, electricity, magnetism, pain and grief, cognitive effort, various biorhythms (circadian, seasonal, hibernation), physiologic states (age, sex, menstrual cycle, pregnancy, lactation), genetics, race, constitution, immunity, hypoxia, hemorrhage, and muscular exercise including athletics. All of the data on the stressor effects of various occupations have been drawn from my encyclopedic treatise, *Stress in Health and Disease* (Reading, Mass.: Butterworths, 1976), where full references to the original publications may be found.

chapter 18

Medical Implications of the Stress Concept

Stress as a common denominator of biologic activity. Basic tenets for a new type of medicine.

Stress as a Common Denominator of Biologic Activity

In the four preceding books of this volume I wanted to tell you how the concept of stress developed and how it has been applied to problems of normal and abnormal life. I tried to show how this abstract idea helped us to learn specific facts about the way stress stimulates the pituitary and the adrenal glands to secrete hormones which diminish the wear and tear of stress; the diseases that may result when such adaptive responses are faulty; how to correct improper adaptive responses by treatment with hormones, their antagonists or the removal of endocrine glands. Much of this is practical and valuable knowledge, but it is not wisdom. Knowledge is the first concern of the scientist, for his principal aim is to find facts; but wisdom is the ultimate intellectual goal of everybody, for wisdom is (as Webster puts it) "the ability to judge soundly and deal sagaciously with facts, especially as they relate to life and conduct." It is about the wisdom to be derived from the study of stress that I should like to speak in this last part of my book.

We have spent quite some time trying to define stress in precise biologic terms; yet, when we finished our laborious analysis of its nature, stress turned out to be something quite simple to understand: the nonspecific response to any demand, including efforts to cope with the *wear and tear* in the body caused by life at any one time.

Whatever we do and whatever is done to us creates demands for function and causes wear and tear. Stress is therefore not the specific result of any one among our actions; nor is it a typical response to any one thing acting upon us from without; it is a common feature of all biologic activities.

The appraisal of virtually every comparable, common characteristic of matter—for instance, color, weight, and temperature—led us not only to discover new scientific facts and laws, but also to gain a like wisdom about ourselves and the world around us. Man can advance from observation to wisdom in many ways—through instinct, for instance by way of faith, intuition, or art. But, if the gap is to be bridged by science, the subject of observation must first be clearly defined and measurable.

That our bodies are constantly active and gradually wear out during life has always been known, but no one could clearly see or measure stress before, because its visage, the stress syndrome (the G.A.S.), had been covered by the fog of all the specific reactions to the agents which evoke stress. You cannot measure outlines through camouflage.

My approach was made possible by an *operational definition of stress*, which helped to clear away the confusing specific reactions. It tells you what must be done to produce and recognize stress. If stress is the common, nonspecific response to the demands and the wear and tear of whatever happens to a living being, you must observe a great many vital reactions and see what happens. Those changes which are specifically induced by only one or another agent must first be rejected; if you then take what is left, that which is nonspecifically induced by many agents, you have unveiled the picture of stress.

This picture expresses itself in the whole body as the G.A.S. Once you know this, you can measure stress objectively in terms of physical and chemical changes characteristic of the G.A.S. For instance, you can measure the enlargement of the adrenals or the shrinkage of the lymphatic tissues in terms of their weights; you can measure with chemical methods the quantities of adaptive hormones produced during stress. In other words, you can objectively assess the magnitude of stress by its measurable effects upon the body. This operational definition also emphasizes that no one measurement can be conclusive in itself. General (systemic) stress is the whole response, not that of any specific system, although it represents the sum of all specific activities throughout the entire body (G.A.S.). Consequently, the more indices you measure, the greater the precision of your appraisal.

Then it was found that the picture of general stress in the body, the G.A.S., has a local counterpart. This is the L.A.S., which can be appraised by exposing many parts of the body selectively to many locally-applied agents. The changes which any agent can produce virtually anywhere in the body constitute the syndrome of local stress. Inflammation and degeneration of cells were found to be the chief components of this picture.

Finally it was discovered that *the G.A.S. and the L.A.S. are interdependent*. General stress can influence local stress reactions, for instance, through hormones (particularly corticoids), which regulate inflammation. Conversely, local stress, if strong enough, can produce general stress and thereby mobilize defensive organs located far from the site of injury. Through chemical messengers (the *alarm signals)* each of the many local stress reactions, which happen to go on in the various parts of the body at any one time, has a voice in determining the extent of the general counterstress measures to be taken (see page 108). This procedure of "regulation by majority decision" is very necessary. For instance, a small splinter entering the skin may create great local demands for anti-inflammatory corticoids, but the limited local inflammation caused by this minor irritant may not justify the exposure of the entire body to an excess of corticoids. The central organs of defense must consider the interests of the whole and, of course, to do so judiciously, they have to be constantly informed of the requirements of all parts. It was chiefly the recognition of these close interac-

tions between the G.A.S. and the L.A.S. which
made it possible to outline a sketch for a unified
theory of medicine (Book IV).

Basic Tenets for a New Type of Medicine

The three most obvious lessons derived from
research on stress are: (1) that our *body can meet
the most diverse aggressions with the same adaptive defensive mechanism;* (2) that we can *dissect
this mechanism* so as to identify its ingredient
parts in objectively-measurable physical and chemical terms, such as changes in the structure of
organs or in the production of certain hormones; (3)
that we need this kind of information to lay the
scientific foundations for a new type of treatment,
whose essence is to *combat disease by strengthening the body's own defenses against stress.* Once we
have learned that in a given situation an excess of
a certain hormone is needed to maintain health, we
can inject that hormone whenever the body is unable to manufacture enough of it. Conversely, once
we have recognized that a disease is due to the
exaggerated adaptive activity of some hormone-
producing gland, we can remove the offending
organ or try to block its activity by drugs.

In other words, we have learned that the body
possesses a complex machinery of self-regulating
checks and balances. These are remarkably effective in adjusting ourselves to virtually anything
that can happen to us in life. But often this
machinery does not work perfectly: sometimes our
responses are too weak, so that they do not offer

adequate protection; at other times they are too strong, so that we actually hurt ourselves by our own excessive reactions to stress.

In order to adjust or repair a machine we first have to know how it works. This is of course also true of the stress machinery with which man combats the wear and tear of whatever he does in this world. Therefore the most obvious, tangible outcome of our work was to show that stress can be dissected into its elements, and that the knowledge derived from this analysis helps us to speed up a part which lags behind or to restrain another which goes too far.

Yet, in some diseases, the physician may help by merely increasing or decreasing the total amount of stress in the body, without attempting to act selectively upon any one part of the stress machinery.

Not only our mental, but even our bodily defense reactions may become stereotyped if we are faced with the same kind of problem again and again. A man can hurt himself by reacting to every proposition according to a set pattern: say, by habitually ridiculing, complaining, agreeing, or disagreeing. Prejudice is the most common basis for such "prejudged," stereotyped mental response patterns. Everybody is aware of this, but it is less well-known that our bodily *defense reactions can also fall into a groove*, for instance, by always responding with the same exaggerated hormonal response, whether it is appropriate to the situation or not.

A child or a hysterical person can snap out of a tantrum if you splash cold water in his face. The body of a patient can also be shaken out of habitually responding in the same senseless manner if you expose it to the stress of some intense shock therapy, such as electroshock, Metrazol shock, insulin shock, or injection of toxic foreign proteins (see page 288).

Another way to deal with essentially the same problems is to provide complete rest, which gives the body time to "forget" stereotyped somatic reactions to stress. Prolonged sleep (e.g., that induced by barbiturates), artificial hibernation, Transcendental Meditation, and treatment with such quieting drugs as chlorpromazine and extracts of the Rauwolfia root appear to act largely through this mechanism.

All we have said up to now helps to guide treatment by a physician; but therapy with hormones and drugs or surgical removal of endocrine glands are certainly not procedures which the patient could prescribe for himself.

In the chapter on the "Diseases of Adaptation," we also spoke about the important role of the diet in conditioning responses to stress. Generally speaking, undernutrition sensitizes the body for anti-inflammatory corticoids, and overeating augments the effect of proinflammatory hormones. An excess of salt aggravates certain renal and hypertensive diseases, which tend to develop when the proinflammatory corticoids are overabundant; and low-salt regimens have a protective effect in such cases. But even dietary treatment must be controlled by a competent physician. All my book can do in this respect is to *help the patient understand why his physician prescribes a certain regimen;* it could not presume to be an adequate preparation for self-treatment along such purely medical lines.

On the other hand, there are many things I have learned from the study of stress which the physician cannot use but the patient can. I particularly want to share these lessons with you because they have helped me with many of my own problems and I am sure they can help others as well. The sociologic and behavioral aspects of our evaluation impressed me as being so complex and important as to warrant dealing with them in a separate book (*Stress without Distress*, Lippincott, 1974) which was devoted entirely to the psychosomatic and philosophic implications of stress. These will be reviewed in the next two chapters. I shall speak to the layman as a layman, for I have had no formal training either in psychosomatic medicine or in philosophy. Yet it may not be inappropriate for an investigator, who has spent most of his life in the laboratory exploring any one aspect of Nature, to pause and contemplate the applicability of his observations to the problems of everyday life. After all—as I said in the introductory passage of this chapter—knowledge is the first concern of the scientist, but wisdom is the ultimate intellectual goal of us all.

Do not take whatever general lessons I have been able to derive from the study of stress more seriously than I do; my technical knowledge is limited to the laboratory. I only ask you to lend me the benevolent ear that the unschooled old mariner deserves when he tries to communicate the wisdom of the sea—not seamanship.

chapter 19

Psychosomatic Implications

To know thyself and be thyself. Dissect your troubles. Somatopsychic vs. psychosomatic. On being keyed up. How to tune down. Stress as an equalizer of activities. The stress quotient. The importance of deviation. Innate vitality must find an outlet. How to sleep.

To Know Thyself and Be Thyself

The ancient Greek philosophers clearly recognized that, with regard to human conduct, the most important, but perhaps also the most difficult, thing was "to know thyself." It takes great courage even just to attempt this honestly. For—as Logan Pearsall Smith said—"How awful to reflect that what people say of us is true!" Yet it is well worth the effort and humiliation, because most of our tensions and frustrations stem from compulsive needs to act the role of someone we are not. Only he who knows himself can profit by the advice of Matthew Arnold:

> Resolve to be thyself: and know that he
> Who finds himself, loses his misery.

Besides, few things earn you more goodwill and love than the gift of always being yourself. Unaffected simplicity is one of the most likeable traits.

It is well-established that the mere fact of *knowing what hurts you has an inherent curative value*. Psychoanalysis has demonstrated the soundness of this principle perhaps better than any other branch of medicine. The psychoanalyst helps you to understand how previous experiences—which may have led to subconscious conflicts, sometimes very early in childhood—can continue almost indefinitely to cause mental or even physical disease. But once you realize the mechanism of your mental conflicts, they cease to bother you. Sigmund Freud's efforts to develop a branch of medicine on the basis of this concept were sharply criticized at first, but now hardly anyone doubts that psychoanalysis can—at least in some cases—help those whose bodily disease manifestations are due to unexplained mental tensions. Of course, here we are also dealing with diseases of adaptation. Our failure to adjust ourselves correctly to life situations is at the very root of the disease-producing conflicts. Psychoanalysis cures because it helps us to adapt ourselves to what has happened.

All this is sufficiently well known as regards mental reactions to deserve no further comment. But "to know thyself" includes the body. Most people fail to realize that "to know thy body" also has an inherent curative value. Take a familiar example. Many people have joints which tend to crack at almost every movement; by concentrating upon this unexplained condition, a person can talk or worry himself into believing he has a crippling arthritis. If, on the other hand, some understanding physician just explains to him that his cracking sensations are caused by slight, inconsequential irregularities in the joint surfaces, and have no tendency to become worse, the disease is practically cured—just by the knowledge of its trifling nature.

Almost everybody has had, at some time or other, some insignificant allergic condition of the skin, cardiac palpitations, or intestinal upsets; any of these can cause serious illness through somato-psychic reactions merely because not knowing what is wrong makes us worry. Every physician knows from experience how much can be done for a patient by just taking time to explain the mechanism of his symptoms which thereby lose the frightening element of mystery. To help with this is one of the principal objectives of this book.

Dissect Your Troubles

We have seen that stress is an essential element of all our actions, in health and in disease. That is why we have analyzed the mechanism of stress so carefully in the preceding sections. Suffice it here to point out once more the principal lesson which we have learned: that most of our troubles have a tripartite origin. The tweezers of stress have three prongs. Whether we suffer from a boil on the skin, a disease of the kidney, or a troubled mind, careful study of the condition usually reveals it to consist of three major elements:

1. The *stressor*, the agent which started the trouble, for instance, by acting directly upon the skin, the kidney, or the mind.

2. The *defensive measures*, such as the hormones and nervous stimuli which encourage the body to

defend itself against the stressor as well as it can.
In the case of bodily injuries, this may be accomplished by putting up a barricade of inflamed tissue
in the path of the invading stressor (the microbe,
allergen, and so forth) or destroying a poison. Mental stressors (orders, challenges, offenses) are met
with corresponding complex emotional defensive
responses, which can be summed up as the attitude
of attacking and not giving in (catatoxic responses).

3. The *mechanisms for surrender*, such as hormonal and nervous stimuli which encourage the
body not to defend itself, for instance, not to put up
barricades of inflamed tissue in the path of invaders nor to destroy them chemically but to ignore
emotional stressors (syntoxic responses).

It is surprising how often a better understanding
of this tripartite mechanism of disease production
(and I use the word *disease* here in its widest sense,
as anything that disturbs mind or body) can help us
to regain our balance, even without having to ask
the advice of a physician. We can often eliminate
the stressor ourselves, once we have recognized its
nature, or we can adjust the proportion between
active defensive attitudes and measures of surrender, in the best interest of maintaining our balance.

Somatopsychic vs. Psychosomatic

An enormous amount of work has been done by
physicians in connection with problems of psychosomatic medicine. In essence, this specialty deals
with the bodily (somatic) changes that a mental

(psychic) attitude can produce. An ulcer of the stomach or a rise in blood pressure caused by emotional upsets are examples in point.

Almost no systematic research has been done, however, on the opposite of this: the effect of *bodily changes and actions upon mentality*. Of course, I do not mean physical damage to the brain, which could evidently influence the mind, but rather, such facts as that looking fit helps one to *be* fit. An unshaven tramp, who wears dirty rags and is badly in need of a bath, probably would not resist either physical or mental stresses as well as he would after a shave, a good bath, and some crisp new clothes have helped to rehabilitate his external appearance.

None of this is new. Intuitively, and merely on the basis of experience throughout centuries, these facts have long been recognized. That is why, to strengthen morale, armies insist on the spotless appearance of their men. That is also why opposite procedures are used (in some countries) for breaking down the physical and mental resistance of prisoners.

I was first introduced to these truths at the age of six by my grandmother, when she found me desperately crying, I no longer recall about what. She looked at me with that particularly benevolent and protective look that I still remember and said, "Anytime you feel that low, just try to smile with your face, and you'll see . . . soon your whole being will be smiling." I tried it. It works.

There is nothing new here. But then, confession had been practised long before Freud; relativity was known before Einstein, and evolution before

Darwin. Man did not need Pavlov's investigations
on conditioned reflexes to find out that, by appropriate reward and punishment, a dog can be
trained to come when you whistle, or a horse to
stop when you say "whoa!" Yet history shows that
only the scientific analysis of these subjects by
these particular men gave the concepts of psychoanalysis, the relativity of all our notions, the evolution of man's body from lower forms, and the conditioned reflexes, that philosophic impact which they
now exercise upon contemporary thinking.

The existence of physical and mental strain, the
manifold interactions between somatic and psychic
reactions, as well as the importance of defensive-
adaptive responses had all been more or less
clearly recognized since time immemorial. But
stress did not become meaningful to me until I
found that it could be dissected by modern research
methods and that individual, tangible components
of the stress response could be identified in chemical and physical terms. This is what helped me to
use the concept of stress, not only for the solution
of purely medical problems, but also as a guide to
the natural solution of many problems presented
by everyday life.

Let us take a few examples of such practical
applications.

On Being Keyed Up

Everybody is familiar with the feeling of being
keyed up from nervous tension; this process is comparable to raising the key of a violin by tightening
the strings. We say that our muscles limber up

during exercise and that we are thrilled by great emotional experiences; all this prepares us for better peak accomplishments. On the other hand, there is the tingling sensation, the jitteriness, when we are keyed up too much. This impairs our work and even prevents us from getting a rest.

Just what happens to us when we are tense? Being keyed up is a very real sensation which must have a physicochemical basis. It has not yet been fully analyzed, but we know that at times of tension our adrenals produce an excess, both of adrenalines and of corticoids. We also know that taking either adrenalines or corticoids can reproduce a very similar sensation of being keyed up and excitable. For example, a person who is given large doses of cortisone in order to treat some allergic or rheumatoid condition often finds it difficult to sleep. He may even become abnormally euphoric, that is, carried away by an unreasonable sense of well-being and buoyancy, which interferes with sleep and is not unlike that caused by being very slightly drunk. Later, somnolence and a sense of deep depression may follow.

We first saw this condition in experimental animals which had been given large doses of corticoids. Here, an initial state of great excitation— corresponding to the euphoria of patients—was followed by depression which might even proceed to complete anesthesia.

It had long been known that not only mental excitement (for instance, that communicated by a rioting mob or by an individual act of violence) but even physical stressors (such as a burn or an infectious fever) could cause an initial excitement, followed by a secondary phase of depression. It is interesting to learn that identifiable chemical compounds—the hormones produced during the acute alarm-reaction phase of the G.A.S.—possess this property of first keying up for action and then causing a depression. Both these effects may be of great practical value to the body: it is necessary to be keyed up for peak accomplishments, but it is equally important to be keyed down by the secondary phase of depression, which prevents us from carrying on too long at top speed.

What can we do about this? Hormones are probably not the only regulators of our emotional level. Besides, we do not yet know enough about their workings to justify any attempt at regulating our emotional key by taking hormones.

Still, it is instructive to know that stress stimulates our glands to make hormones which can induce a kind of drunkenness. Without knowing this, no one would ever think of checking his conduct as carefully during stress as he does at a cocktail party. Yet he should. The fact is that *a person can be intoxicated with his own stress hormones.* I venture to say that this sort of drunkenness has caused much more harm to society than the alcoholic kind.

We are on our guard against external toxicants, but hormones are parts of our bodies; it takes more wisdom to recognize and overcome the foe which fights from within. In all our actions throughout the day we must consciously look for signs of being keyed up too much—and we must learn to stop in time. To watch our critical stress level is just as important as to watch our critical quota of cocktails. More so. Intoxication by stress is sometimes unavoidable and usually insidious. You can quit alcohol and, even if you do take some, at least you can count the glasses; but it is impossible to avoid stress as long as you live, and your conscious thoughts often cannot gauge its alarm signals accurately. Curiously, the pituitary is a much better judge of stress than the intellect. Yet, you can learn to recognize the danger signals fairly well if you know what to look for (pages 171-178).

How to Tune Down

It is not easy to tune down when you have exceeded your stress quota. Many more people are the helpless slaves of their own stressful activities than of alcohol. Besides, simple rest is no cure-all. Activity and rest must be judiciously balanced, and *every person has his own characteristic requirements for rest and activity.* To lie motionless in bed all day is no relaxation for an active person. With advancing years, most people require increasingly more rest, but the process of aging does not progress at the same speed in everybody. Many a valuable person, who could still have given several years of useful work to society, has been made physically ill and prematurely senile by the enforced retirement at an age when his requirements and abilities for activity were still high. This psychosomatic illness is so common that it has been given a name: *retirement disease.*

All work and no play is certainly harmful for anyone at any age; but then, what is work and what is play? Fishing is relaxing play for the business executive, but it is hard work for the professional fisherman. The former can go fishing to unwind, but the latter will have to do something else, or simply take a rest, in order to relax.

What has research on stress taught us about the way *to reach a healthy balance between rest and work?* Are there objective physiologic facts which could guide our conduct in this respect? I emphatically believe that there are, but, in order to grasp their lesson, we must turn back to what we have learned about the most general tissue reactions to stress: cellular fatigue and inflammation. This may seem odd; you may feel that there is no conceivable relationship between the behavior of our cells (for instance, in inflammation) and our conduct in everyday life. I do not agree. All the reactions of our body are governed by general biologic laws, and the simplest way to understand these is to examine how they affect the simplest tissue reactions.

Stress as an Equalizer of Activities

It seems to be one of the most fundamental laws regulating the activities of complex living beings that no one part of the body must be disproportionately overworked for a long time. Systemic stress seems to be the great equalizer of activities within a person; *it helps to prevent one-sided overexertion.*

To carry a heavy suitcase for a long time without fatigue, you have to shift it from one arm to the other occasionally. Here, local stress, manifested as muscular fatigue, is the equalizer; it acts by way of the nervous system which experiences the feeling of fatigue and thereby suggests the change-over.

In other instances, general stress may arrange the proper equalization of local activities through the intermediary of the adaptive hormones. Sup-

pose a person has a severe infection in his left knee
joint. An arthritis develops with all the characteristic manifestations of inflammation. A strong
inflammatory barricade is constructed around the
joint to delimit the trouble; then, various cells and
enzymes will enter the joint cavity in order to
destroy the causative germs. Now, suppose both
knees are infected. There develops an inflammation on both sides, but its degree will be less severe.
Why? Because local stress of the inflamed territory
sends out alarm signals, via the pituitary, to
stimulate the production by the adrenals of anti-
inflammatory corticoids through systemic stress.

This arrangement is also a useful defense mechanism, because there is a limit to how much inflammation the body can tolerate. If only a small region
is injured, a strong inflammatory reaction will be
the best response, since inflammation has a local
protective value; but if several parts of the body
are simultaneously injured, the patient may not be
able to stand maximal inflammatory reactions
everywhere. Thus it is often in the best interests of
the body as a whole to cut down local defensive
activities.

This situation is quite comparable to that of a
country which, when attacked on one front only,
can send all its armies to the endangered region,
but cannot do so when several frontiers are simultaneously invaded.

Now, since stress is a common attribute of all
biologic activities, these considerations apply not
only to inflammation, but to all types of biologic
work. For instance, the intensity of inflammation
in a knee joint may be diminished, not only by
inflammation in other regions, but also by exces-

sive muscular work, nervous activity, or anything else that requires effort. This is so because any part under stress sends out alarm signals to coordinate resistance. For the same reason, any intense reaction in one part can influence (and, to some extent, equalize) all kinds of biologic activities in other parts of the same body.

The Stress Quotient

These facts, which have been established by laboratory experiments on rats, are also remarkably true when applied to the daily problems of human beings, including even our purely mental activities. In analyzing our stress status, we must always think, not only of the total amount of stress in the body, but also of its proportionate distribution between various parts. To put this into the simplest terms, we might say that the stress quotient to be watched is:

$$\frac{\text{local stress in any one part}}{\text{total stress in the body}}$$

If there is proportionately too much stress in any one part, you need diversion. If there is too much stress in the body as a whole, you must rest.

The Importance of Deviation

Deviation or diversion is the act of turning something (for instance, a biologic mechanism) aside from its course. It is not necessarily a pleasant and relaxing diversion. We have seen, for instance, how severe shock (electroshock, drug shock) can— through its general stress effect upon all parts— deviate the body's somatic or psychic defense reactions from a habitual stereotyped course.

When the concentration of effort in any one part of our body or mind is not very intense and chronic, as we all know from experience, milder types of deviation are often quite effective (sports, dancing, music, reading, travel, whisky, chewing gum or even smoking, gambling and, last but not least, sex). These do not have to act primarily through the stress mechanism and the pituitary-adrenal axis—nor do I unconditionally recommend them— but they always cause a decentralization of our efforts, which often helps to restore a lopsided stress quotient toward normal.

The rich executive would not think of moving his heavy furniture, yet he will go regularly for a "workout" to the gym of his expensive club. The body is not built to take too much stress always on the same part; we need work but it should be diversified.

Deviation is particularly important in combating purely mental stress. Everyone knows how much harm can be caused by worry. The textbooks of psychosomatic medicine are full of case reports describing the production of peptic ulcers, hypertension, arthritis, and many other diseases by chronic worry about moral and economic problems. *Nothing is accomplished by telling such people not to worry*. They cannot help it. Here again, the best remedy is deviation, or general stress. By highlighting some other problem, through deviation, or by activating the whole body, by general stress, the source of worry automatically becomes less important in proportion.

I like to remember an old recommendation that I learned as a child from an Austrian peasant woman:

> Imitate the Sundial's Ways
> Count Only the Pleasant Days.

This can be practiced consciously. Of course, for a person who is to undergo a very dangerous surgical operation, or who finds himself on the verge of economic disaster, it is impossible to stop worrying just by deciding not to—especially if he is the worrying kind. *You must find something to put in the place of the worrying thoughts to chase them away.* This is deviation. If such a person undertakes some strenuous task which needs all his attention, he may still not forget his worries, but they will certainly fade. Nothing erases unpleasant thoughts more effectively than conscious concentration on pleasant ones. Many people do this subconsciously, but unless you know about the mechanism of diversion, it is difficult to do it well.

Some neurotics compulsively concentrate on the most extraordinary and harmful things in the course of subconscious efforts to divert themselves from sexual frustrations. Psychoanalysts call this *sublimation*, which is defined as "the act of directing the energy of an impulse from its primitive aim to one that is culturally or ethically higher." I would not know about that; but it is deviation.

Incidentally, another practically important

aspect of deviation is the development of a competition between memory and learning power. It seems that to some extent *newly-learned facts occupy the place of previously-learned or subsequently learnable ones.* Consequently there is a limit to how much you can burden your memory; and trying to remember too many things is certainly one of the major sources of psychologic stress. I make a conscious effort to forget immediately all that is unimportant and to jot down data of possible value (even at the price of having to prepare complex files). Thus I manage to keep my memory free for facts which are truly essential to me. I think this technique can help anyone to accomplish the greatest simplicity compatible with the degree of complexity of his intellectual life.

Innate Vitality Must Find an Outlet

I have described elsewhere in this book the animal experiments which showed that every living being has a certain innate amount of *adaptation energy* or vitality. This can be used slowly for a long and uneventful life, or rapidly during a shorter and more stressful, but often also more colorful and enjoyable existence. Let me add now that the choice is not entirely ours. Even the optimum tempo at which we are to consume life is largely inherited from our predecessors. Yet, what is in us must out; otherwise we may explode at the wrong places or become hopelessly hemmed in by frustrations. *The great art is to express our vitality through the particular channels and at the particular speed which Nature foresaw for us.*

This is never very easy, but here again, intelli-

gent self-analysis helps. We have seen, for
instance, how deviation, not complete rest, may be
the best solution for a person who feels generally
tired although he has temporarily overworked only
one channel of self-expression. In some such cases,
rather paradoxically, even general stress (for
instance, shock therapy or muscular exercise) can
help by equalizing and decentralizing activities
which habitually have become concentrated in one
part of our being.

There are various ways of self-expression. The
one which I have found most consistent with biologic laws and most effective in practice will be
described later in Chapter 20 in the section on
"altruistic egoism."

Man must work, but to do it most efficiently he
also has to relax periodically. If we are just doing
too much—in general, not too much of any one
thing—the problem is one of excessive general
stress. It cannot be handled either by deviation or
by more stress; the great remedy here is to learn to
relax as quickly and completely as possible. This is
not as easily done as said, but a number of techniques have been developed which help us to diminish both mental and physical activity to the absolute minimum still compatible with survival. Their
efficacy can be judged by a variety of highly objective physiologic indexes, such as pulse rate, blood
pressure, respiration, the electroencephalogram,
and the basal metabolic rate.

Among the methods of achieving self-induced
states of altered consciousness are: Transcendental Meditation (TM—the alleged basis of the Science of Creative Intelligence, or SCI), Yoga, Zen,

Subud, Nichiren Sho Shu, Hare Krishna, Scientology, Black Moslemism, self-hypnosis, the "relaxation response" (Benson), and many others. Some of these are, others are not, associated with religious cults, but all of them are strongly enforced by following certain traditions or mystic rites which help to induce a state of altered consciousness in which total relaxation is accompanied by increased mental alertness. The monotonous repetition of certain words, concentration on a single sound, a source of light or even the hypnotist's eyes help to bring about this state, presumably by deflecting attention from disturbing stimuli. None of these, however, should be overdone.

Maharishi Mahesh Yogi was chiefly responsible for introducing into the Western world the old Eastern practice of Transcendental Meditation, which has met with considerable success in the Americas and Europe. Dr. H. Benson of Harvard University has developed a modified form of it under the name of the "relaxation response" which is divested of the mystic elements. Both of these techniques, however, involve the induction of the deepest possible relaxation, with eyes closed for about twenty to thirty minutes twice daily, and permit awakening, whenever desired, in a completely relaxed state, which appears to facilitate creative thinking.

The basic elements of such techniques have been known for centuries, usually as religious rituals. We find them in the stereotyped repetition of prescribed prayers or litanies, the obligatory "contemplation" sessions of Carmelite nuns, the mystic contemplation of God's presence. After a while these become totally mechanical and soothing and thereby also help to cut out all exacting mental or physical activity which might demand adaptation to change or other types of performance that require attention. Although the biologic mechanism of all these practices remains to be clarified, they do manifestly offer much-needed relaxation to many people and can be even more efficient in this respect than deep sleep.

As we have often said, complete absence of stress is incompatible with life since only a dead man makes no demand upon his body or mind. Yet even the most agreeable, intense eustress cannot be kept up indefinitely and should be interrupted by periods of rest. Apparently, the various forms of the relaxation responses permit us to diminish activity to the lowest tolerable level.

Of course, those who like to lead a lazy life are less in need of such special techniques to help them relax, but only at the cost of losing the delights of eustress and creative accomplishment. I have often tried to enjoy laziness, but I have never succeeded. I suppose it is just not in my nature. I am afraid, if you want to learn this art, you will have to read another author. But, for a long time, I have suffered from insomnia, and I did learn how to sleep, so perhaps I might say a few words about this now.

How to Sleep

The stress of a day of hard work can make you sleep like a log or it can keep you awake all night. This sounds contradictory, but if you come to analyze the work that helps you to sleep and the work that keeps you awake, there is a difference. *Muscular activity or mental work which leads to a definite solution prepares you for rest and sleep; but intellectual efforts which set up self-maintaining tensions keep you awake.* The fatigue of work well accomplished gets you ready for sleep but, during the night, you must protect yourself against being awakened by stress. Everybody knows the value of protection against noise, light, variations in temperature, or the difficulties of digesting a heavy meal taken before retiring. We need not speak about such protective measures here. But what can you do to regulate psychologic stress so it will not keep you awake?

If you suffer from insomnia, there is no point in telling yourself, "Forget everything and relax; sleep will come by itself." It does not.

Sheep-counting, warm milk, hot baths, and so forth are also of little value, since they only help those who have faith in them. The fact is that by the time you retire it is too late for anything except the sleeping pill. *It is during the whole day that you must prepare your dreams;* for, whatever you do during the day, your next night's sleep depends largely on how you have spent your previous day.

The recipe for this preparation can be deduced from the following passages:

Do not let yourself get carried away and keyed up more than is necessary to acquire the momentum for the best performance of what you want to do in the interest of self-expression. If you get keyed up too much, especially during the later hours of the day, your stress reaction may carry over into the night.

Keep in mind that the hormones produced during acute stress are meant to alarm you and key you up for peak accomplishments. They tend to combat sleep and to promote alertness during short periods of exertion; they are not meant to be used all day long. If too much of these hormones is circulating in your blood, they will keep you awake, just as a tablet of amphetamine would. (Incidentally, amphetamine is chemically related to adrenaline.) Your insomnia has a chemical basis, which cannot easily be talked away after it has developed; and at night in bed it is too late to prevent it from progressing.

Try not to overwork any one part of your body or mind disproportionately by repeating the same actions to exhaustion. Be especially careful to avoid the senseless repetition of the same mental task when you are already exhausted. A moment of objective self-analysis will suffice to convince you that this work could be done much more easily after a good night's sleep, or even after only a few hours of doing something else (deviation). If you get yourself deep in a rut, you may not be able to stop, and mentally you will keep on repeating your routine throughout the night.

Nature likes variety. Remember this, not only in planning your day, but in planning your life. Our civilization tends to force people into highly specialized occupations which may become monotonously repetitive. Remember that stress is the great equalizer of biologic activities and if you use the same parts of your body or mind over and over again, the only means Nature has to force you out of the groove is general (systemic) stress.

Remember also that insomnia is a powerful stressor in itself. If a sleepless night follows a day of overexertion, next day your usual work will have to be done while you are sleepy. The stress of it may mean another sleepless night and the development of a vicious circle which is difficult to break. Fortunately, this complication will rarely develop if you follow my prescription; but if it does, the best way out is to sleep during the day if you can, or to take a mild sleeping pill at night.

To summarize: protect yourself against stress at night, not only by cutting out too much light, noise, cold, or heat, but particularly by never allowing yourself to be under the kind of stress during the day that may automatically go on throughout the night. This self-perpetuating kind of stress may be the result of a heavy meal, whisky, emotional upsets, and many other things. Watch for them. So, remember: stress keeps you awake while it lasts (even when it outlasts its cause) but it prepares you for sleep later when your reaction to it is finished.

chapter 20

Philosophic Implications

*Facing the demands of life: defense, offense,
wear and tear. To die of old age. The origin of
individuality. The need for self-expression.
What are man's ultimate aims? Greatness and
excellence. The philosophy of gratitude. The
principle of altruistic egoism. Success formula?*

Facing the Demands of Life: Defense, Offense, Wear and Tear

For our scientific research in the laboratory we
needed an operational definition of stress, that is,
one which showed us what to do in order to see
stress. It is only by the intensity of its manifestations—the adrenal enlargement, the increased corticoid concentration in the blood, the loss of weight,
and so forth—that we can recognize the presence
and gauge the intensity of stress. The fact that you
cannot see it directly or otherwise demonstrate it
as such does not make stress less real. After all, as
Christina L. Rosetti put it:

Who has seen the wind?
Neither you nor I
But when the trees bow down their heads
The wind is passing by.

For the present discussion, our short Aristote-
lian definition—which merely classifies stress as
one aspect of wear and tear throughout life, at any
one time—is most satisfactory. When so defined,
the close relationship between defense, offense,
work, aging, and stress becomes particularly evident. General systemic stress is the sum of all the
nonspecific effects of any vital reaction. That is
why it can act as a common denominator of all the
biologic changes which go on in the body; it is a
kind of "speedometer of life."

Now, in discussing my experiments, I have often
had occasion to point out that aging, at least true
physiologic aging, is not determined by the time
elapsed since birth, but by the total amount of wear
and tear to which the body has been exposed. There
is, indeed, a great *difference between physiologic
and chronologic age.* One man may be much more
senile in body and mind, and much closer to the
grave, at forty than another at sixty. True age
depends largely on the rate of wear and tear, on the
speed of self-consumption; for life is essentially a
process which gradually spends the given amount
of adaptation energy that we inherited from our
parents. Vitality is like a special kind of bank
account which you can use up by withdrawals but
cannot increase by deposits. Your only control over
this most precious fortune is the rate at which you
make your withdrawals. The solution is evidently
not to stop withdrawing, for this would be death.
Nor is it to withdraw just enough for survival, for
this would permit only a vegetative life, worse than
death. The intelligent thing to do is to withdraw

and expend generously, but never wastefully for worthless efforts.

Many people believe that, after they have exposed themselves to very stressful activities, a rest can restore them to where they were before. This is false. Experiments on animals have clearly shown that each exposure leaves an indelible scar, in that it uses up reserves of adaptability which cannot be replaced. It is true that immediately after some harassing experience, rest can restore us almost to the original level of fitness by eliminating acute fatigue. But the emphasis is on the word *almost*. Since we constantly go through periods of stress and rest during life, even a minute deficit of adaptation energy every day adds up—it adds up to what we call *aging*.

Apparently, there are *two kinds of adaptation energy:* the superficial kind, which is ready to use, and the deeper kind, which acts as a sort of frozen reserve. When superficial adaptation energy is exhausted during exertion, it can slowly be restored from a deeper store during rest. This gives a certain plasticity to our resistance. It also protects us from wasting adaptation energy too lavishly in certain foolish moments, because acute fatigue automatically stops us. It is the restoration of the superficial adaptation energy from the deep reserves that tricks us into believing that the loss has been made good. Actually, it has only been covered from reserves—and at the cost of gradually depleting the latter. We might compare this feeling of having suffered no loss to the careless optimism of a spendthrift who keeps forgetting that whenever he restores the vanishing supply of dollars in his wallet by withdrawing from the invisible stocks of his bank account, the loss has not really been made good: there was merely a transfer of money from a less accessible to a more accessible form.

I think, in this respect, the lesson of animal experimentation has a great practical bearing upon the way we should live; it helps us to translate knowledge into wisdom.

The lesson is a particularly timely one. Due to the great advances made by classic medicine during the last half century, premature death caused by specific disease producers (microbes, malnutrition, etc.) has declined at a phenomenal rate. As a result of this, the *average human life-span* increased in the United States from 48 years in 1900 to about 72 years by 1973. But since everybody still has to die sometime, more and more people are killed by pathogens which cannot be eliminated using the methods of classic medicine. An ever-increasing proportion of the human population dies from the so-called wear-and-tear diseases, diseases of civilization, or degenerative diseases, which are primarily due to stress.

In other words, the more man learns about ways to combat external causes of death (germs, cold, hunger), the more likely is he to die from his own voluntary, suicidal behavior. I am not competent to speak about wars—though these are also signs of maladaptation—but perhaps my experiments can teach us something about the way to conduct our personal lives in keeping with natural laws. Life is a continuous series of adaptations to our surroundings and, as far as we know, our reserve of adaptation energy is an inherited finite amount, which cannot be regenerated. On the other hand, I am sure we could still enormously lengthen the average human life-span by living in better harmony with natural laws.

In chemical terms one might view adaptation energy as the ability to remove the chemical scars of life. Each biologic process leads to some chemical changes whose end-products are usually soluble or subject to destruction and elimination. Whenever this form of restoration is rapid, and recovery complete, our tissues undergo little change and we remain "young." However, an infinitesimally small percentage of all biologic reaction-products are insoluble, or at least less rapidly removable than their rate of deposition. The so-called "aging pigments," calcium deposits, cross-linked proteins, and many other products of biologic activity belong to this class. Mere excessive accumulation suffices to block the machinery. It could induce the changes we consider characteristic of aging by the mere presence of ever larger amounts of inert waste products and the consequent inability to produce indispensable vital ingredients at the proper rate.

To Die of Old Age

What makes me so certain that the natural human life-span is far in excess of the actual one is this:

Among all my autopsies (and I have performed well over one thousand), I have never seen a person who died of old age. In fact, *I do not think anyone has ever died of old age yet.* To permit this would be the ideal accomplishment of medical research (if we disregard the unlikely event of someone discovering how to regenerate adaptation energy). To die of old age would mean that all the organs of the body had worn out proportionately, merely by having been used too long. This is never the case. We invariably die because one vital part has worn out too early in proportion to the rest of the body. Life, the biologic chain that holds our parts together, is only as strong as its weakest vital link. When this breaks—no matter which vital link it be—our parts can no longer be held together as a single living being.

You will note I did not say "our parts die," because this is not necessarily so. In tissue cultures, isolated cells of a human being can go on living for a long time after the body as a whole has died. It is only the complex organization of all our cells into a single individual that necessarily dies when one indispensable part breaks down. An old man may die because one worn-out, hardened artery breaks in his brain, or because his kidneys can no longer wash out the metabolic wastes from his blood, or because his heart muscle is damaged by excessive work. But *there is always one part which wears out first and wrecks the whole human machinery*, merely because the other parts cannot function without it.

This is the price we pay for the evolution of the human body from a simple cell into a highly complex organization. In principle, *unicellular animals never need to die* save through accidents. They just divide, and the parts live on.

The lesson seems to be that, as far as man can

regulate his life by voluntary actions, he should seek to equalize stress throughout his being, by what we have called *deviation*, the frequent shifting-over of work from one part to the other. The human body—like the tires on a car, or the rug on a floor—wears longest when it wears evenly. We can do ourselves a great deal of good in this respect by just yielding to our natural cravings for variety in everyday life. We must not forget that the more we vary our actions, the less any one part suffers from attrition.

We have seen in a previous passage through what mechanisms stress itself can act as an equalizer of biologic activities (see page 414); but it is equally true that stress, perhaps precisely due to its equalizing effect, gives an excellent chance to develop innate potential talents, no matter where they may be slumbering in the mind or body. In fact, *it is only in the heat of stress that individuality can be perfectly molded.*

The Origin of Individuality

In 1859, when Charles Darwin published *The Origin of Species*, he promised that in his book "light would be thrown on the origin of man and his history." This volume marked a new epoch in scientific, philosophic, and religious thought because it described observations suggesting that the animal species had developed "by means of natural selection or the preservation of favored races in the struggle for life." In many respects, there is a curious resemblance between the means employed by Nature in evolving species and individuals. Limita-

tions of food and space restrict the development of
species to the strongest ones. Similar limitations of
nutrition and anatomy, within each individual,
force stress to develop (through preferential usage)
those organs, aptitudes and attitudes which are
best suited to maintain life.

The features of a species reflect the cumulative
memories of past generations; individuality results
from the gradual engraving upon this inherited
background of personal memories (including "biochemical memories") as they are acquired during a
single life-span. In the course of the development of
a species, every member of each successive generation must relive—as an embryo before entering
this world—the entire history of its ancestors from
the primeval ameba up to the contemporary newborn stage. Then, after birth, each individual,
indeed every organ in his body, again goes through
innumerable adaptive reactions, to develop those
personal characteristics which distinguish him
from all other individuals. *Just as among the races,
so among the organs and aptitudes of each person
only the favored survive in the struggle for existence.* We have seen that within the individual this
is accomplished largely through the stress mechanism which also regulates behavior.

When too much is going on in any one place
within the body, that part is temporarily put out of
action, by tissue breakdown, acute inflammation,
or mere fatigue—which comprise essentially the
alarm phase of the L.A.S. This forces other parts
to take over, and thereby gives them a chance to
develop as far as they can.

But even without there being excessive activity

in any one part, too much may be going on in the body as a whole. Then, the central coordinators of adaptation (the nervous system and the endocrine glands) are informed of this by the sum of the alarm signals arriving from all parts at any one time. When general stress is excessive the whole organism needs a rest; it cannot afford a struggle anywhere. This provides an opportunity to try again and again, even after repeated failures, until the best distribution of organ development is reached. Thus the individual can be molded in harmony with his inherited potentialities and the demands made upon him by his surroundings. Of course, congenital aptitudes form the baseline of adaptability. They depend upon evolution and inheritance from ancestors and parents, but the manifest features of a person are largely the result of the stresses to which this adaptability is then exposed during the individual's own lifetime.

If we are to learn something by observing stress in Nature, if we are to derive some lesson that could guide our conduct in daily life, we must again ask ourselves, "What can we do about all this?" The development of fatigue or inflammation in an overworked organ, the production of ACTH and corticoids during stress, are obviously beyond voluntary control. So is our genetic make-up. There is something compulsive, something strictly obligatory, even in our "voluntary activities." It is all very well to say that our vitality (our adaptation energy) should be used wisely, at a certain rate, and for certain tasks, but all this is theory. In practice, when it comes to guiding human conduct, it seems that we must all bow to the great law

which says that what is in us must express itself; in
fact it must express itself at a speed and in directions predetermined by our own inherited structure. This is largely true, but not quite—and on the
little untruth in this dictum rests my whole philosophy of conduct.

The Need for Self-expression

After a pilot has left the ground in a plane—unless
he wants to kill himself—he cannot stop his motor
for a nice long rest before he gets back to earth
again. He must complete his mission back to earth.
Yet there is very much he can do, through voluntary choice of conduct, to get as far as possible with
a given airplane and fuel supply under given cli-
matic conditions. For instance, he can fly at a speed
and on a course best suited to his machine under
the prevailing weather conditions. The two great
limiting factors over which, once in flight, he has no
control are: his initial fuel supply and the structure
of his plane, particularly the amount of wear and
tear its weakest vital part can tolerate.

When a human being is born—unless he wants to
kill himself—he cannot stop either, before he has
completed his mission on earth. Yet he too can do
much, through voluntary choice of conduct, to get
as far as possible with a given bodily structure and
supply of adaptation energy, under given social
conditions. For instance, he can live and express
his personality at a tempo and in a direction best
suited to his inherited talents, under the prevailing
social conditions. The two great limiting factors—
which are fixed once a man is born—are: his supply

of adaptation energy and the wear and tear that the weakest vital part of his body can tolerate.

So, actually, we can accomplish a great deal by living wisely in accordance with natural laws. We can determine our optimum speed of living, by trying various speeds and finding out which one is most agreeable. We can determine our course and part of our destiny by the same empirical method, keeping in mind, however, that occasional deviations have a virtue of their own: they equalize the wear and tear throughout the body, and thereby give overworked parts time to cool down.

In my analogy you will find two weak points which are particularly instructive because they highlight the difference between an inanimate and a living machine.

First, the real strength of life is not the fuel (food) we take, but adaptability, because the living machine can make considerable repairs and adjustments *en route*, as long as it has adaptation energy. With this it can assimilate caloric energy from its surroundings. Consequently, resting an overworked part in the body helps not only by "cooling it down" but also by permitting it to make major repairs and even improvements in its structure.

Second (I say "second" as a physician, but would have said "first" as a human being), the object of man is not to keep going as long as possible. This is rather charmingly expressed by the motto on the masthead of the *Journal of Gerontology*, a medical journal devoted to the study of old age: "To add life to years, not just years to life."

Man certainly does not get the feeling of happiness, of having completed his mission on earth, just by staying alive very long. On the contrary, a long life without the feeling of fulfillment is very tedious. And yet, when (and if) they analyze their lives, most people get the feeling of merely muddling through, of drifting aimlessly, from one day to another. Just staying alive, no matter how comfortably and securely, is no adequate outlet for man's vital adaptation energy. Comfort and security make it easier for us to enjoy the great things in life, but they are not, in themselves, great and enjoyable aims.

What Are Man's Ultimate Aims?

Philosophers, psychologists, and mystics have argued about this since time immemorial. We have heard many noble and many vulgar answers: to please God, to obtain power, love, or sexual satisfaction, to receive recognition and approval from others or from ourselves, to achieve creative expression—or simply, happiness. All these answers ring true to some people and none of them to all. Looking at this list gives me the same feeling I had when, as a young medical student in Prague, I first examined patients suffering from various diseases: there must be some common denominator here.

It is a very fundamental human need, for instance, to work for some reward, and to judge and enjoy our success in proportion to the magnitude of the compensations we can accumulate. They may be dollars, titles, medals, or any other possession. They may even be fellow human beings who become our slaves—because of our dollars, titles or other possessions. They may be good deeds for which God will repay us. But one thing is certain: they *must be additive.* How else could we count our gains? How else could we know whether we have accomplished enough to be secure and happy?

I found my answer to these problems in what I like to call *the philosophy of altruistic egoism.** It helped me to form my personal attitude toward stress in life. It may help you, too. But then, I realize, that it may not; for you might not see things my way. Here I am outside my element, the laboratory, where a proven fact is binding for everyone. Here, I have ventured into pure philosophy: a very dangerous thing for a medical scientist to do, and a thing for which I shall no doubt be severely rebuked by some of my more reserved and reticent colleagues! But, you see, it is part of my philosophy that I must express myself, so I cannot help it. It was indeed very stressful to spend all my adult life in the laboratory, working on stress; it was perhaps even more stressful to express my thoughts in the form of this book and of the many lectures I gave about its substance. But well do I know that not to express all this would have

*In the first edition of this book I called essentially the same attitude "the philosophy of gratitude" and although I have received many letters showing that most readers found the basic idea satisfactory as a guide for motivation, they felt uncomfortable about admittedly doing things only in order to gain gratitude. I think the problem lies mainly in the connotations of narrow-minded vanity the word has received, whereas "altruistic egoism" offers essentially the same reward and is more readily defensible on the basis of unavoidable biologic laws, as we shall see later.

deprived me of much eustress and caused me much more distress.

It is strange that what I value most, as my personal reward for the time spent on dissecting the stress mechanism, is not a medical but a philosophic lesson. And yet this lesson is not even very new; vaguely, most people have always felt it. The scientific analysis of how the body reacts to stress has only helped to translate, into terms of intellect, what the instinctive wisdom of the emotions had always dimly appreciated. Still, in an age so largely governed by intellect as ours, it is gratifying to learn that much of what religions and philosophies have taught as doctrines to guide our conduct is based on scientifically-understandable biologic truths. It is not easy to put this lesson into words, but I really want to try.

Is the need for self-expression the common denominator of man's ultimate aims? Do we always look for rewards because we need some cumulative indicator of success which tells us to what extent we have accomplished self-expression? If this were so, it would explain why purely sensual satisfaction—the enjoyment of any among the pleasures of the flesh—has never been a truly satisfactory long-range aim for man. No matter how acute the happiness they give, the pleasures of the flesh are ephemeral; they cannot be accumulated in the form of any kind of capital. They cannot give us the sense of a life mission well accomplished or of having earned some type of wealth which assures our security throughout life.

Goodwill, whether you receive it or give it, is in itself very enjoyable. But there are many pleasing things which do not seem to be logically related to the incitement of gratitude or to altruistic egoism. The passive receipt of rewards, for instance. The enjoyment of food and drink, of a beautiful sunny day, of a magnificent painting, or the purely sensual pleasures of sex, are certainly not sought to inspire goodwill or gratitude in others. But let us not forget that the actual receipt of rewards—no matter how great the delight they can give us—is also quite unsuitable as an ultimate aim in life. Why? Simply because it is too transient. It can be ardently sought to enrich a moment; but we cannot accumulate these sensations into a treasure assuring our security and peace of mind in the future. Still, striving toward gratitude and goodwill is so deeply rooted in man's nature that we feel the instinctive urge somehow to connect even these values with thankfulness: to say grace before dinner, to ennoble sex with grateful love, to feel indebted to the maker of every enjoyable thing—be it a poem, a health-restoring drug, or a sunny day—has its roots in this feeling.

We have said these passive pleasures are disqualified from being ultimate aims; but they can still be very important aims. To a certain extent, some of them even have a measure of a stabilizing (homeostatic) effect, and at least their afterglow can be stocked and accumulated. The passive enjoyment of great art or of the great wonders of Nature does help us to achieve a degree of equanimity; and while, to the mere onlooker, they give no means for self-expression, they do help to provide self-sufficiency. In this sense, a great capacity to derive pleasure out of feelings can steady our inter-

personal relations, because it makes us less dependent upon society. But, in analyzing the relationship between passive and active attitudes toward
pleasure—between means and ends, between work
and reward, between satisfying the impulse to
express ourselves and our feeling of having accomplished this—we must give special attention to the
afterglow of pleasure, which can be stocked. Its
benefits are cumulative because the better we
learn to enjoy greatness—be it in art or in
Nature—the more we profit from contemplating it.
To learn how to enjoy this kind of greatness can be
a very exacting task, and, since it involves activity,
it is in itself an outlet for self-expression. This can
be learned, and it is well worth learning.

Besides the wish to earn the gratitude and goodwill of others through the medical applications of
the stress concept, it was the purely selfish desire
to enjoy Nature better, by learning to understand
one of its fundamental mechanisms, that acted as
the strongest motive for my investigations. In fact,
one of the principal inducements to write this book
was the wish to share with others the serene and
elevating satisfaction which comes from understanding the inherent, harmonious beauty of
Nature.

No sensitive person can look at the sky on a
cloudless night without asking himself where the
stars came from, where they go, and what keeps
the universe in order. The same questions arise
when we look at the internal universe within the
human body, or even just at that pair of sensitive
and searching human eyes which constantly strive
to bridge the gap between these two universes.

The capacity to contemplate, at least with some

degree of understanding, the harmonious elegance in Nature's manifestations, is one of the most satisfactory experiences of which man is capable. To attain even a small measure of it is a noble and gratifying aim in itself, quite apart from any material advantages it may offer. But actually it does also help us in our everyday life, very much in the same way as a deep religious faith or a well-balanced philosophic outlook can help us. Looking at something infinitely greater than our conscious selves makes all our daily troubles appear to shrink by comparison. There is an equanimity and a peace of mind which can be achieved only through contact with the sublime.

> The fairest thing we can experience [said Einstein] is the mysterious. It is the fundamental emotion which stands at the cradle of true art and true science. He who knows it not and can no longer wonder, no longer feel amazement, is as good as dead, a snuffed-out candle.

You do not have to be a professional scientist to experience the great melodious creations of Nature, any more than you have to be a composer to enjoy music. The most harmonious and mysterious creations are those of Nature; and to my mind, it is the highest cultural aim of the professional scientist to interpret them so that others may share in their enjoyment.

As children we all had what it takes to enjoy wonderful and mysterious things. When a child points out something unusual which he has never seen before—a colorful butterfly, an elephant, or a sea shell—just watch his eyes as he cries out with

enthusiasm, "Look, Mummy!" and you will know
what I mean.

We all had this priceless talent for pure enjoyment when we were young, but as time goes by,
most of us—not all—lose this gift. We lose it
because, gradually, we have seen most of the
things that we are likely to encounter in everyday
life, and custom stales variety. The petty routine of
daily problems also tends to blunt our sensitivity to
the detached enjoyment of greatness and wonder.
It is a pity that nowadays most people are so anx-
iously bent on being practical, on getting ahead in
life, that they no longer find time to make sure
where they really want to go. After a while, the
prosperous businessman, the efficient administra-
tor, the up-and-coming young lawyer begin to get
that lost feeling of aimlessly drifting from day to
day—toward retirement. So many people work
hard and intelligently for some immediate objective which promises leisure to enjoy life tomorrow;
but tomorrow never becomes today. There is
always another objective which promises even
more leisure in exchange for just a little more
work. Hence, very few people in the usual walks of
life retain the ability really to enjoy themselves:
that wonderful gift which they all possessed as
children. But it hurts to be conscious of this defect,
so adults dope themselves with more work (or other
things) to divert attention from their loss. Some
people nowadays even speak of "workaholism" for
the behavior of those who work merely as a means
of escape from a life which became stale.

The inspired painter, poet, composer, astronomer, or biologist never grows up in this respect; he

does not tend to get the feeling of aimlessly drifting, no matter how poor or old he may be. He
retains the childlike ability to enjoy the impractical
by-products of his activity. Pleasures are always
impractical, they can lead us to no reward. They
are the reward. It is commonplace to say that
money is no ultimate aim, but few people seem to
live as though they understood this. The labors of
the artist who succeeds in expressing some hidden
aspect of his soul in painting, or of the physician
who learns how a hitherto inexplicable disease
develops, may have practical advantages for him—
benefits which can be expressed in dollars—but
this is not the kind of reward that can make his life
a real success. The great financier must also seek
his final compensation elsewhere. To find it he
must stop worrying about the success of his enter-
prises, at least long enough to think of his own
success. *He must first find a way of life which can
assure him the equanimity necessary for enjoyment, and then he must learn to distinguish between
what can give him pleasure and what are only
means to buy pleasure.*

The most acquisitive person is so busy reinvest-
ing that he never learns how to cash in. "Realistic
people" who pursue "practical aims" are rarely as
realistic and practical, in the long run of life, as the
dreamers who pursue only their dreams.

Greatness and Excellence

Greatness or excellence in any field can become a
very satisfactory aim in itself.

In Webster's dictionary "great" is defined as

"that which is particularly noted or notable for superiority of accomplishment especially in a particular field of activity." The meaning of the word is also discussed in relation to the terms: elaborate, ample, numerous, heavy, forceful, intense, extreme, marked, prominent, renowned, eminent, distinguished, important, significant, weighty, effective, favorite, friendly, main, principal, lofty, noble, magnanimous, assiduous, persistent, wonderful, admirable, and many other concepts. All of these (even the "perfect crime") are customarily regarded as having the characteristics of greatness or excellence.

The adjective is also applied to such different inanimate things as Mount Everest, famines, wars, revolutions, epidemics, the Amazon River, the Taj Mahal, the laws that govern natural phenomena, from the movement of the planets to the behavior of submicroscopic cell particles. In addition it is used to designate those divine or human beings to whom the creation of these things is attributed.

This list is so vast that it is difficult to define just what can make a person deserve this adjective.

Most people stand in awe of greatness, and for many the possibility of achieving it through excellence is a major force motivating conduct.

To show the complexity of the problem, let us mention the names of some people who have been considered great in one sense or another: Albert Einstein, Adolf Hitler, Bertrand Russell, Benito Mussolini, Bernard Shaw, Charlie Chaplin, Sarah Bernhardt, Laurence Olivier, Richard Wagner, Napoleon Bonaparte, Genghis Khan, Leonardo da Vinci, Karl Marx, Pablo Picasso, I. P. Pavlov, Al

Capone, Alexander the Great, Galina Ulanova, Jack Dempsey, Moses, Confucius, Jeanne d'Arc, Copernicus, Mao Tse-tung, Attila the Hun, Queen Victoria, Jesus Christ, and Mohammed. To this same unusually dissimilar group also belong the Pharaohs who built the pyramids, the religious martyrs, the great organizers of the Mafia, billionaires, and record-breakers in any field. All of them have been considered great whether their achievements were good or bad, constructive or destructive. Napoleon certainly showed greatness as a conqueror, but undoubtedly caused more suffering than pleasure both to his fellow Frenchmen and to the people he conquered. The same is true of many religious, political and philosophic leaders.

One main motivator for achievement is to avoid monotony, ennui, aimlessness, which are terribly difficult to bear for any length of time. The second inducement is our respect for excellence as such. Certainly, greatness, as the ultimate of achievement, is one of the leading motivators of human endeavor; like its prerequisite, excellence, it is an aim in itself.

Our admiration for it explains the success of all the bards who sang the glory of greatness and excellence, irrespective of its final product, from *The Iliad* to *Jonathan Livingston Seagull* or *The Old Man and the Sea;* to *The Great Train Robbery* and *Blue Beard*. It is not the accomplishment of the heroes but the greatness of their efforts that moves us. From time to time we need to be lifted out of the mediocrity and monotony of our life, and this can be done by tales of greatness, by the quiet and elevating atmosphere of a cathedral, the sight

of a majestic panorama, or the glory of having
accomplished a seemingly unattainable aim.

The Philosophy of Gratitude

Could, and should, consciously planned striving for
gratitude become the basis of a practical philosophy—a way of life? Working for any kind of reward
seems rather unworthy of becoming the ultimate
aim of our existence. Most people would not like to
admit, even to themselves, that they do what they
do just in order to make other people grateful.

When you ask an artist why he paints, an author
why he writes, a soldier why he risks his life in
battle, they may give you all kinds of answers
(some idealistic, some mercenary) but they would
laugh at the suggestion that what they really want
is gratitude.

The scientist who sacrifices his private life in
favor of exacting laboratory work may admit that
he does it only "for fun" or out of a purely altruistic
wish "to be of service"; and, if he is more reserved,
he may recite the ready-made slogan of "science for
science's own sake." But he would be very much
surprised, and indeed ashamed, if you succeeded in
convincing him that he actually works to earn the
gratitude of his fellow men. Most scientists would
consider this a very selfish, if not naive, justification for their efforts. And yet, if you come to think
of it, which is more selfish and more naive: working
"for fun" and such intangibles as "science's own
sake," or for the inspiration in others of well-
earned gratitude?

My suggestion seems even more preposterous

when you think of people who do things which could not be of any material or spiritual help to anybody. Do they also work for gratitude? Take the gunman, whose life is nothing but a chain of brutal robberies and murders. And what of the kind-hearted, deeply religious man, who gives anonymously to the poor, precisely because—by not asking for gratitude—he wants to please God?

Yet, if you look a little closer, in the final analysis are not all these varied forms of self-expression subconsciously planned to earn gratitude and approval from one source or another? Where is the gratitude of those who are inspired by a great painting or a great idea, the thankfulness of men who have been saved from catastrophe by the valor of soldiers or the genius of scientists? And does not even the most debased thug commit his brutal crimes because all his earlier attempts to express himself in a manner which would earn gratitude have failed? And does not even the saintly giver remain anonymous because he prefers the grateful approval of a divine being to the gratitude of men?

The Principle of Altruistic Egoism

From what the laboratory and the clinical study of somatic diseases has taught us concerning stress, we have tried to arrive at a code of ethics based, not on traditions of our society, inspiration, or blind faith in the infallibility of any particular prophet, religious leader or political doctrine, but on the scientifically-verifiable laws that govern the body's reactions in maintaining homeostasis and living in satisfying equilibrium with its surroundings. When you meet a helpless drunk who showers you with insults but is obviously quite unable to do you any harm, nothing will happen if you take a "syntoxic attitude"—go past and ignore him. However, if you respond catatoxically and fight, or even only prepare to fight, the consequences may be tragic. You will discharge adrenalines that increase blood pressure and pulse rate, while your whole nervous system becomes alarmed and tense in anticipation of combat. If you happen to be a coronary candidate, the result may be a fatal heart accident. In this case, who is the murderer? The drunk didn't even touch you. This is biologic suicide! Death was caused by choosing the wrong reaction. If, on the other hand, the man who showers you with insults is a homicidal maniac with a dagger in his hand, evidently determined to kill you, you must take an aggressive catatoxic attitude. You must try to disarm him, even at the calculated risk of injury to yourself from the physical accompaniments of the alarm reaction in preparation for a fight. It is clear that, contrary to common opinion, Nature does not always know best because, on both the cellular and the interpersonal level, we do not always recognize what is and what is not worth fighting for.

Yet, it is a biologic law that—like all the lower animals—man has to fight and work for some goal that he considers worthwhile. He must use his innate capacities to enjoy the eustress of fulfillment. Only through effort, often aggressive egoistic effort, can he maintain his fitness and assure his homeostatic equilibrium with the surrounding society and the inanimate world. To achieve this

state, his activities must earn lasting results; the
fruits of his work must be cumulative and must
provide a capital gain to meet future needs. To
succeed, we have to accept the scientifically-estab-
lished fact that man has an inescapable, natural
urge to work egoistically for things that can be
stored to strengthen his homeostasis in unpredictable situations with which life may face him. These
are not instincts we should combat or be ashamed
of. We can do nothing about having been built to
work and work primarily for our own good. Organs
that are not used (muscles, bones, even the brain)
undergo inactivity atrophy. Every living being
looks out for itself first of all. There is no example
in Nature of a creature guided exclusively by altruism and the desire to protect others. In fact, a code
of universal altruism would be highly immoral,
since it would expect others to look out for us more
than for themselves.

"Love thy neighbor as thyself" is a command full
of wisdom but, as originally expressed, it is incompatible with biologic laws; no one ought to develop
an inferiority complex if he cannot love all his fellow men on command. Neither should we feel guilty
because we work for treasures that can be stored to
ensure our future homeostasis. Hoarding is, as we
have said, a vitally important biologic instinct that
we share with all animals, such as ants, bees, squir-
rels and beavers.

How could we develop a code of ethics which
accepts, as morally correct, egoism and working to
hoard personal capital? The "philosophy of altruistic egoism" advocates the creation of feelings of

accomplishment and security through the inspiration in others of love, goodwill and gratitude for what we have done or are likely to do in the future.

As explained in *Stress without Distress* (page iii), the basic concepts and guidelines are:

1. *Find your own natural stress level.* People differ with regard to the amount and kind of work they consider worth doing to meet the exigencies of daily life and to assure their future security and happiness. In this respect, all of us are influenced by hereditary predispositions and the expectations of our society. Only through planned self-analysis can we establish what we really want; too many people suffer all their lives because they are too conservative to risk a radical change and break with traditions.

2. *Altruistic egoism.* The selfish hoarding of the goodwill, respect, esteem, support, and love of our neighbor is the most efficient way to give vent to our pent-up energy and to create enjoyable, beautiful, or useful things.

3. *EARN thy neighbor's love.* This motto, unlike love on command, is compatible with man's natural structure and, although it is based on altruistic egoism, it could hardly be attacked as unethical. Who would blame anyone who wants to assure his own homeostasis and happiness by accumulating the treasure of other people's benevolence towards him? Yet, this makes him virtually unassailable, for nobody wants to attack and destroy those upon whom he depends.

Man is a social being. Avoid remaining alone in the midst of the overcrowded society which surrounds you. Trust people, despite their apparent untrustworthiness, or you will have no friends, no support. If you have earned your neighbor's love, you will never be alone.

These three main principles are derived from observations on the basic mechanisms that maintain homeostasis in cells, people, and entire societies, and that help them to face the stressors encountered in their constant fight for survival, security, and well-being. They have developed into instincts during evolution but evolution has not yet reached its final completion; it is still in progress. In the meantime we can best use this principle by conscious understanding and voluntary control.

However, there remain many techniques whose value in improving the quality of life has been established beyond doubt by purely empirical observations, although they are not directly related to attaining any particular goal; they help us indirectly by improving our physical and mental fitness. Among these we have mentioned muscular exercise, hot baths, saunas, and a number of psychologic techniques such as those of Transcendental Meditation, Yoga, or Zen, whose beneficial effects upon general well-being and mental performance cannot yet be fully explained in somatic terms. Yet, with time, this will undoubtedly become possible, since our brain is also part of our body and hence, of necessity, it must be subject to the eternal laws of Nature that govern somatic functions.

In view of the advances made in our knowledge of the role played by chemical compounds (adrena-

lines, 5–HT, psychotropic drugs) and nervous processes, it is in this field that we can see the greatest
future for the further development of a code of
behavior based on biologic laws.

Success Formula?

Despite all we have just said it must be clearly
understood that *there is no ready-made success
formula which would suit everybody*. We are all
different. The only thing we have in common is our
obedience to certain fundamental biologic laws
which govern all men. I think the best the professional investigator of stress can do is to explain the
mechanism of stress as far as he can understand it;
then, to outline the way he thinks this knowledge
could be applied to problems of daily life; and,
finally, as a kind of laboratory demonstration, to
describe the way he himself applied it successfully
to his own problems.

It was the dissection of stress and the analysis of
its structure which helped me most with my own
problems; and I do not think there is any better way
to learn more about something that, of necessity,
must be done differently by every person. It is
manifestly *impossible to construct a rigid "procedure manual" applicable to any problem that may
come up;* besides, this would make life intolerably
monotonous, by leaving no scope for individual
ingenuity in problem solving. No previous code of
ethics—religious, philosophic, or political—has
provided specific prescriptions for each possible
event that may be met in life, since even the same
problem must be solved differently depending upon

a person's genetic background, previous experiences, state of health, etc. Reactivity is as important as activity. Christianity, communism, or patriotism cannot tell you precisely what to do in each specific situation. Many times you should not "do unto others what you would like them to do unto you," because the requirements of others may not be the same as yours. The decision of how to be useful to different people must remain a problem for your own ingenuity.

What is the use, for example, of dissecting a sentence and explaining its structure? In actual speech you would never have the time to apply the rules of syntax and grammar by conscious intellectual processes. Still, people who know something about syntax and grammar use better language, thanks to this knowledge. You cannot teach a man how to express himself because it is the first rule of the game that his speech must reflect his personality, not yours. Moreover, few of the rules of syntax and grammar are absolute; the most unpolished slang is often more effective and picturesque than the King's English. All formal teaching can do is to explain the basic elements of language, so as to make them available for translation from conscious intellectual appraisal—which is impersonal, slow, and cold—into instinct—which is personal, quick, and warm.

I intended to do, and could do, no more in these pages than to present the syntax and grammar of stress, illustrating its application to the philosophy of life by one example: my own. A single case does not prove much; but, against my laboratory background, one actual experiment proves a great deal more than volumes of pure speculation. In such an experiment the indexes of success are purely subjective; therefore, I could not repeat the test on others and still vouch for the veracity of my findings. All I can say is that the philosophy of stress has helped me enormously in achieving equanimity and a personally satisfactory program for the way I want to go through life. I rather think if you tried it, it might help you too.

But, after all, I am no philosopher and certainly not a prophet! So, let me finish this book by giving an outline of what I think are the most important avenues opened up by stress research in its *strictly medical applications*, the new directions that we should follow in the study of disease: the road ahead.

chapter 21

The Road Ahead

Now that we have a blueprint of the body's own nonspecific general methods to combat disease, it is largely a matter of time and money to fill in the gaps. For this *organized research teamwork* is necessary. Although this is expensive, the cost will be trivial in comparison with the relief of human suffering that can be expected from it.

One major avenue for future research will be the scientific analysis of *adaptation energy*. We have seen (pages 36-38) that the stress syndrome develops in three stages, eventually leading to the depletion of adaptability or adaptation energy. This final exhaustion by stress is strikingly similar to senility; it is a kind of accelerated, premature aging. By learning more about the body's adaptation energy, the *life-span* could probably be greatly prolonged and health during old age improved. The diseases of old age become constantly more important as more and more people live to be old, thanks to medical progress. According to the estimates of the Twentieth Century Fund, and the U.S. Census, there were 14 million people aged 65 or more in the United States in 1956, when the first edition of this book appeared, and that means three times as many as in 1920. In 1974, there were 22 million people aged 65 or more, or almost five times the figure for 1920. Their number, and hence, the national importance of their problems, continues to increase rapidly.

Adaptation energy seems to be something of which everybody has a given amount at birth, an inherited capital to which we cannot add, but which we can use, more or less thriftily, in fighting the stress of life. Still, we have not fully excluded the possibility that adaptation energy could be regenerated to some extent, and perhaps even transmitted from one living being to another, somewhat like a serum. If its amount is unchangeable, we may learn more about how to conserve it. If it can be transmitted, we may explore means of extracting the carrier of this vital energy—for instance, from the tissues of young animals—and transmitting it to the old and aging.

Another fascinating field for future research is the study of stress in relation to *cancer*. It is well known that a large variety of cancers do not grow well in animals or people subjected to severe stress. In fact, some types of cancer have undergone considerable (though incomplete) regression under the influence of ACTH, cortisone, and other stress hormones. To what extent could we, by learning more about the mechanism of such regressions, help in the fight against this, the most terrible among human ailments?

We still know very little about the role of *catatoxic hormones* in the treatment of disease. They appear to be as powerful in increasing resistance as are the syntoxic hormones (such as cortisone), but their field of application is entirely different. What is their normal function in the body and how could they be used as drugs for treatment?

Many of these possibilities are still very remote, but so was treatment with the antibiotics from molds or the hormonal treatment of rheumatoid arthritis, not so many years ago. It may be well for the general public to realize that definite research plans for this type of study do now exist, and are handicapped mainly by the lack of adequate support.

Perhaps the most fascinating aspect of medical research on stress is its *fundamentally permanent value* to man. Even the most powerful drugs (chemicals which have curative value, but are not normally produced by the body) are of importance to us only for a certain time. Sooner or later, they are replaced by still more effective remedies and then they become uninteresting.

Take the arsenic derivative, Salvarsan, that Paul Ehrlich—the Father of Chemotherapy—introduced around 1910 for the treatment of syphilis. Until then this venereal disease was one of the greatest scourges of mankind. That a significant number of cures could be obtained with certain arsenicals had been justly hailed as one of the most important medical discoveries of all time. Yet now, after less than half a century, this treatment has lost its importance because penicillin has proved to be even more effective. The same fate awaits any of our potent drugs, as soon as still more effective ones will be found.

The study of stress differs essentially from research with artificial drugs because it deals with *the defensive mechanisms of our own body*. The immediate results of this budding new science are not yet as dramatic in their practical applications as are those of many drugs, but what we learn

about Nature's own self-protecting mechanisms
can never lose its importance. Such defensive measures as the production of adaptive hormones by
glands are built into the very texture of the body;
we inherited them from our parents and transmit
them to our children, who, in turn, must hand them
on to their offspring, as long as the human race
shall exist. *The significance of this kind of research
is not limited to fighting this or that disease. It has a
bearing upon all diseases and indeed upon all
human activities,* because it furnishes knowledge
about the essence of THE STRESS OF LIFE.

Yet, today, looking back upon 40 years of
research on stress, my greatest hope lies in the
possibilities it offers of arriving at a code of conduct
based upon natural laws. For the greatest problem
of our time is not atmospheric pollution, nor over-
population, nor even the atomic bomb, but the lack
of motivation by generally acceptable and
respected ideals. Science has shaken our blind faith
in virtually every traditional value and "infallible
authority." Our young are no longer willing to
believe blindly in the sanctity of purity in soul or
body, of the family structure and responsibilities,
the fatherland, the security offered by capital,
social status, or the loyal submission to the will of
our prophets and rulers, whether the divine rulers
of the east or our western kings and presidents.
The authority of the clergy, and indeed the existence of God, have been called into question. An
attitude of pessimism and doubt seems to have
settled upon mankind; violence, drug abuse, and
aimless destructive aggression appear more and
more to replace constructive behavior as an out-

let for our need of self-expression and creation. Virtually every code of law inspired by human logic or divine inspiration has been flaunted with contempt, and often impunity, at some time, by some people, except one: the code of the eternal laws of Nature. To develop and disseminate this code strikes me as the greatest contribution that research on the stress of life could make to humanity.

Glossary

A more detailed discussion of the concepts mentioned in this glossary will be found in the text at the pages indicated in parentheses.

abscess. A localized collection of pus within a capsule of connective tissue, as for instance, a boil.

AC. Abbreviation for anti-inflammatory corticoid.

ACTH. Abbreviation for adrenocorticotrophic hormone.

adaptation energy. The energy necessary to acquire and maintain adaptation, apart from caloric requirements. (See pp. 81, 162, 307.)

adaptive hormones. Hormones produced for adaptation to stress. (See p. 250.)

adrenaline. One of the hormones of the adrenal medulla. (See pp. 117–118.)

adrenalines. This designation is used as synonymous with "catecholamines," a technical term which we wanted to avoid for the sake of simplicity. It is described in the Glossary under that heading.

adrenals. Endocrine glands which lie (one on each side) just above the kidneys. They have a triangular, or Y-shaped form on cross section, and consist of a whitish outer cortex, or bark, and a dark brown medulla, or marrow. (See p. 100.)

adrenocorticotrophic hormone (ACTH). A pituitary hormone which stimulates the growth and function of the adrenal cortex. (See pp. 140–143.)

alarm reaction. The first stage of the adaptation syndrome. In the G.A.S. it affects the body as a whole; in the L.A.S. it is limited to a part. Correspondingly, we speak of a general and of a local alarm reaction. (See pp. 36–38.)

aldosterone. One of the proinflammatory corticoids. (See p. 295.)

angiotensin. A vasopressor substance generated by renin.

antagonist. An agent which acts against another agent.

antibiotics. Antibacterial substances, most of which are prepared from molds or fungi (e.g., penicillin, streptomycin).

anti-inflammatory corticoids. Adrenocortical hormones which inhibit inflammation, for example, cortisone or cortisol. They have a marked effect upon glucose metabolism and are therefore also known as *glucocorticoids*. (See p. 218.)

atrophy. See *involution*.

catatoxic. (From the Greek prefex *cata* = down or against.) Catatoxic substances increase the destruction and/or excretion of potentially toxic substances.

catecholamines. Adrenaline and noradrenaline (also known as epinephrine and norepinephrine), as well as some of their derivatives, are technically described as "catecholamines." However, we shall just refer to this group as the "adrenalines," to avoid unnecessary complications of terminology which could confuse the reader.

cell. A relatively autonomous, circumscribed, small mass of living material, visible under the microscope. The tissues of all living beings consist mainly of cells.

central nervous system (CNS). That portion of the nervous system consisting of the brain and spinal cord.

CNS. Abbreviation for central nervous system.

COL. Abbreviation for cortisol.

CON. Abbreviation for cortisone.

conditioning factors. Substances or circumstances which influence the response to an agent, for instance, a hormone. (See p. 123.)

connective tissue. A tissue consisting of cells and fine fibers; it is a kind of living cement which connects and reinforces all other tissues. Inflammation develops mainly in connective tissue. (See p. 154.)

corticoids. Hormones of the adrenal cortex. It is customary to subdivide them into the anti-inflammatory glucocorticoids and the proinflammatory mineralocorticoids. (See pp. 106, 119.)

corticotrophic. Stimulating the growth of the adrenal cortex and of the production of its hormones, the corticoids.

corticotrophin releasing factor (CRF). A substance produced by the hypothalamus which stimulates the production of ACTH.

cortisol (COL). One of the anti-inflammatory corticoids. (See pp. 224-226.)

cortisone (CON). One of the anti-inflammatory corticoids. (See pp. 119-120.)

CRF. Abbreviation for corticotrophin releasing factor.

crossed resistance. Resistance to one agent produced by pretreatment with another agent. (See p. 329.)

desoxycorticosterone (DOC). One of the proinflammatory corticoids. (See pp. 183-187.)

developmental adaptation. A simple progressive adaptive reaction, accomplished by mere enlargement and multiplication of preexisting cell elements, without qualitative change. In technical language: homotropic adaptation. (See p. 330.)

diagnosis. Recognition; for instance, the recognition of a disease.

direct pathogen. An agent causing disease through its direct effect (e.g., a burn).

diseases of adaptation. Maladies which are principally due to imperfections of the G.A.S., for example, to an excessive or insufficient amount, or an improper mixture, of adaptive hormones. (See p. 169.)

distress. Unpleasant or disease-producing stress.

DOC. Abbreviation for desoxycorticosterone.

duodenum. The first part of the small intestine, which comes immediately after the stomach.

electrolyte. Any solution which conducts electricity by means of its ions (e.g., potassium or sodium).

endocrines. Ductless glands which secrete their products, the hormones, directly into the blood. (See p. 20.)

enzyme. A naturally-occurring substance, formed by living cells, which accelerates certain chemical reactions (formerly called *ferment*).

eosinophils. Certain white blood cells which can readily be stained by the dye eosin. They play an important part in allergy. (See p. 23.)

epinephrine. Same as adrenaline.

eustress. Pleasant or curative stress.

extract. A preparation obtained by mixing tissue, e.g., liver, ovary, etc., or constituents of a drug, with solvents (water, alcohol, etc.) and then separating the soluble from the insoluble material. (See pp. 21–22.)

focal infection. Infection (in a more or less circumscribed region) which causes disease manifestations in distant parts of the body through mechanisms other than the mere spreading of bacteria or their poisons. (See p. 227.)

Formalin. An irritating aqueous solution of formaldehyde. (See p. 27.)

G.A.S. Abbreviation for general adaptation syndrome.

GC. Abbreviation for glucocorticoid.

general adaptation syndrome (G.A.S.). The manifestations of stress in the whole body, as they develop in time. The G.A.S. evolves in three distinct stages: alarm reaction, stage of resistance, stage of exhaustion. (See pp. 36–38, 55.)

glucagon. A hormone of the pancreas which stimulates glucose release (sugar).

glucocorticoids. See *anti-inflammatory corticoids*.

granuloma pouch. An experimental example of a stand-
ardizable inflammation. It is produced by making a
sac through the subcutaneous injection of air, followed by some irritant which produces an inflammatory barrier or wall ("granuloma"). It has
approximately the size and shape of a small egg
under the skin of the rat. The solid inflammatory
tissue of the wall surrounds the inflammatory fluid
("exudate") which accumulates in the cavity. Thus,
both constituents of inflammation (solid and fluid)
can be separately measured. (See pp. 216–218.)

growth hormone. Same as somatotrophic hormone.

heterostasis. The artificially-induced stimulation of the
body's defense mechanisms, e.g., syntoxic and catatoxic hormones. (See p. 85.)

heterotropic adaptation. See *redevelopmental adaptation.*

histology. The study of the microscopic structure of tissues.

homeostasis. The body's tendency to maintain a steady
state despite external changes; physiologic stability. (See pp. 12, 480.)

homotropic adaptation. See *developmental adaptation.*

hormones. Chemical substances released into the blood
by the endocrine glands to stimulate and coordinate distant organs. Bodily growth, metabolism,
resistance to stress, and sexual functions are
largely regulated by hormones. (See pp. 21, 218–
221.)

5-HT. Abbreviation for 5-hydroxytryptamine.

5-Hydroxytryptamine (5-HT). A substance which regulates brain activity.

hypophysis. Same as *pituitary.* A little endocrine gland
embedded in the bones of the skull just below the
brain. (See pp. 26, 476.)

hypothalamus. A part of the brain immediately above
the hypophysis, which regulates the hormone
secretion of the latter.

indirect pathogen. An agent causing disease by stimulating an inappropriate or excessive defensive response (e.g., immune reactions, inflammation).

inflammation. The typical reaction of tissue (particularly of connective tissue) to injury. Its main purpose is to barricade off and to contain the injurious agent by which it was elicited. (See pp. 129–143.)

insulin. The antidiabetic hormone produced by the pancreas.

involution. Same as *atrophy*. Natural shrinkage or decline of an organ.

L.A.S. Abbreviation for local adaptation syndrome.

local adaptation syndrome (L.A.S.). The manifestations of stress in a limited part of the body as they develop in time. The L.A.S. evolves in three stages, characterized mainly by inflammation, degeneration, or death of cell groups in the directly-affected part. (See pp. 81, 142.)

lymphatic tissues. Tissues containing mainly lymphocytes, for example, the thymus, the lymph nodes. (See p. 22.)

lymph nodes. Nodular organs, consisting of lymphatic tissue, in the groins, under the armpits, along the neck, and in various parts of the body. (See p. 22.)

lymphocytes. The smallest white blood cells. They make up the lymphatic tissue, but can also circulate freely in the blood. (See p. 23.)

MAD. Abbreviation for methylandrostenediol.

MC. Abbreviation for mineralocorticoid.

metabolism. The transformation of foodstuffs into tissue and energy which occurs in the body.

methylandrostenediol (MAD). An artificial virilizing hormone. (See p. 294.)

milieu intérieur. The internal environment of the body; the soil in which all biologic reactions develop. (See p. 51.)

mineralocorticoids. See *proinflammatory corticoids*.

nephritis. Inflammation of the kidney. (See p. 186.)

nephrosclerosis. A kidney disease often causing hypertension. (See p. 186.)

nephrosis. A kidney disease which leads to dropsy and loss of protein through the urine. (See p. 186.)

nonspecific. A *nonspecifically-formed* change is one which affects all or most parts of a system without selectivity. It is the opposite of a specifically-formed change, which affects only one or, at least, few units within a system. A *nonspecifically-caused* change is one which can be produced by many or all agents. (See p. 67.)

nonspecific therapy. Treatment which is beneficial in various kinds of diseases.

noradrenaline. A close relative of adrenaline, the principal hormone of the adrenal medulla. Unlike the latter hormone, noradrenaline is mainly produced at nerve endings to transmit impulses to various tissues. (See pp. 117–118.)

norepinephrine. Same as noradrenaline.

ovaries. The female sex glands.

pancreas. A gland whose endocrine parts produce insulin.

pathogen. A disease-producing agent.

pathology. The study of disease.

pathos. Greek for suffering, disease. (See p. 11.)

PC. Abbreviation for proinflammatory corticoid.

peptic. Aiding digestion (as in peptic juice), or caused by digestion (as in peptic ulcer). (See pp. 259–263.)

pituitary. Same as *hypophysis.*

placenta. The vascular organ with which the embryo is attached to the mother's womb; the afterbirth.

pónos. Greek for toil, stress. (See p. 11.)

pressor substances. Hormones or hormone-like products which raise the blood pressure. (See p. 155.)

proinflammatory corticoids. Adrenocortical hormones which stimulate inflammation, as for example, aldosterone, desoxycorticosterone. They have a marked effect upon mineral metabolism, and are therefore also known as *mineralocorticoids*. (See p. 220.)

prolactin. Same as luteotrophic or lactogenic hormone (LTH) which stimulates lactation and, in some species, such as the rat, growth and function of the corpus luteum or the "yellow body" of the ovary.

psychoanalysis. The method of analyzing an abnormal mental state by having the patient review his past emotional experiences and relating them to his present mental life. The technique furnishes hints for psychotherapeutic procedures.

reaction. In biology, the response of the body, or of one of its parts, to stimulation.

reacton. The smallest possible biologic target. It is the primary subcellular unit in living matter, which still exhibits the property of responding selectively to stimulation. (See p. 338.)

redevelopmental adaptation. Adaptation in which a tissue, organized for one type of action, is forced to readjust itself completely to an entirely different kind of activity. In technical language: heterotropic adaptation. (See p. 330.)

renal blood pressure regulators. Substances produced by the kidney that regulate blood pressure. (e.g., renin, angiotensin).

renin. An enzyme of the kidney which raises blood pressure by making angiotensin.

renal pressor substances (RPS). Endocrine substances produced by the kidney to raise the blood pressure. (See p. 147.)

rheumatic fever. An acute and often recurring disease, most common in children and young adults. It is characterized by fever with inflammation of the joints and the heart valves. It often follows upon focal infection in the tonsils. (See p. 236.)

rheumatism. A vague term which includes rheumatic

fever, rheumatoid arthritis, and several allied conditions. (See p. 236.)

rheumatoid arthritis. A more or less chronic disease, characterized by an inflammation of the joints, with swelling, pain, stiffness, and deformity. There are several variants in which one or the other among these manifestations predominates. (See p. 236.)

RPS. Abbreviation for renal pressor substances.

shock therapy. Treatment with shocks elicited by drugs or electricity. (See p. 288.)

somatic. Pertaining to the body.

somatotrophic hormone (STH). A pituitary substance which stimulates the growth of the body in general and of inflamed connective tissue in particular. Also known as *growth hormone*. (See pp. 141–142.)

specific. A *specifically-formed* change is one which affects only a single, or at least, few units within a system, with great selectivity. A *specifically-caused* change is one which can be produced only by a single, or at least, by few agents. The term *specific* has no meaning unless we indicate whether it refers to the change itself or to its causation. (See p. 67.)

specific resistance. Resistance to an agent induced by pretreatment with the same agent. (See p. 329.)

stage of exhaustion. The final stage of the adaptation syndrome. It may be general or local, depending upon whether the whole body or only a region has been exposed to stress. (See pp. 37, 329.)

stage of resistance. The second stage of the adaptation syndrome. It may be general or local, depending upon whether the whole body or only a region has been exposed to stress. (See pp. 37, 331.)

STH. Abbreviation for somatotrophic hormone.

stimulus. In biology, anything that elicits a reaction in the body or in one of its parts.

stress. The *state manifested by the specific syndrome which consists of all the nonspecifically-induced changes within a biologic system.* Thus stress has its own characteristic form, but no particular specific cause. A detailed analysis of this fundamental definition will be found on pp. 61 and 491. However, for general orientation, it suffices to keep in mind that by *stress* the physician means the common results of exposure to anything. For example, the bodily changes produced, whether a person is exposed to nervous tension, physical injury, infection, cold, heat, x-rays or anything else, are what we call *stress*. This is what is left when we abstract from the specific changes that are produced only by one or few among these agents. In my earlier writings I had defined stress, somewhat more simply but less precisely, as "the sum of all nonspecific changes caused by function or damage," or "the rate of wear and tear in the body." Its simplest and most generally-accepted definition is: *the nonspecific response of the body to any demand.*

syndrome. A group of symptoms and signs which appear together.

synergist. An agent which facilitates the action of another agent.

syntoxic. (From the Greek prefix *syn* = with or together.) Syntoxic hormones induce a peaceful coexistence of the organism with the toxic agent. They are anti-inflammatory, immunosuppressive hormones.

stressor. That which produces stress. (See p. 78.)

target area. The region upon which a biologic agent acts.

thalamus. The part of the brain immediately above the hypothalamus.

therapy. Treatment.

thymicolymphatic organs. The thymus and lymph nodes.

thymus. A large lymphatic organ in the chest. (See p. 23.)

thyroid. An endocrine gland in the neck, which regulates metabolism in general. (See p. 150.)

tissue. An aggregate of cells and intercellular substances forming one of the structural materials of the body. Each type of tissue (nervous, muscular, connective) has a different specific structure.

triad. A syndrome consisting of three manifestations. (See pp. 22–24.)

tripartite. Having three parts.

triphasic. Having, or developing in three stages, as does the G.A.S.

ulcer. Inflammation and erosion on a surface.

vasopressor. An agent that stimulates contraction of the muscular tissue of the capillaries and arteries.

viruses. Living agents, even smaller than bacteria, which can cause infectious diseases. For instance, measles, mumps, poliomyelitis, and the common cold, are produced by viruses.

white blood cells. Cells which circulate freely in the blood and do not contain the coloring matter characteristic of the red blood cells. The lymphocytes, eosinophils, and other leukocytes belong to this group. (See p. 100.)

Annotated References

In this volume we could mention only the highlights of what is known about stress. For those interested in more information in lay or technical language on specific aspects, I have chosen and annotated the following key references from among the approximately 110,000 titles in my stress library. Most of these are books or reviews which quote much additional literature on special topics. Inclusion of a title does not imply approval. On the contrary, many of the references were selected purposely to represent different, and sometimes conflicting, points of view. Among these titles, students and teachers will find detailed texts on stress in relation to virtually every aspect of life in health and disease.*

Alexander, F. *Psychosomatic Medicine*, p. 300. New York: W. W. Norton & Co., Inc., 1950.
    Simple textbook on psychosomatic medicine in relation to psychoanalysis and the G.A.S. (260 references).

Appley, M. H., Trumbull, R., eds. *Psychological Stress. Issues in Research*, p. 471. New York: Appleton-Century-Crofts, 1967.

*Some of the following Annotated References have been drawn from *Stress without Distress* by Hans Selye, M.D. Copyright © 1974 by Hans Selye. Reprinted by permission of J. B. Lippincott Company.

Conference on psychologic stress, with the participation of numerous specialists who gave papers on
the technical aspects of the G.A.S. in relation to
psychosomatic medicine.

Bajusz, E., ed. *Physiology and Pathology of Adaptation
Mechanisms*, p. 583. Oxford, London, Edinburgh:
Pergamon Press, 1969.

Technical monograph with independent articles
by numerous specialists in adaptation. One large
section deals with "the pituitary-adrenocortical
system, its regulation and adaptive functions," and
another with "regulation of 'adaptive hormones'
other than ACTH." Additional presentations are
concerned with neuroendocrine regulatory adaptation mechanisms and adaptation to changes in
environmental temperature.

Baker, G. W., Chapman, D. W. *Man and Society in Disaster*, p. 442. New York: Basic Books, 1962.

Symposium on the roots and consequences of various catastrophes in war and peace. Somatic stress
reactions have been considered only by some con-
tributors, but the book does contain interesting
observations on the behavior of individuals and
groups during disasters.

Baron, R. A. *The Tyranny of Noise*, p. 294. New York,
Evanston, San Francisco, London: Harper & Row,
Publishers, 1971.

Easily understandable summary of the price you
pay for the stressor effect of various types of noise
characteristic of our civilization. Special attention
is given to the noise of urban life, the abusive use of
technology, and aviation. Statistics on noise in
terms of health and dollars. Technical means to
avoid or minimize noise.

Barton, A. H. *Communities in Disaster. A Sociological
Analysis of Collective Stress Situations*, p. 352. Garden City, N.Y.: Doubleday and Co., 1969.

Detailed sociologic study of behavior at times of catastrophe in war and peace. The author speaks of "collective stress" in referring to extreme disaster situations in entire communities, but the purely medical, especially biochemical, aspects of stress reactions are not considered. The volume is of greater value to sociologists than to physicians.

Basowitz, H., Persky, H., Horchin, S.J., Grinker, R. R. *Anxiety and Stress*, p. 320. New York, Toronto, London: McGraw-Hill Book Co., Inc., 1954.

Monograph on anxiety, especially in relation to stress and the G.A.S. (numerous references).

Benson, H. "Your Innate Asset for Combating Stress." *Harv. Business Rev.* July–Aug., 1974, pp. 49–60.

Detailed description of the "relaxation response" as a prophylactic measure, especially against the stress of modern executive life. It is based on a combination of relaxation in a quiet environment, taking up a passive attitude in a comfortable position, and repeating silently, or in a low gentle tone, a single-syllable sound or word (e.g., "one," "God"). The technique is closely related to Transcendental Meditation, Zen, Yoga, autogenic training, progressive relaxation, hypnosis with suggested relaxation, and sentic cycles, with which its effects upon oxygen consumption, respiratory rate, heart rate, α-waves, blood pressure, and muscle tension are compared. Its elements have been known for centuries, usually as religious rituals, but they are presented here in a noncultic factual manner and described in a language easily acceptable to the modern executive. The technique is recommended for the alleviation of certain toxicomanias, including alcoholism and cigarette smoking, and such diseases of adaptation as hypertension, peptic ulcers, and some mental disturbances. It is suggested that the relaxation response be induced once or twice daily for about twenty to thirty minutes. "When the response is elicited more frequently—for example, for many hours daily over a period of several days—some individuals have experienced a withdrawal from life and have developed symptoms which range from insomnia to hallucinatory behavior. These side effects of excessive elicitation of the relaxation response are difficult to evaluate on a retrospective basis, since many people with preexisting psychiatric problems might be drawn to any technique which evangelistically promises relief from tension and stress. However, it is unlikely that the twice daily elicitation of the response would do any more harm than would regular prayer."

Benson, H., Beary, J. F., Carol, M. P. "The Relaxation Response." *Psychiatry* **37**, 37–46 (1974).

Various self-induced states of altered consciousness (Transcendental Meditation, Zen, Subud, Nichiren Sho Shu, Hare Krishna, Scientology, Black Muslimism, Meher Baba, Shintoism, and other religious practices consisting of sitting quietly and inspiring through the nose, then expiring through the mouth) are reviewed as potential antistress measures. "Subjective and objective data exist which support the hypothesis that an integrated central nervous system reaction, the 'relaxation response,' underlies this altered state of consciousness." When elicited for periods of twenty to thirty minutes once or twice daily, they do not appear to have any adverse effect. However, "when elicited more frequently, some subjects experience a withdrawal from life and symptoms which range in severity from insomnia to psychotic manifestations, often with hallucinatory behavior."

Blythe, P. *Stress Disease. The Growing Plague*, p. 175. New York: St. Martin's Press, 1973.

A very readable description of the role of stress in various diseases as well as in interpersonal relations, particularly family difficulties and social habits.

Bourne, P. G. *The Psychology and Physiology of Stress: With Reference to Special Studies of the Viet Nam War,* p. 242. New York, London: Academic Press, 1969.

A symposium.

Broadbent, D. E. *Decision and Stress,* p. 522. New York, London: Academic Press, 1971.

Monograph on decision-making in relation to stress with a chapter on "the arousal theory of stress." Comparatively little reference has been made to the hypothalamus-pituitary-adrenal system (about 100 references).

Buck, V. E. *Working Under Pressure,* p. 252. London: Staples Press, 1972.

Monograph on job pressure by a professor of organizational behavior and administrative theory. Written mainly from a behavioral science perspective, the volume does not deal only with purely somatic aspects, but gives advice to management and lower level employees alike regarding job pressure and satisfaction. Interpretation of numerous questionnaires and statistics (over 150 references).

Buckley, J. P. "Physiological Effects of Environmental Stimuli." *J. Pharm. Sci.* **61,** 1175–1188 (1972).

Highly constructive and critical evaluation of the present status of the stress concept, based on technical literature (158 references).

Calloway, D. H., ed. *Human Ecology in Space Flight II,* p. 285. New York: New York Academy of Sciences, 1966.

Conference on the medical aspects of space flight, with special emphasis on the stressor effect of high G forces, motion sickness, variations in temperature, toxic gases, ionizing rays, life in a magnetic field, and emotional factors, and particularly on the combined stressor action of several among these factors.

Cannon, W. B. *The Wisdom of the Body*, p. 332. New York: W. W. Norton & Co., Inc., 1932.

A classic monograph written in semipopular style, but with many detailed descriptions of experiments which led to the concept of "homeostasis."

Cannon, W. B. *Bodily Changes in Pain, Hunger, Fear and Rage* (2nd ed.), p. 404. Boston: Charles T. Branford Co., 1953.

Excellent summary of the author's classic observations on the somatic manifestations of acute emotions, particularly with regard to the effect of fear, rage, hunger, and thirst upon the sympathetic nervous system and adrenaline secretion.

Cohen, B. M., Cooper, M. Z. *A Follow-up Study of World War II Prisoners of War*, p. 81. Washington, D.C.: Veterans Administration Medical Monograph, 1954.

Statistical analysis by the U.S. Army of white male survivors of imprisonment by the Japanese and Germans during World War II. Special emphasis is placed on after-effects (morbidity, mortality) following liberation or escape. Although extensive data suggest lasting unfavorable after-effects, evaluation of the role of stress as such or of more specific factors (malnutrition, infection, trauma) is difficult.

Corcoran, A. C. *A Mirror Up to Medicine*, p. 506. Philadelphia, New York, Montreal: J. B. Lippincott Co., 1961.

Essentially a philosophic analysis of the history of medicine, primarily based on excerpts or direct quotations from the most important contributions of a variety of philosophers and physicians, includ-

ing Aristophanes, Aristotle, Sir Francis Bacon, W.
B. Cannon, H. Cushing, E. Darwin, Hippocrates, O.
W. Holmes, Maimonides, Sir William Osler, Paracelsus, Albert Schweitzer, and several others. The
book makes very interesting and instructive reading, and offers a most judicious selection of aphor-
isms and pithy sentences about medicine in general. Four pages are devoted to an analysis of the
first edition of _The Stress of Life._

Curtis, H. J. _Biological Mechanisms of Aging_, p. 133.
Springfield, Ill.: Charles C Thomas, Publisher, 1966.

Discussion of the biochemical basis of aging, with
a special section on the stress theory.

Dill, D. B., and others, eds. _Handbook of Physiology_,
Section 4. "Adaptation to the Environment," p.
1056. Washington, D.C.: American Physiological
Society, 1964.

Encyclopedic treatise on adaptation to various
environmental changes. Several sections deal with
the role of the G.A.S.

Dohrenwend, B. S. "Life Events As Stressers: a Method-
ological Inquiry." _J. Hlth. Soc. Behav._ 14, 167–175
(1973).

"Stressfulness is better conceived as life change
than as undesirability of life events," as judged by
extensive statistical studies based on questionnaires.

Dohrenwend, B. S., Dohrenwend, B. P., eds. _Stressful
Life Events: Their Nature and Effects_, p. 340. New
York, London, Sydney: John Wiley & Sons, 1974.

An excellent anthology on the role played by
stress in the most varied events encountered in
daily life. Among the numerous outstanding con-
tributors apart from the editors themselves, are,
for example: L. E. Hinkle, Jr., T. H. Holmes, R.
Rahe, D. Mechanic, T. Theorell, and several other
internationally-recognized experts.

Dubos, R. *Man Adapting,* p. 527. New Haven, London:
    Yale University Press, 1965.

    Scientifically well-founded monograph on adapta-
tion, with many sections referring to Cannon's
"emergency reaction" and the G.A.S. The volume
formed the subject of the Silliman Lectures at Yale
University.

Dunn, J. P., Cobb, S. "Frequency of Peptic Ulcer among
    Executives, Craftsmen, and Foremen." *J. Occup.
    Med.* 4, 343–348 (1962).

    Statistical studies on several Pittsburgh compa-
nies showed that foremen suffered from peptic
ulcer more frequently than craftsmen or executives. The data do not support the widely-held
notion that ulcer disease is unusually high among
executives.

Eitinger, L., Strøm, A. *Mortality and Morbidity After
    Excessive Stress: A Follow-up Investigation of Nor-
    wegian Concentration Camp Survivors,* p. 153. New
    York: Humanities Press, Inc., 1973.

    Evaluation of the population described in the
title led to the conclusion that "the most natural
explanation of the ex-prisoners' higher mortality
and morbidity is that the excessive stress they
experienced during imprisonment lowered their
resistance to infection and lessened their ability to
adjust to environmental changes. . . . Other forms
of stress may have similar effects on the organism
and may contribute to the increase of 'stress
diseases' in the modern world."

Eliot, R. S., ed. *Stress and the Heart.* Volume 1, p. 415.
    New York: Futura Publishing Co., 1974.

    Report on a highly technical congress concerning
the effect of stress upon cardiovascular disease,
with contributions from numerous specialists in
this field.

Engle, E. T., Pincus, G., eds. *Hormones and the Aging Process*, p. 323. New York, London: Academic Press, 1956.

Proceedings of a symposium at which experts discussed the literature on hormones and aging in fairly technical language, well-documented by references. One section, by D. J. Ingle, is specifically devoted to the role of stress in aging and the hormones produced during the G.A.S.

Farber, S. M., Mustacchi, P., Wilson, R. H. L., eds. *Man under Stress*, p. 173. California: University of California Press, 1964.

Proceedings of a symposium organized by the University of California. A group of physicians, surgeons, and basic research men (among them Brock Chisholm, René Dubos, Seymour Farber, Stanley Sarnoff, Hans Selye, Paul Dudley White) discussed the various aspects of stress, particularly in relation to the philosophy of life, social environment, cardiovascular disease, space medicine, etc. Most of the speakers refrained from highly technical discussions, but key references to scientific papers are given.

Fraser, T. M.: "Men under Stress." *Sci. Technol.* No. 73, 38–44, 82 (1968).

Semipopular review on men under stress with special reference to environmental factors.

Friedman, M., Rosenman, R. H. *Type A Behavior and Your Heart*, p. 276. New York: Alfred A. Knopf, 1974.

Detailed discussion of the authors' definition of Type A and Type B behavior as influencing predisposition to coronary heart disease. Emphasis is placed upon the fact that Type A, the coronary-prone patient, is overambitious and is exposed to much more stress than Type B (no references).

Friedrich, R., ed. *Frontiers of Medicine*, p. 320. New
    York: Liveright Publishing Corporation, 1961.
      Popularization of several new concepts in medi-
    cine (antibiotics, artificial hibernation, sleep ther-
    apy, etc.) with one section entitled "A New System:
    Selye's Theories of Stress and Adaptation."
Funkenstein, D. H., King, S. H., Drolette, M. E. *Mastery
    of Stress*, p. 329. Cambridge: Harvard University
    Press, 1957.
      Observations on stress-inducing situations and
    their prophylaxis in man and experimental ani-
    mals. Main emphasis is laid upon psychologic fac-
    tors, but the somatic aspects of the G.A.S. are also
    considered.
Galdston, I. *Beyond the Germ Theory*, p. 182. New York,
    Minneapolis: Health Education Council, 1954.
      Very readable book with major emphasis upon
    the disease-producing effects of "deprivation
    stress" in relation to the G.A.S. Special sections on
    deprivation of food and emotional stimuli.
Glass, D. C., Singer, J. E. *Urban Stress: Experiments on
    Noise and Social Stressors*, p. 182. New York, Lon-
    don: Academic Press, 1972.
      Monograph on the stressor effect of noise, mainly
    as a function of predictability and subject control.
    Despite the title, little is said about other stressors
    in urban life, but the book—which earned its
    authors the 1971 Socio-Psychological Prize of the
    American Association for the Advancement of Sci-
    ence—undoubtedly contains many valuable data
    on human responses to psychosocial stressors
    (about 120 references).
Graham-Bonnalie, F. E. *The Doctor's Guide to Living
    with Stress*, p. 148. New York: Drake Publishers,
    1972.
      Monograph on the physiologic basis of stress, and

particularly the hypothalamus-pituitary-adreno-cortical axis, with special reference to psychosomatic illness.

Grinker, R. R., Spiegel, J. P. *Men under Stress*, p. 484. Philadelphia: The Blakiston Co., 1945.

Detailed study on the stressor effects of combat upon U.S. troops during World War II. Special sections deal with genetic predisposing factors, the environment of combat, combat morale, reactions after combat, and applications to civilian psychiatry.

Gross, N. E. *Living with Stress*, p. 207. Foreword by Hans Selye. New York, Toronto, London: McGraw-Hill Book Co., Inc., 1958.

Summary, in lay language, of the stress concept and its application to daily life.

Gunderson, E. K. E., Rahe, R. H., eds. *Life Stress and Illness*, p. 264. Springfield, Ill.: Charles C Thomas, Publisher, 1974.

Review on a symposium held by NATO in 1972, at which 15 comparatively independent papers were presented on stress in relation to psychosomatic medicine. Highly recommended reading.

Hambling, J., ed. *The Nature of Stress Disorder*, p. 298. Springfield, Ill.: Charles C Thomas, Publisher, 1959.

Proceedings of the Conference of the Society for Psychosomatic Research (Royal College of Physicians, London). Several experts discussed the G.A.S. on the basis of animal experiments and observations in man. Special sections deal with stress in aviation, skin disorders, gastrointestinal disease, industry, the family setting, and genetic predisposition.

Hanlon, J. J. "Environmental Hazards." *Fed. Proc.* **31**, TF101–TF120 (1972).

Review on physical, biologic, psychologic, and

chemical environmental hazards to man, with brief sections on noise and the roles of adaptive hormones (65 references).

Janis, I. L. *Psychological Stress*, p. 439. New York, London, Sydney: John Wiley & Sons, 1958.

Psychoanalytic and behavioral studies on surgical patients. Interviews before and after operations are reported, and practical lessons to be drawn from them are pointed out.

Jensen, J. *Modern Concepts in Medicine*, p. 636. St. Louis: The C. V. Mosby Co., 1953.

Voluminous treatise which attempts to reinterpret virtually the whole of physiology, biochemistry, and medicine using the G.A.S. as a unifying concept. Very painstaking compilation of data interpreted in a somewhat daringly speculative manner.

Kearns, J. L. *Stress in Industry*, p. 160. London: Priory Press, 1973.

Monograph on the workaday aspects of dealing with stress in industry, mainly from the standpoint of interpersonal relations. The terms "stress" and "stressors" are used but not defined, and the biologic basis of the G.A.S. is excluded from consideration. Even such words as adrenal, adrenaline, corticoids, hypothalamus, and nervous system are not to be found in the index. The book aims primarily at giving practical advice concerning behavior and, being illustrated by many humorous drawings, is easy to read.

Kennedy, J. A. *Relax and Live*, p. 205. Englewood Cliffs, N.J.: Prentice-Hall, Inc., 1953.

Notes on how to relax and avoid disease, given in lay language. One section is devoted to the relationship between aging and the G.A.S.

Kerner, F. *Stress and Your Heart*, p. 237. Introduction

by Hans Selye. New York: Hawthorn Books, Inc., 1961.

Practical advice on the avoidance of cardiovascular disease resulting from stress, based mainly on the technical monographs of Hans Selye.

Kiev, A. *A Strategy for Handling Executive Stress*, p. 178. Chicago, Ill.: Nelson-Hall, 1974.

The author uses as a motto for this monograph these words from Emerson's essay on self-reliance: "It is easy in the world to live after the world's opinion; it is easy in solitude to live after our own; but the great man is he who in the midst of the crowd keeps with perfect sweetness the independence of solitude." The book is replete with practical advice which can be characterized by a few quotations: "Every communication holds a stress." "Business is a battle." "Stress and the drives of life are inseparable." The bodily manifestations of stress and its biochemical mechanism are given little attention.

Klausner, S. Z. *Why Man Takes Chances*, p. 267. Toronto: Doubleday and Co., 1968.

Experience of people who deliberately seek stress in the form of adventure, excitement, challenge, and opportunity worthy of their mettle and who enjoy it. The author was probably the first to use the expression "eustress."

Kositskii, G. I., Smirnov, V. S. *The Nervous System and "Stress,"* p. 265. Washington, D.C.: National Aeronautics and Space Administration, 1972.

A well-documented technical monograph on the relationship between the role played by the nervous system (Pavlov) in resistance phenomena, and hormonal reactions to stress (Selye). The nonhormonal aspects (including nervous mediation) of the G.A.S. are not considered. The extensive bibliog-

raphy in this English translation of the Russian
original will be a valuable source of references to
the pertinent Soviet literature for those not speaking Russian. [The original Russian edition was published by Nauka in 1970, under the same title.
(H.S.)]

Kraus, H. *Backache, Stress and Tension: Their Cause,
Prevention and Treatment*, p. 183. New York: Simon
& Schuster, Inc., 1965.

Well-illustrated book on the role of stress in causing backache, with advice concerning physical therapy—mainly exercise—to combat this complication.

Kroes, W. H., Margolis, B. L., Hurrell, J. J., Jr. "Job
Stress in Policemen." *J. Police Sci. Admin.* **2**, 145–
155 (1974).

This statistical study on 100 policemen of the
Cincinnati force revealed, through questionnaires,
that their most significant stressors were those circumstances which threatened their sense of professionalism. There is much interesting material on
the stressors that cause greatest job dissatisfaction
among policemen, but adequate statistical evaluation of their predisposition to stress diseases is still
lacking.

Laszlo, E. *Introduction to Systems Philosophy—Toward
a New Paradigm of Contemporary Thought*, p. 328.
Foreword by Ludwig von Bertalanffy. New York,
Evanston, Ill., San Francisco, London: Harper
Torchbooks, 1973.

Excellent review of systems philosophy as
applied to natural and artificial systems. Special
attention is given to "system-cybernetics," adaptive self-stabilization, adaptive self-organization
and intra- and inter-systemic hierarchies. The
endocrine feedback in biologic rhythms is used as
an example of adaptability in relation to homeosta-

sis and the G.A.S. The bibliography contains an extensive list of the most important key references.

Lazarus, R. S. *Psychological Stress and the Coping Process,* p. 466. New York, Toronto, London: McGraw-Hill Book Co., Inc., 1966.

Detailed and very competent discussion of stress in relation to psychology, with special reference to the problem of coping with threatening situations. Correlations between the adaptive mechanisms of the CNS and the G.A.S. are given adequate attention throughout this volume.

Lazarus, R. S., Opton, E. M., Jr. "The Study of Psychological Stress: A Summary of Theoretical Formulations and Experimental Findings." In Spielberger, C. D. *Anxiety and Behavior,* pp. 225–262. New York, London: Academic Press, 1966.

Detailed description of the authors' use of films, occasionally combined with tape recordings, in order to produce psychogenic stress. Galvanic skin resistance and heart rate proved to be helpful objective indicators of autonomic activity, yet the two were not necessarily parallel. This may be due to differences in endocrine sensitivity.

Levi, L. *Stress. Sources, Management, and Prevention,* Foreword by Hans Selye, p. 192. New York: Liveright Publishing Corporation, 1967.

Very readable volume on the sources, management, and prevention of distress, emphasizing both the purely medical and the psychologic aspects of everyday experiences.

Levi. L., ed. *Society, Stress and Disease. Volume 1. The Psychosocial Environment and Psychosomatic Diseases,* p. 485. New York, Toronto, London: Oxford University Press, 1971.

International Interdisciplinary Symposium sponsored by the University of Uppsala and the W.H.O. The principal subjects for discussion were: definition of problems and objectives of stress research, relationships between the G.A.S. and social adjustment, neuroendocrine function, potentially pathogenic psychosocial stressors in today's society, epidemiologic evidence for diseases produced by stressors, and possible ways of modifying or preventing psychosomatic diseases through social action. First formulation of the definition: "biologic stress is the nonspecific response of the body to any demand made upon it." An excellent overview of contemporary ideas on the different somatic and psychic manifestations of stress. Rich source of useful references.

Levine, S., Scotch, N. A., eds. *Social Stress*, p. 295. Chicago, Ill.: Aldine Publ. Co., 1970.

An anthology on social stress with contributions by numerous specialists.

Levinson, H. *Executive Stress*, p. 289. New York, Evanston, San Francisco, London: Harper and Row, Publishers, 1970.

Monograph describing the social stress situations characteristic of executive work. No attempt is made to correlate these with confirmed data on the physiologic and, particularly, the somatic mechanisms regulating stress responses.

Margetts, E. L. "Historical Notes on Psychosomatic Medicine." In Wittkower, E. D., Cleghorn, R. A. *Recent Developments in Psychosomatic Medicine*, pp. 41–68. London: Pitman Medical Publ. Co., Ltd., 1954.

Motto of C. H. Parry (1755–1822): "It is much more important to know what sort of a patient has a disease, than what sort of a disease a patient has." The history of ideas about correlations between man, body, and cell is traced back to antiquity and followed through up to the publication in 1950 of Selye's first detailed monograph on stress.

Mason, J. W. "A Re-evaluation of the Concept of 'Nonspecificity' in Stress Theory." *J. Psychiat. Res.* 8, 323–333 (1971).

Brief but excellent analysis of the evidence contradicting Selye's definition of stress. Mason states that stress "may simply be the psychological apparatus involved in emotional or arousal reactions to threatening or unpleasant factors in the life situation as a whole."

McGrath, J. E. *Social and Psychological Factors in Stress*, p. 352. New York, Chicago, San Francisco: Holt, Rinehart and Winston, Inc., 1970.

A collection of papers on stress in man, based mainly on a conference on social and psychologic stressors which took place in 1967 under the auspices of the Air Force Office of Scientific Research. It includes contributions by 12 conference participants.

McKenna, M. *Revitalize Yourself! The Techniques of Staying Youthful*, p. 276. Foreword by J. A. Bailey. New York: Hawthorn Books, Inc., 1972.

Practical advice, in popular terms, on how to stay fit. A special section deals with "Stress and Its Aging Effects" in the light of the G.A.S., and throughout the well-illustrated text, frequent attention is called to the beneficial effects of the revitalizing stressors, especially exercises.

McLuhan, M. *Understanding Media*, p. 365. New York, Toronto, London: McGraw-Hill Book Co., Inc., 1964.

Monograph on the author's much-discussed and rather unique philosophy, with many references to the possible implications of the stress theory in human behavior.

McQuade, W. "What Can Stress Do to You." *Fortune*, Jan., 1972, pp. 102–141.

Excellent popular review of the stress concept. Both the physiologic mechanisms and the implications in daily life, particularly its relationship to diseases, are discussed on the basis of interviews

with various North American specialists in this
field.

McQuade, W., Aikman, A. *Stress. What It Is, What It Can
Do to Your Health, How to Fight Back*, p. 243. New
York: E. P. Dutton and Co., Inc., 1974.

Popular monograph on stress with a brief chapter on the underlying mechanisms and many examples of stress and the diseases of adaptation as they
appear in everyday life.

Mechanic, D. *Students under Stress. A Study in the
Social Psychology of Adaptation*, p. 231. Glencoe,
Ill.: Free Press, 1962.

An instructive monograph on the stress problems
encountered by students. However, here stress is
defined not in the medical sense, but as "the dis-
comforting responses of persons in particular situations."

Page, R. C. *How to Lick Executive Stress*, p. 176. New
York: Simon & Schuster; An Essandess Special
Edition, 1966.

A medical consultant to several governmental
and industrial management groups and former
Chairman of the Board of the Occupational Health
Institute gives advice in lay language on how to
apply the stress theory to problems of executives in
overcoming the constant pressures of their occupations. No reference is made to technical literature.

Papaikonomou, E. *Biocybernetics, Biosystems, Analysis
and the Pituitary Adrenal System*, p. 334. Purmer-
end: Nooy's Drukkerij, 1974.

A monograph which combines insight and wit in
applying the principles of systems analysis strategy and biocybernetics to the study of the pituitary-adrenocortical apparatus in relation to the
G.A.S.

Scharrer, E., Scharrer, B. *Neuroendocrinology*, p. 289.
New York, London: Columbia University Press,
1963.

Very technical study of the relationships between endocrine glands and the nervous system. A separate chapter is devoted to the stress concept based on the works of Cannon and Selye. Extensive bibliography.

Schindler, J. A. *How to Live 365 Days a Year*, p. 222. Englewood Cliffs, N.J.: Prentice-Hall, Inc., 1959.

Recommendations on how to avoid psychosomatic illness, based primarily on the stress concept. Written exclusively for the lay reader.

Schwartz, H. S., ed. *Mental Health and Chiropractic. A Multidisciplinary Approach*, p. 300. New York: Sessions Publ., 1973.

Monograph mainly concerned with stress-induced psychologic disturbances and the role of the G.A.S. in chiropractic.

Selye, H. *Hormones and Resistance*, 2 vols., p. 1140. New York, Heidelberg, Berlin: Springer-Verlag, 1971.

Very extensive technical encyclopedic treatise on the role of various hormones in resistance to specific and stressor agents. First detailed description of the difference between syntoxic and catatoxic hormones and the results of extensive screenings of steroids for these actions. Among all compounds tested, pregnenolone-16α-carbonitrile (PCN) proved to be the most active catatoxic substance.

Selye, H. *Stress without Distress*, p. 171. Philadelphia, New York: J. B. Lippincott Co., 1974.

Very concise description of the medical basis and historical evolution of the stress concept, followed by a detailed analysis of its psychosocial implications. An attempt is made to develop a code of behavior based exclusively upon natural laws of resistance, such as emerged from somatic stress research.

Selye, H. *Stress in Health and Disease*. Reading, Mass.: Butterworths, 1976.

The most extensive encyclopedic treatise of the

entire literature on stress in medicine and daily
life. Cites and evaluates about 7,500 references,
carefully selected from the world's largest collection of pertinent books and original articles (about
110,000 entries) in the author's library.

Snyder, S. H. *Madness and the Brain*, p. 295. New York,
Toronto, London: McGraw-Hill Book Co., Inc., 1974.

Monograph on the mechanisms of mental illness,
with special reference to schizophrenia. The so-
called "acute schizophrenics" often appear quite
well-adjusted until they suddenly deteriorate as a
result of some stressful life event. "Acute schizophrenia does not seem to run in families. Perhaps it
is some sort of reaction to extreme stress, which
could conceivably afflict almost anyone exposed to
an overwhelmingly traumatic situation. For example, it is well-known that many soldiers, otherwise
normal, become psychotic in the battlefield, but
recover rapidly when removed from the battlefront
and do not become mentally ill thereafter."

Sorenson, S. *The Quest of Wholeness*, p. 138. Reykjavik:
Prentsmidja Jóns Helgasonar, 1971.

Painstaking efforts by a physician, conversant
with the original Sanskrit text on yoga, to explain
its effects upon the body and psyche in modern
medical terms. A special section is devoted to the
relief of distress by yoga (70 references).

Sos, J., Gáti, T., Csalay, L., Dési, I. *Pathology of Civilization Diseases*, p. 174. Budapest: Akadémiai Kiadó,
1971.

Many illnesses due mainly to stress are considered to be "diseases of civilization." A special section is devoted to the role of corticoids and stress in
the development of peptic ulcers.

Spencer, J. *Stress and Release in an Urban Estate. A
Study in Action Research*, p. 355. London: Tavistock
Publ., 1964.

Very practical discussion of the stress of urban life and the means to avoid it. However, little attention is given to the purely somatic aspects of the stress mechanism.

Spielberger, C. D. *Anxiety and Behavior*, p. 414. New York, London: Academic Press, 1966.

Monograph on anxiety with extensive sections on its relationship to psychogenic stress. Little attention is given to the hypothalamus–pituitary–adrenal system.

Timiras, P. S. *Developmental Physiology and Aging*, p. 692. New York: The Macmillan Co., 1972.

A textbook on aging, with a chapter on "Decline in Homeostatic Regulation" having special reference to the G.A.S.

Toffler, A. *Future Shock*, p. 505. New York: Random House, Inc., 1970.

Popular book about the stressor effect of the continuous changes in modern society and the way in which we adapt—or fail to adapt—to the future (359 references).

Torrance, E. P. "A Theory of Leadership and Interpersonal Behavior under Stress." In Petrullo, L., Bass, B. M. *Leadership and Interpersonal Behavior*, pp. 100–117. New York, Toronto, San Francisco: Holt, Rinehart and Winston, 1961.

A theory of the relationship between the G.A.S., leadership, and interpersonal behavior is developed and summarized in tabular form.

Torrance, E. P. *Constructive Behavior: Stress, Personality and Mental Health*, p. 432. Belmont, Calif.: Wadsworth, 1965.

Monograph on the psychologic implications of the G.A.S., with reference to performance and the development of a healthy personality. Particular chapters are devoted to constructive responses to stress, personality resources which help such responses, how groups cope with stress, and individual resources and strategies in coping with stress (350 references).

Welch, B. L., Welch, A. S., eds. *Physiological Effects of Noise*, p. 365. New York, London: Plenum Press, 1970.

Extensive text on the pathogenic effect of noise upon animals and man, with numerous references to the stressor action of sound which can cause "diseases of adaptation." Rich source of pertinent literature.

Wilkinson, R. "Some Factors Influencing the Effect of Environmental Stressors upon Performance." *Psychol. Bull.* **72**, 260–272 (1969).

Review of the literature on the effect of various stressors (particularly heat, sleep deprivation, noise, hypoxia, and vibration) upon the performance of man, as judged by a number of tests.

Wolff, H. G. *Stress and Disease*, 2nd ed., p. 199. Edited by S. Wolf and H. Goodell. Springfield, Ill.: Charles C Thomas, Publishers, 1968.

In this revised, expanded edition, the editors emphasize protective adaptive reactions, which can play a decisive role in the resistance of man to the common stressors of modern life. Special sections are devoted to "stress interviews" and the part played by stress in headache, migraine, and respiratory, cardiovascular, and digestive diseases, in relation to social adjustment and a healthy philosophy of life.

Zatykó, J. "Is Selye's Stress Theory Applicable to Plants?" *Az élet és Tudomány Kalendáriuma* **73**, 37–41 (1973).

Brief summary in lay language of scientific evidence indicating that stress can occur in plants. In Hungarian.

Zuckerman, M. "Perceptual Isolation as a Stress Situation." *Arch. Gen. Psychiat.* **11**, 255–276 (1964).

Systematic analysis of the literature on biochemical and physiologic responses to isolation produced by various techniques in normal and abnormal individuals. "Sensory deprivation" (darkness and quiet) is compared with "perceptual deprivation" (unpatterned light and constant "white noise") (68 references).

Index

This Index would have been much more concise and easier to read had it been based completely on the Symbolic Shorthand System (SSS) (see p. 94, and H. Selye: *Journal of the American Medical Association* **161**, 1411, 1956). However, this could not have been done without asking the reader to study all the rules of our complex code.

In the SSS there are no synonyms, and every symbol reminds us what it stands for (e.g., DOC = desoxycorticosterone; COL = cortisol; STH = somatotrophic hormone; ACTH = adrenocorticotrophic hormone). Furthermore, connecting sentences or words are replaced by signs. A colon indicates an interrelationship (as in aging: adaptation energy, showing the interrelationship of the two factors). An arrow is used to indicate effect of one agent upon another (e.g., ACTH → inflammation, for effect of ACTH upon inflammation; blood vessels ← corticoids, for effect of corticoids upon blood vessels). Only such simple signs will be used here.

Since the entire book deals with stress, it would defeat the purpose of this Index if we were to place "stress" constantly as the first keyword. Therefore, entries are indexed in alphabetic order of the factors concerned with stress. Boldface numerals refer to principal discussions of a subject. Figures illustrating a particular topic are marked by their number, followed (in parentheses) by the number of the page on which they appear.

About the Author

Dr. Hans Selye is without question one of the great pioneers of medicine. His famous and revolutionary concept of stress opened countless new avenues of treatment through the discovery that hormones participate in the development of many degenerative diseases, including coronary thrombosis, brain hemorrhage, hardening of the arteries, high blood pressure and kidney failure, arthritis, peptic ulcers and even cancer. At present, most of his research is concerned with formulating a code of behavior based on the laws governing the body's stress resistance.

Dr. Selye has served since 1945 as Professor and Director of the Institute of Experimental Medicine and Surgery at the University of Montreal. Born in Vienna in 1907, he studied in Prague, Paris, and Rome. He received his medical degree and his Ph.D. from the German University in Prague. He is the author of 32 books and more than 1500 technical articles. He holds earned doctorates in medicine, philosophy and science, as well as 19 honorary degrees from universities around the world. He is a Fellow of the Royal Society of Canada and an Honorary Fellow of 42 other scientific societies throughout the world. A recipient of numerous honorary citizenships and medals, including the Starr Medal (the highest distinction of the Canadian Medical Association); the Prix de l'Oeuvre Scientifique (the highest award of the Association des Médecins de Langue Française du Canada), he has been made a Companion of the Order of Canada (the highest decoration awarded by his country). Dr. Selye makes his home in Montreal with his wife and four children.